D1524616

New Techniques in Cardiothoracic Imaging

New Techniques in Cardiothoracic Imaging

Edited by

Phillip M. Boiselle

Beth Israel Deaconess Medical Center
Boston, Massachusetts, USA

Charles S. White

University of Maryland Medical Center
Baltimore, Maryland, USA

informa
healthcare

New York London

Informa Healthcare USA, Inc.
52 Vanderbilt Avenue
New York, NY 10017

Printed in the United States of America on acid-free paper
10 9 8 7 6 5 4 3 2 1

International Standard Book Number-10: 0-8493-9019-2 (Hardcover)
International Standard Book Number-13: 978-0-8493-9019-7 (Hardcover)

Library of Congress Cataloging-in-Publication Data

New techniques in cardiothoracic imaging / edited by Phillip M. Boiselle, Charles S. White
p. ; cm.
Includes bibliographical references and index.
ISBN-13: 978-0-8493-9019-7 (hardcover : alk. paper)
ISBN-10: 0-8493-9019-2 (hardcover : alk. paper)
1. Heart–Imaging. 2. Chest–Imaging. I. Boiselle, Phillip M. II. White, Charles S.
[DNLM: 1. Diagnostic Imaging–methods. 2. Thoracic Diseases–diagnosis. WF 975 N5315 2007]

RC683.5.I42N49 2007
616.1′20754–dc22 2007018865

Visit the Informa Web site at www.informa.com

and the Informa Healthcare Web site at www.informahealthcare.com

To my wife, Ellen, and my mother, Dee
—PMB

To my wife, Ellen, and my three children,
Billy, Rachel, and Danny
—CSW

Preface

Five years ago, we had the privilege to edit the first edition of *New Techniques in Thoracic Imaging*, a text that aimed to provide a compendium of the state of the art in imaging of thoracic disorders and to familiarize the reader with new and emerging technologies in the field. When approached to edit a second edition, we marveled at how much has changed in just five years. For example, the field of thoracic imaging has expanded into cardiothoracic imaging, prompting a change in the title of this edition to *New Techniques in Cardiothoracic Imaging*. Additionally, important technological advances have occurred in all imaging modalities, continuously improving and expanding our ability to diagnose cardiothoracic disorders.

Although the field has expanded and technologies have changed in the past five years, the primary goals of this text have remained constant. The first is to provide a pragmatic compendium of the state of the art in imaging of disorders that are encountered in daily practice. Toward this end, there are updated chapters on the subjects of the solitary pulmonary nodule, diffuse lung disease, pulmonary embolism, and aortic disorders. Additionally, a new chapter has been added on the role of computed tomography and magnetic resonance in imaging a variety of acute and chronic cardiac diseases. The second goal is to familiarize the reader with new technologies that are playing an increasingly important role in our field. In order to meet this objective, we have included chapters devoted to 64-multi-detector-row computed tomography, computed tomography-positron emission tomography, and digital radiography. The final goal is to introduce the reader to emerging techniques that are not yet widely used in practice but will play an important role in the near future. Toward this end, there are chapters on the subjects of functional magnetic resonance imaging, radiofrequency ablation, lung cancer screening, and functional airway imaging.

This book is a collaborative project that has greatly benefited from the contributions of many expert authors. We are especially grateful to our contributing authors for sharing their time, expertise, and talents: Drs. Prachi Agarwal, Talissa Altes, Suzanne Aquino, Cesario Ciccotosto, Jeremy Erasmus, Matthew Freedman, Larry Goodman, Curtis Green, Ella Kazerooni, Jeff Klein, Vikram Krishnasetty, David Levin, Page H. McAdams, Jonas Rydberg, Bradley Sabloff, Kumar Sandrasegaran, Amita Sharma, Jo-Anne Shepard, and Lacey Washington. We would also like to acknowledge the support and guidance of Sherri R. Niziolek and Alyssa K. Fried of Informa Healthcare publishing. Finally, we would like to thank our wives, families, and colleagues for their ongoing encouragement and support.

The intended audience for this book is primarily radiologists, but we anticipate that this material will also prove useful to pulmonologists, cardiologists, and other physicians who are involved in the care of patients with cardiothoracic disorders. It is our hope and intent that this book will prove valuable to its readers in the imaging evaluation of patients with cardiothoracic disorders now and in the future.

Phillip M. Boiselle
Charles S. White

Contents

Contributors

Prachi P. Agarwal Division of Cardiothoracic Radiology, Department of Radiology, University of Michigan, Ann Arbor, Michigan, U.S.A.

Talissa A. Altes Department of Radiology, Children's Hospital of Philadelphia, Philadelphia, Pennsylvania, U.S.A.

Suzanne L. Aquino Department of Radiology, Massachusetts General Hospital, Harvard Medical School, Boston, Massachusetts, U.S.A.

Phillip M. Boiselle Department of Radiology, Beth Israel Deaconess Medical Center and Harvard Medical School, Boston, Massachusetts, U.S.A.

Cesario Ciccotosto U.O.C. Radiologia, Ospedale S. Donato, Arezzo, Italy

Jeremy J. Erasmus Department of Diagnostic Imaging, M. D. Anderson Cancer Center, University of Texas, Houston, Texas, U.S.A.

Matthew Freedman Department of Oncology, Lombardi Comprehensive Cancer Center, Georgetown University, Washington, D.C., U.S.A.

Lawrence R. Goodman Departments of Diagnostic Radiology and Pulmonary Medicine and Critical Care, Section of Thoracic Imaging, Medical College of Wisconsin and Froedtert Memorial Lutheran Hospital, Milwaukee, Wisconsin, U.S.A.

Curtis E. Green Department of Radiology, Section of Cardiothoracic Radiology, University of Vermont College of Medicine, Fletcher Allen Health Care, Burlington, Vermont, U.S.A.

Ella A. Kazerooni Division of Cardiothoracic Radiology, Department of Radiology, University of Michigan, Ann Arbor, Michigan, U.S.A.

Jeffrey S. Klein Department of Radiology, Section of Cardiothoracic Radiology, University of Vermont College of Medicine, Fletcher Allen Health Care, Burlington, Vermont, U.S.A.

Vikram Krishnasetty Department of Radiology, Massachusetts General Hospital, Harvard Medical School, Boston, Massachusetts, U.S.A.

David L. Levin Department of Radiology, Mayo Clinic, Rochester, Minnesota, U.S.A.

Page H. McAdams Department of Radiology, Duke University Medical Center, Durham, North Carolina, U.S.A.

Jonas Rydberg Department of Radiology, Indiana University School of Medicine, Indianapolis, Indiana, U.S.A.

Bradley S. Sabloff Department of Diagnostic Imaging, M. D. Anderson Cancer Center, University of Texas, Houston, Texas, U.S.A.

Kumaresan Sandrasegaran Department of Radiology, Indiana University School of Medicine, Indianapolis, Indiana, U.S.A.

Amita Sharma Department of Radiology, Massachusetts General Hospital, Boston, Massachusetts, U.S.A.

Jo-Anne O. Shepard Department of Radiology, Massachusetts General Hospital, Boston, Massachusetts, U.S.A.

Lacey Washington Department of Radiology, Section of Thoracic Imaging, Duke University, Durham, North Carolina, U.S.A.

Charles S. White Department of Diagnostic Radiology, University of Maryland Medical Center, Baltimore, Maryland, U.S.A.

1

Fundamentals of Multislice CT Scanners

Kumaresan Sandrasegaran and Jonas Rydberg
Department of Radiology, Indiana University School of Medicine, Indianapolis, Indiana, U.S.A.

INTRODUCTION

In the last decade CT has undergone tremendous technical advances. In 1992, the first dual-slice CT scanner (CT Twin, formerly Elscint Technologies, Haifa, Israel) was introduced. In 1998, 4-slice CT scanners were introduced. Coronary CT angiography became possible with 4-slice scanners. The number of detector-rows in CT scanners continued to increase, and the 16-slice scanner was introduced in 2002. In 2004, the first 64-slice CT scanners became available. The progression of CT technology is not only about an increase in the number of detector-rows and the speed of gantry rotation. Long held ideas regarding pitch, radiation dose, and noise have had to change. Newer technological features, such as cone-beam reconstructions, automatic tube current modulation (ATCM), isotropic imaging, and automatic multiplanar reformations, have been introduced as an adjunct to the superior capabilities of multislice CT scanners. In this chapter we discuss these newer developments in multislice CT scanners.

TECHNICAL SPECIFICATIONS OF MULTISLICE CT SCANNERS

The technical specifications of the 16- and 64-slice CT scanners from the four main CT vendors are given in Tables 1 and 2. In the 64-slice mode, the beam coverage of GE (LightSpeed Pro, GE Medical Systems, Waukesha, Wisconsin, U.S.A.) and Philips (Brilliance 64, Philips Medical Systems, Cleveland, Ohio, U.S.A.) scanners is

Table 1 Technical Aspects of 16-Slice CT Scanners[a]

	GE LightSpeed Pro[d]	Philips Brilliance-16[e]	Siemens Sensation-16[f]	Toshiba Aquilon-16[g]
Detector configuration (inner rows)	16 x 0.625 mm	16 x 0.75 mm	16 x 0.75 mm	16 x 0.5 mm
Detector configuration (outer rows)	8 x 1.25 mm	8 x 1.5 mm	8 x 1.5 mm	12 x 1 mm
Z-axis detector length (16-slice mode) (mm)	10	12	12	8
Fastest gantry rotation (s)	0.40	0.40	0.37	0.50
Helical acquisition widths in 16-slice mode (mm)	0.625, 1.25	0.75, 1.5	0.75, 1.5	0.5, 1, 2
Widest coverage in 1 s, with pitch=1, in 16-slice mode (mm)	25	30	32.4	16
Maximum field of view (mm)	50 (option to 65)	50	50 (option to 70)	50
X-ray generator power (kW)	100	60	60	60
Anode heat capacity (MHU)	8	8	Equivalent to 30	7.5
Maximum mA at 120 kV	800	500	500	500
Matrix	512	512, 768, 1028	512	256, 512
Automatic dose reduction	3D Dose modulation	DoseRight	CareDose 4D	SureDose
Simultaneous ATCM in x-, y-, and z-planes	Yes	Yes	Yes	No
Cone-beam reconstruction algorithm	2D	3D	2D	3D
Simultaneous functions[b]	Yes	Yes	Yes	Yes
Speed of reconstruction (s)[c]	9	6	4	2.5

[a] The specifications may not represent upgrades installed after February 2006.
[b] Simultaneous scanning, reconstruction, archiving, and hardcopy filming.
[c] Time from start of scanning to appearance of 30th image in helical abdominal scan.
[d] GE Medical Systems, Waukesha, Wisconsin, U.S.A.
[e] Philips Medical Solutions, Cleveland, Ohio, U.S.A.
[f] Siemens Medical Solutions, Forchheim, Germany.
[g] Toshiba Medical Systems, Tustin, California, U.S.A.
Abbreviations: ATCM, automatic tube current modulation; 2D, two-dimensional algorithm; 3D, three-dimensional algorithm (see text).
Source: Modified from Ref. 22.

Table 2 Technical Aspects of 64-Slice CT Scanners[a]

	GE LightSpeed Pro[d]	Philips Brilliance-64[e]	Siemens Sensation-64[f]	Toshiba Aquilon-64[g]
Detector configuration (inner rows)	64 x 0.625 mm	64 x 0.625 mm	32 x 0.6 mm	64 x 0.5 mm
Detector configuration (outer rows)	NA	NA	8 x 1.2 mm	NA
Z-Axis detector length (64-slice) (mm)	40	40	19.2	32
Helical acquisition widths in 64-slice mode (mm)	0.625	0.625	0.6	0.5
Fastest gantry rotation (s)	0.35	0.40	0.33	0.40
Scan field of View (mm)	25, 50	25–50	50 (option to 70)	18, 24, 32, 40, 50
Widest coverage in 1 s, with pitch of 1 in 64-slice mode (mm)	114.3	100	58.2	80
X-ray generator power (kW)	100	60	80	60
Anode heat capacity (MHU)	8	8	Equivalent to 30	8
Maximum mA at 120 kV	800	500	665	500
Matrix	512	512, 768, 1028	512	512
Automatic dose reduction	3D Dose modulation	DoseRight	CareDose 4D	SureDose
Simultaneous ATCM in x-, y-, and z-planes	Yes	Yes	Yes	Yes
Cone-beam reconstruction algorithm	3D	3D	3D	3D
Automatic reformation in multiple planes	Source axial images	Source axial images	Raw data	Source axial images
Simultaneous functions[b]	Yes	Yes	Yes	Yes
Speed of reconstruction[c]	22	14	2	2

[a] The specifications may not represent upgrades installed after February 2006.
[b] Simultaneous scanning, reconstruction, archiving, and hardcopy filming.
[c] Time from start of scanning to appearance of 30th image in helical abdominal scan(s).
[d] GE Medical Systems, Waukesha, Wisconsin, U.S.A.
[e] Philips Medical Solutions, Cleveland, Ohio, U.S.A.
[f] Siemens Medical Solutions, Forchheim, Germany.
[g] Toshiba Medical Systems, Tustin, California, U.S.A.
Abbreviations: ATCM, automatic tube current modulation; 3D, three-dimensional algorithm (see text for details); NA, not applicable; S, R, A, and H, simultaneous scanning, reconstruction, archiving, and hardcopy filming.
Source: Modified from Ref. 23.

40 mm, while the Toshiba 64-slice scanner (Aquilion 64, Toshiba Medical Systems, Tustin, California, U.S.A.) has a coverage of 32 mm. The Siemens 64-slice scanner (Somatom Sensation 64, Siemens Medical Solutions, Forchheim, Germany) has 32 inner detector-rows that are 0.6 mm wide in the *z*-axis, that are activated in the "64-slice mode." The beam coverage of this scanner is the least among 64-slice scanners.

Dual-Source CT Scanner

In 2005, a dual-source CT scanner (Somatom Definition, Siemens Medical Solutions) became available (Fig. 1). The experience with this scanner is limited, and at the time this chapter was written there were only a handful of publications based on this scanner (1–6). Possible advantages of this scanner include evaluation of coronary arteries without need for beta blockage (2), lower radiation dose during cardiac examinations (5,6), better image quality in obese patients, and the ability to perform dual kV studies (as described in detail below) (1). The disadvantages include the substantial additional cost of a second X-ray tube and the limited beam coverage of 19.2 mm per gantry rotation.

Dual-Energy CT

Dual-source CT scanners were initially designed to increase the temporal resolution of CT. Recently, however, exciting new CT imaging options have become available with this technology by concurrently running two orthogonal tubes at different energy levels (80 and 140 kVp) (1,7). This imaging method is also referred to as "dual-energy" CT. By exploiting differences in the mass attenuation coefficients of different materials as a function of energy, this technique provides enhanced discrimination and quantification between different tissue elements, providing greater tissue characterization than traditional CT techniques (1,7). Because the 80 and 140 kVp data sets are acquired simultaneously, there is no misregistration between the data sets. This allows for precise subtraction or fusion of the data sets that may be utilized to highlight specific substances or anatomy (Fig. 2). For example, by discriminating between calcium and iodine, CT angiography can be performed without bone overlay. Moreover, contrast medium within vessels and calcified vascular plaque can be readily differentiated. Material-specific quantitative perfusion (iodine) and ventilation

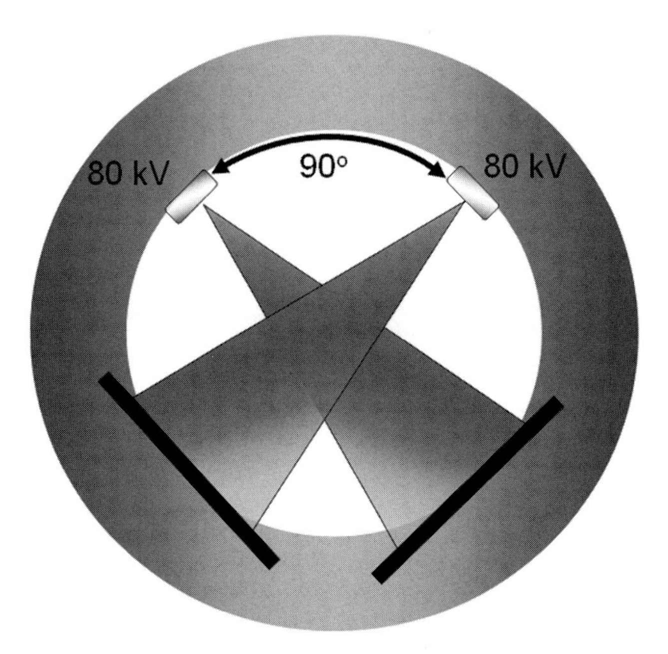

Figure 1 Simplified diagram of dual-source CT scanner (Somatom Definition, Siemens Medical Solutions, Forchheim, Germany). The two X-ray tubes are in the same axial plane and are separated by 90°. The gantry rotation is 330 ms, the same as Sensation-64 CT scanner (Siemens Medical Solutions). The temporal resolution in coronary CT angiography is the time taken to acquire 180° of data. Each gantry has to rotate only 90° to acquire this information from the two sets of detectors. Thus, the temporal resolution of this scanner is only 83 ms (330/4), allowing assessment of coronary arteries with heart rates of 80–90 beats per minute. Note that the temporal resolution of catheter coronary angiography is about 20 ms.

(xenon) imaging may also be possible. At the time of this writing, the potential applications for this exciting new technology are only beginning to be explored. We anticipate that dual-energy CT will play an important role in thoracic imaging in the near future.

SLICES, DETECTOR-ROWS, AND CHANNELS

The 16-slice CT scanner does not acquire 16 image slices per gantry rotation or per second. In this type of scanner, 16 rows of detectors are activated during scanning. This number is often less than the total number of detector-rows. For instance, most 16-slice CT scanners have at least 24 detector-rows (Table 1). In the 16-slice mode, only the central 16 detector-rows are used to collect data. In addition, the 32- and 64-slice Toshiba CT scanners have 64 detector-rows of 0.5 mm width. If the 32-slice scanner is purchased, only 32 channels are activated. On upgrading to a 64-slice CT, a software "key" is used to activate all channels.

The number of electronic channels that are activated gives the most accurate indicator of the scanner's potential. The flow of information from the detector through the hardware of a Brilliance-16 CT scanner (Philips Medical System) is shown in Figure 3. Note that the number of slices that may be derived from a scan has little to do with the number of electronic channels that are activated. Therefore, some believe that the term 16-channel CT scanner (or 64-channel CT scanner) is a more accurate descriptor than 16-slice or 16-detector row CT scanner. In this chapter, we have chosen to use the more widely accepted term "multislice CT."

RECONSTRUCTION ALGORITHMS

In single-slice CT scanners the X-ray beams are almost parallel. With multislice CT scanners the X-ray beam is cone shaped. As a result newer reconstruction algorithms are required. The traditional two-dimensional filtered back projection reconstructions, such as 180° linear interpolation reconstruction, assume that all of the rays used to reconstruct an image lie entirely within the axial plane of that image (Fig. 4A), and are unable to handle an X-ray beam that spans several detector-rows in the *z*-axis (Fig. 4B). Various reconstruction techniques have been proposed to deal with this cone-beam problem in 16- and higher slice scanners (4-slice CT scanners use traditional reconstruction algorithms). These cone-beam reconstructions can be broadly classified into two- and three-dimensional types. It should be noted that, due to complexity of calculations, reconstructions are not exact and use approximations (a potential source of artifacts).

Two-dimensional cone beams reconstruct a series of intermediate tilted image planes based on the trajectory of these gantry around the patient. The tilted image planes are used to create axial slices (Fig. 5): this technique is used in some 16-slice CT scanners (Table 1). In contrast, all 64-slice scanners use three-dimensional cone-beam reconstructions. These algorithms back project each ray along its true path through the three-dimensional volume, and reconstruct each voxel independently based on multiple projections. Three-dimensional techniques are less prone to artifacts, and have a higher degree of accuracy than the two-dimensional algorithms (8).

PITCH, NOISE, AND RADIATION DOSE

In a single-slice scanner, the pitch of the helical scan refers to the ratio of the table movement per gantry rotation to the slice width (or detector width). This definition is not entirely satisfactorily when applied to multislice CT scanners. For instance, the Brilliance-16 CT scanner (Philips Medical Systems) can be used as a 16-slice scanner in two different modes (Fig. 3). In the 12 mm collimation mode, slice widths ranging from 0.8 to 3 mm and results in different pitch for the same table movement

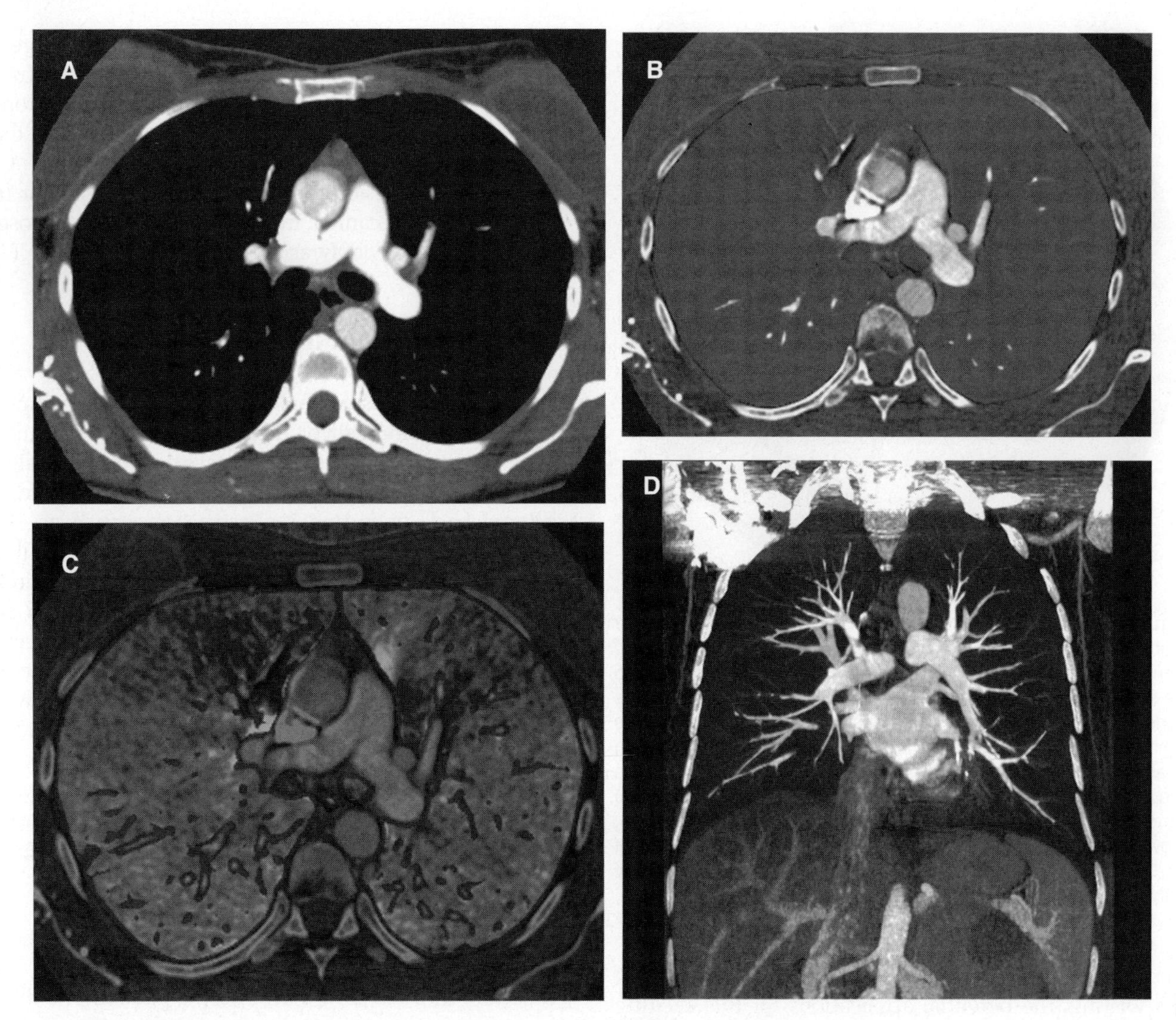

Figure 2 Normal CT pulmonary angiography study using single acquisition dual-energy technique. (**A**) Conventional 2 mm collimation image at level of central pulmonary arteries generated from a dual-energy acquisition. (**B**) Subtraction 2 mm collimation image generated at the same level by dual-energy processing, demonstrating vascular enhancement only, simulating an angiographic sequence. (**C**) CT perfusion imaging. Conventional image (as in **A**) fused with color-coded calculated map of iodine distribution in the lung parenchyma. This technique has the potential to enhance detection of pulmonary embolism (PE) by allowing simultaneous visualization of direct (endovascular filling defects) and indirect (perfusion defects) signs of PE. (**D**) 20 mm coronal maximal intensity projection (MIP) image of angiographic data (also shown in axial plane on **B**). *Source*: Photo courtesy of Dr. Ioannis "Johnny" Vlahos. (*See color insert for* **C**.)

speed may be obtained. A better definition of pitch in multislice CT is the ratio of table movement per gantry rotation to the X-ray beam width. Using this definition, the lengths of volume scanned by 64-slice CT scanners, when a pitch of 1 is chosen, are given in Table 2.

In single-slice CT, the gantry always has to rotate through a certain angle, depending on the reconstruction algorithm used, in order to acquire the projection information needed to create an axial image (9). Thus, the number of photons that are used to produce an axial image (the principle determinant of image noise) depends on the tube current–time product and not on the pitch. However, as the pitch increases, radiation dose reduces, since each part of the scanned volume spends less time in the X-ray beam.

The relationship between pitch, noise, and radiation dose is not the same with current multislice scanners (10). In the noncardiac mode, as the pitch is increased, 64-slice scanners automatically increase the tube current to maintain a relatively constant noise level. With higher pitch, the larger focal spot may be automatically chosen. These secondary effects negate any reduction of radiation dose that is intuitively expected with an increase in pitch (10,11). Therefore, changing the pitch, per se, in current multislice CT scanners does not result in alteration of the radiation

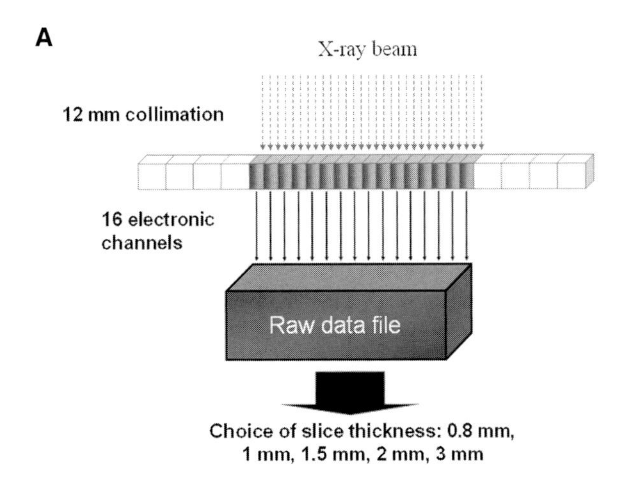

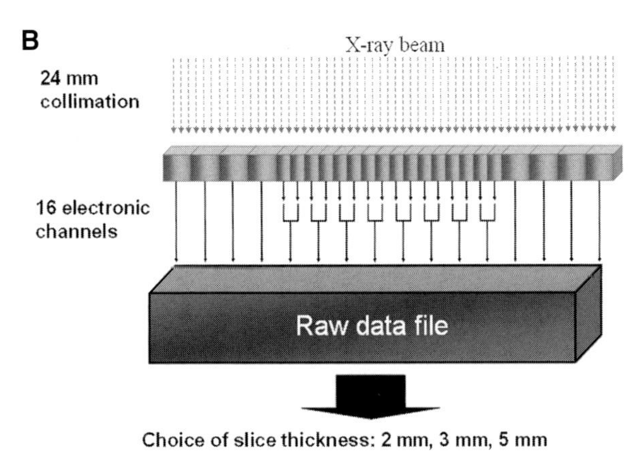

Figure 3 Flow of information through 16-slice CT scanner (Brillince-16, Philips Medical Solutions, Cleveland, Ohio, U.S.A.). (**A**) In the "thin" slice mode, e.g., for angiography, only the central detectors (16 x 0.75 mm) are activated. These result in 16 channels of electronic information, and slice thickness ranging from 0.8 to 3 mm. (**B**) In the routine chest CT, all 24 detector-rows are activated. The information from the 16 central detectors is grouped into 8 channels giving a channel configuration of 16 x 1.5 mm. Slice thickness of 2 to 5 mm are possible.

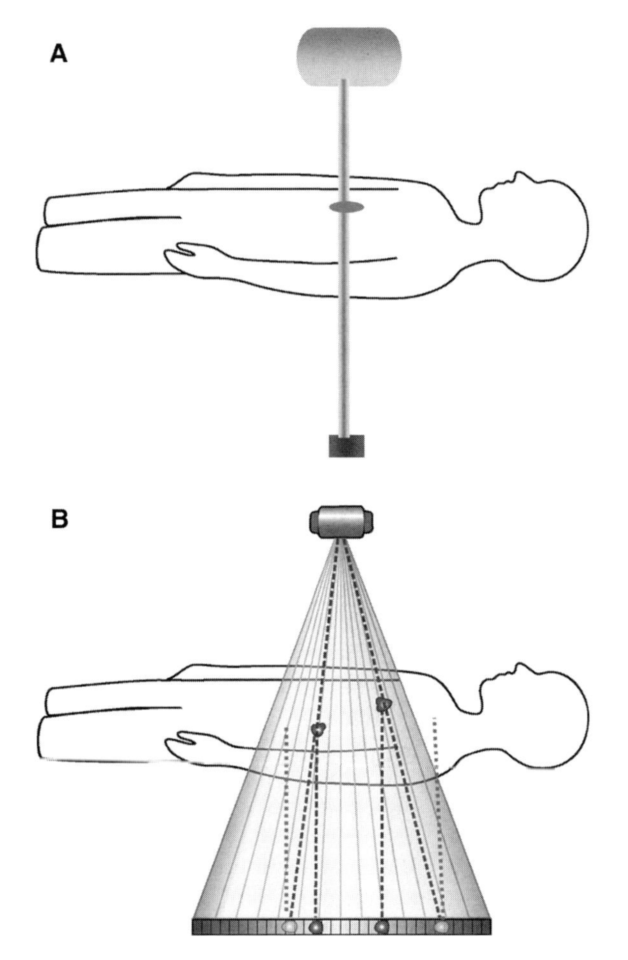

Figure 4 Linear interpolation algorithm. (**A**) Traditional two-dimensional filtered back projection reconstructions (180° linear interpolation) assume that all rays used to reconstruct an image lie entirely within plane. (**B**) In 64-slice CT the beam is cone shaped. Linear interpolation algorithms may lead to incorrect positioning of lesions (as shown by gray-dashes). New reconstruction techniques are required.

dose or a significant change in noise. In addition, with multislice CT, the pitch does not have a significant effect on the slice sensitivity profile (12). However, as the pitch is increased, insufficient data may be collected for accurate reconstructions leading to artifacts termed windmill or splay artifacts (Fig. 6).

In the cardiac mode of multislice CT, the minimum data required to reconstruct an image is acquired over a rotation of 180° plus the angle subtended by the X-ray beam in the x–y plane (known as the fan angle) (13). As a result, as is the case with single-slice CT scanners, noise is dependent on the tube current and not on the pitch. A major driving force in cardiac CT technology is the attempt to "freeze" the cardiac motion with the development of scanners with faster gantry rotation. With faster gantry rotation, the pitch has to be reduced to eliminate gaps in anatomic coverage in images reconstructed from consecutive heartbeats. This results in increased radiation dose.

REDUCING RADIATION DOSE

CT examination is responsible for about 70% of the radiation dose received by the general population from imaging tests (14). The risk of cancer death from a single-phase abdominal CT is estimated at 12.5 per 10,000 (15). The decision to use ionizing radiation should always be made from a risk versus benefit perspective, and knowledge of methods of limiting radiation is important.

The use of multislice CT scanners has resulted in a rapid increase in radiation dose to the general population. There are several reasons for this increase in radiation. Thin overlapping slices are acquired by these scanners. The indications for multislice CT constantly increase and now include the diagnosis

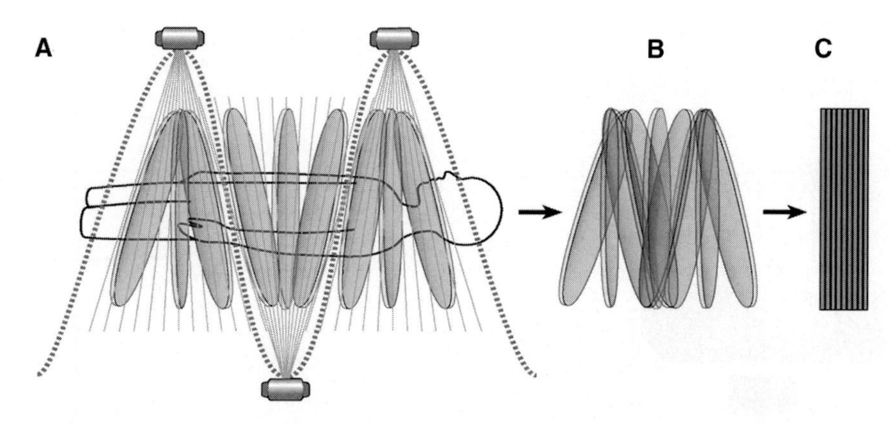

Figure 5 Two-dimensional cone-beam reconstruction. This reconstruction method uses back projection to create slices in tilted planes (**A**), which are used to create overlapping projections (**B**), which are then filtered in the *z*-axis to make axial slices (**C**). *Source*: Visual Media, Indiana University School of Medicine.

or evaluation of vascular disease, acute chest pain, and abdominal pain. For some indications, such as CT urography, multiphasic examinations are routine. However, when comparisons are made for single-phase scans using the same slice width, multislice CT scanners are more dose efficient than single-slice scanners. One reason is the reduction in the nonimage contributing penumbra radiation (Fig. 7).

Modern scanners also employ techniques to reduce radiation dose. ATCM changes the tube current to produce an acceptable noise level for each slice. The tube current modulation may be in the radial (x–y) plane (Fig. 8A), or in the z-axis (Fig. 8B). Though the modulation techniques work differently in each scanner, in general the mA is altered to maintain a selected noise level throughout the scanned volume. In some scanners, such as Sensation 64 (Siemens Medical Solutions), the tube current is constantly varied using dosimetry reading from prior gantry rotations. In others, the localizer image is used to calculate regions requiring higher and lower X-ray tube currents. It is possible on most 64-slice scanners to simultaneously use both radial and z-axis ATCMs leading to an overall reduction in dose of 40–60% compared with fixed mAs scanning. The use of ATCM has been shown to maintain image quality in the assessment of structures with high inherent contrast differences, such as in chest CT and CT colonography (16,17). However there is a potential of ATCM to increase noise and adversely affect image quality in studies where the differences in tissue contrast is low (18).

In cardiac imaging, other methods of dose reduction may be used. As mentioned above the dose from coronary CT angiogram has increased from about 8 mSv with 16-slice CT scanners to about 15 mSv with 64-slice CT scanners. The effective dose is higher in females due to breast radiation and should be compared to the dose of 2–5 mSv from catheter coronary angiography. This increase is mainly due to lower pitch values used in 64-slice CT scanners. Dual-source CT scanner (Somatom Definition, Siemens

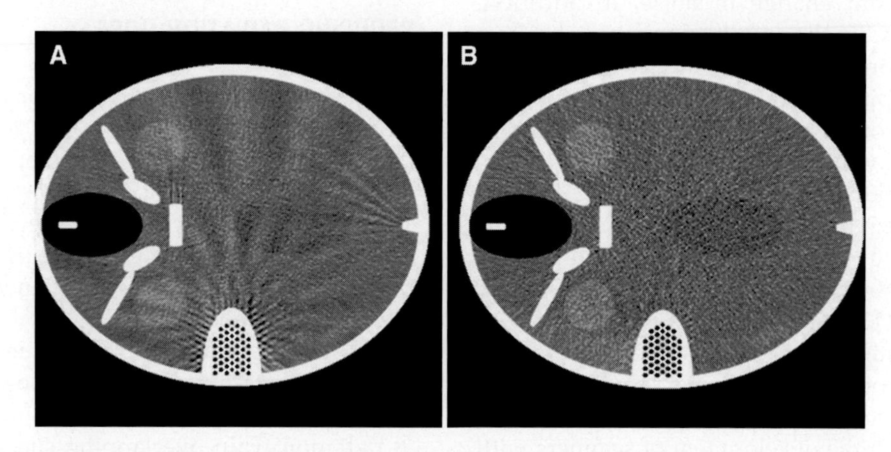

Figure 6 Windmill artifact. The alternating windmill-like dark and light bands are less prominent with lower pitch due to better sampling in the z-axis. The left image (**A**) is a scan of a head phantom using 16 x 1.5 mm configuration, pitch of 1.5, and 2 mm slice width. The right image (**B**) was obtained using same parameters, except for a 0.5 pitch.

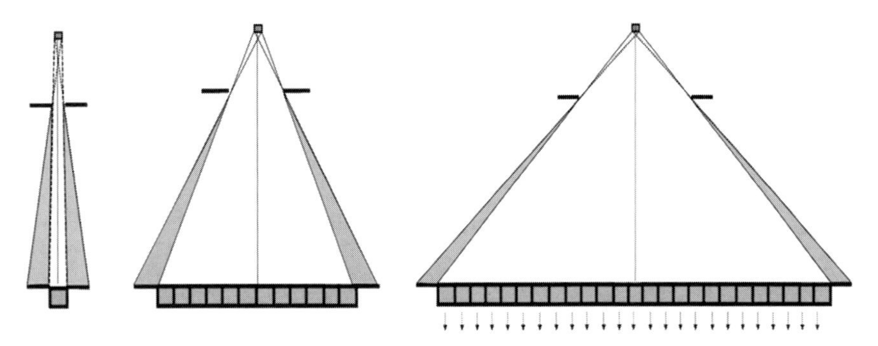

Figure 7 Penumbra radiation. Figure shows that as the X-ray beam becomes wider, the proportion of wasted penumbra radiation (shown as gray bands of radiation falling outside the active detectors) becomes smaller.

Medical Solutions) are reported to have lower radiation dose, since higher pitch values may be used (5). ECG modulation is one method of reducing dose. Most of the images reconstructed from a cardiac study are obtained in diastole, about 60–80% of the time duration from one R wave to the next R wave (so-called 60–80% of cardiac cycle). Images from systole are usually not necessary for image reconstruction when the heart rate is less than 65 beats per minute. By reducing the dose during systole it is possible to substantially decrease the total radiation dose (Fig. 9). ECG gating, however, is not useful when the heart rate is high since images in systole may be required, particularly for assessing the right coronary artery, and because there may be insufficient time to ramp the tube current up and down during the cardiac cycle.

ISOTROPIC IMAGING AND HANDLING LARGE DATA SETS

For over 30 years, nearly all CT applications have been acquired and reported in the axial plane. Two of the main hurdles to using nonaxial planes were the poor spatial resolution of reformations in these planes and the time required to create these reformations. However, good quality coronal and sagittal reformations may increase the confidence of diagnosis or demonstrate findings that may be missed on axial images (Fig. 10). A study comparing axial and nonaxial reformations of a heterogeneous group patients undergoing isotropic chest CT found that in 11% there were significant findings (those that impacted on management) that were better seen on nonaxial images (19). Other studies have shown the usefulness of coronal reformations in a wide variety of clinical situations, such as diagnosing the etiology of infiltrative lung diseases (20), and in staging of lung cancer (21).

To ensure that nonaxial reformations have the same resolution as axial images, the voxels have to be cubic, a situation termed isotropic imaging. When examining large parts of the body such as the thorax, a field of view of 40–45 cm is typically selected. Given a 512 x 512 matrix, the dimension of the voxels in the x- and y-directions is less than 1.0 mm. If the voxels are to be cubic the slice width of the source images,

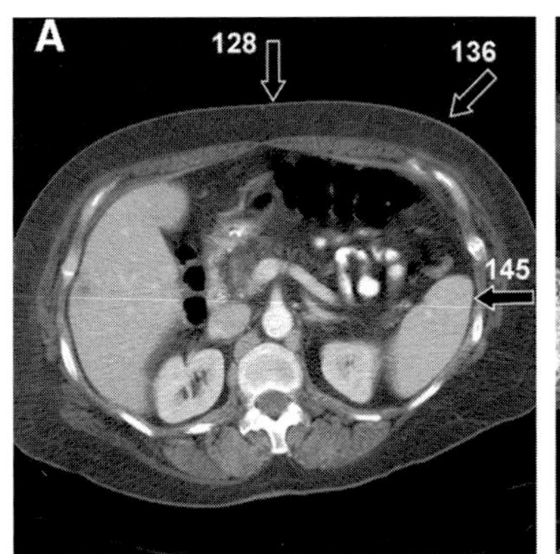

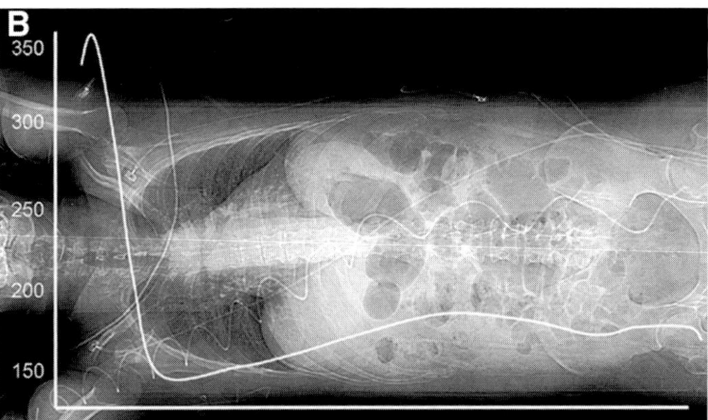

Figure 8 Automatic tube current modulation. (**A**) Angular (x–y axis or radial) tube current modulation works by changing the tube current during a gantry rotation (numbers in mA, shown at different angles). (**B**) Simplified diagram of z-axis modulation shows the tube current is constantly changed (*white curve*) through the scan. It is high when scanning through the shoulders, low through the lungs, and higher through the abdomen. If extremities are scanned, the tube current reduces. The parameters used to alter the tube current vary for each vendor. In general the tube current is constantly altered to maintain noise within a small range.

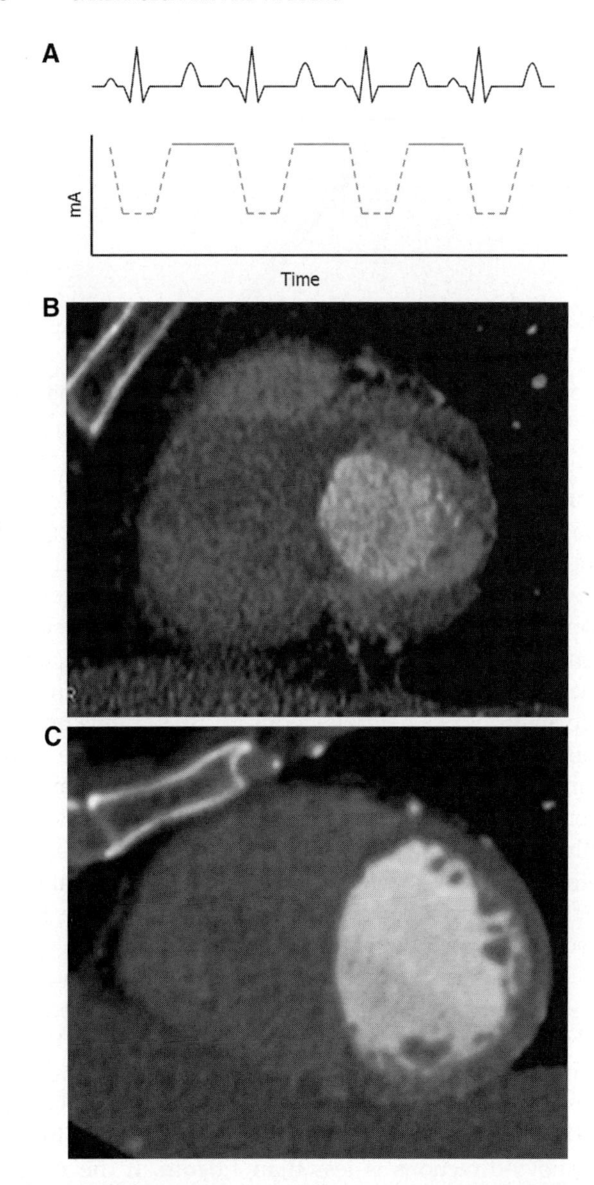

Figure 9 ECG tube current modulation. (**A**) Diagram showing how the tube current is reduced to 20–30% during systole (*dashed lines*). In diastole, the normal tube current (*solid gray lines*) is maintained. This results in an overall reduction in radiation dose of about 40–50%. (**B, C**) Reformation of images in systole (**B**) and diastole (**C**). Note the increased noise in liver dome in the systolic image, due to reduced tube current.

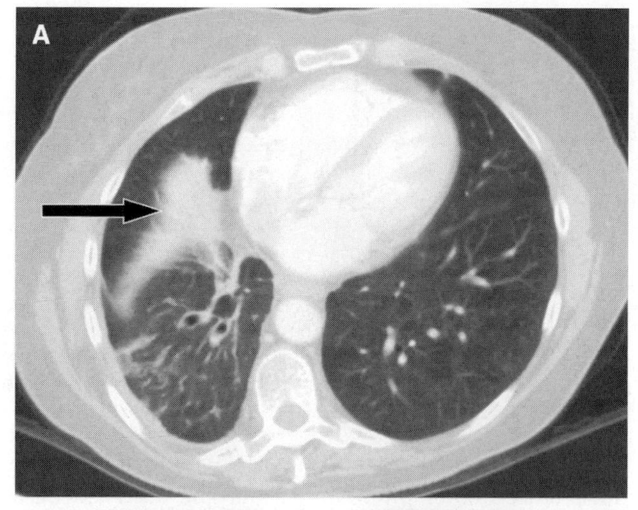

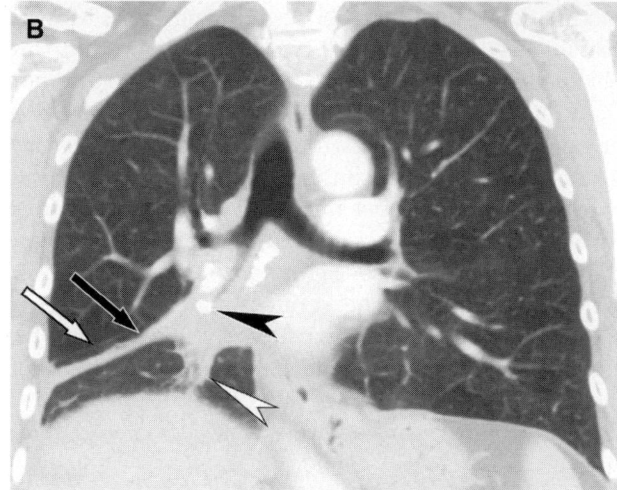

Figure 10 Value of coronal reformations in 67-year-old female with calcified nodes due to histoplasmosis causing bronchial obstruction. (**A**) Axial CT shows triangular increased density (*arrow*) in what was thought to be segmental collapse of right lower lobe. (**B**) Coronal reformation shows location of segmental collapse more accurately. There is collapse of medial segment of right middle lobe (*black arrows*). Note aerated lung inferior to minor fissure (*white arrows*) indicating patent bronchus to lateral segment of middle lobe. Calcified lymph nodes are seen in the mediastinum and the right hilum, including node causing bronchial obstruction (*black arrowhead*). There is atelectasis of superior segment of right lower lobe (*white arrowhead*).

which represents the *z*-axis dimension of the voxel, has to be of similar size.

The thorax in an average adult is about 40 cm long. If isotropic imaging is performed with 0.45 mm reconstruction intervals, approximately 900 images will constitute an average examination. It is easy to become overloaded with images unless a strategic plan exists to handle these large image numbers. In our experience, the best method of reducing the number of images viewed is to reformat the thin axial source images into thicker axial and coronal reformats, and only use these thicker reformats for reporting. The time to review the multiplanar image sets has not significantly increased (Fig. 11).

In the past, reformations were created, in a time-inefficient manner, at a workstation. With all 64-slice CT scanners it is possible to automatically plan nonaxial reformats on the scanner console using the localizer (scout) image (Fig. 12). Reformations are directly created from raw data in Siemens 64-slice CT scanner, while other scanners produce an intermediate data set of submillimeter source images that are

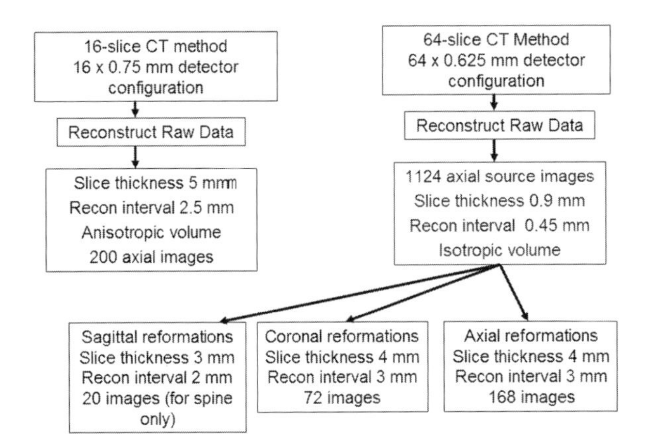

Figure 11 Line diagram showing workflow changes at our institution on switching from 16-slice CT (Brilliance-16, Philips Medical Systems, Cleveland, Ohio, U.S.A.) to 64-slice CT (Brilliance-64, Philips Medical Systems). With 16-slice CT, anisotropic axial images were obtained and in a typical chest CT about 200 such images were reviewed. With 64-slice CT an intermediate step has been introduced. The raw data are reconstructed into submillimeter isotropic axial source images. Such images are not used for image review. Reformations of these thin source images are produced in all three planes and used for image review. The total number of images to be reviewed has not substantially increased.

used to create thicker multiplanar reformations. In our experience of 3 years of using this technique, it was not necessary to retrieve the submillimeter source images for additional review, once the report dictation was completed. Therefore, it is acceptable to discard these source images, like the raw data, and not send them to long-term storage on picture archiving and communications systems (PACS).

Instead of using multiplanar images created at the scanner console, it may be possible to use advanced features available on current PACS. Such systems allow creation, within a few seconds, of reformations in any orthogonal plane, and of any slice thickness. This method is more versatile than using reformations from the scanner since the radiologist need only create reformations in patients in whom these are thought to be of value. However, to obtain high-quality nonaxial reformations it is necessary to transfer to PACS the large volume of thin isotropic source images, which may cause the network to slow down, and increases the memory requirements for archiving.

CONCLUSION

Several technical issues related to 64-slice CT scanners have been discussed. Knowledge of these features help in pushing the limits of these versatile scanners, like obtaining good quality images in the obese patients or reducing the dose in a pediatric patient. There are some technical differences between the 64-slice CT scanners from the different vendors, though these variations are small compared to the similarities they share.

ACKNOWLEDGMENT

The authors gratefully acknowledge Drs. Phillip Boiselle and Ioannis "Johnny" Vlahos for the contribution of text and images related to dual-energy CT.

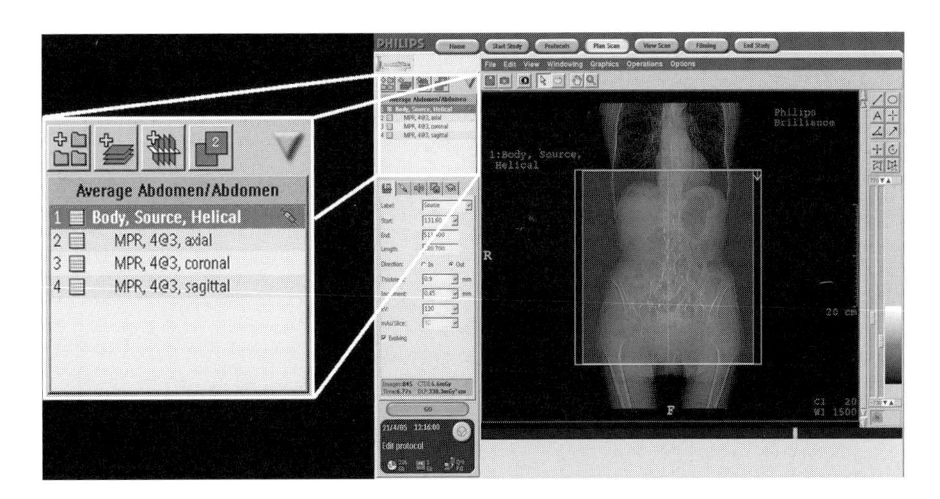

Figure 12 Automatic multiplanar reformations at scanner console. The volume to scan is shown on the scout (localizer) image on a 64-slice CT scanner (Briliance-64, Philips Medical Systems, Cleveland, Ohio, U.S.A.) console. The source images are automatically reformatted in multiple planes according to the preset protocol shown on the left. The reformations are completed within a few seconds at the end of the study and sent to the picture archiving and communications system (PACS). All 64-slice CT scanners have software that semiautomatically creates reformations in any orthogonal plane.

REFERENCES

1 Johnson TR, Krauss B, Sedlmair M, et al. Material differentiation by dual energy CT: initial experience. Eur Radiol 2007; 17(6):1510–17.
2 Scheffel H, Alkadhi H, Plass A, et al. Accuracy of dual-source CT coronary angiography: first experience in a high pre-test probability population without heart rate control. Eur Radiol 2006; 16(12):2739–47.
3 Johnson TR, Nikolaou K, Wintersperger BJ, et al. Dual-source CT cardiac imaging: initial experience. Eur Radiol 2006; 16:1409–15.
4 Achenbach S, Ropers D, Kuettner A, et al. Contrast-enhanced coronary artery visualization by dual-source computed tomographyinitial experience. Eur J Radiol 2006; 57:331–5.
5 Flohr TG, McCollough CH, Bruder H, et al. First performance evaluation of a dual-source CT (DSCT) system. Eur Radiol 2006; 16:256–68.
6 Reimann AJ, Rinick D, Birinci-Aydogan A, et al. Dual-source computed tomography: advances of improved temporal resolution in coronary plague imaging. Invest Radiol 2007; 42:196–203.
7 Kalender W. Dual energy CT: Is there escape from the Hounsfield unit cage? In: GlazerGM, RubinGD, eds. Stanford Radiology. Eighth Annual International Symposium on Multidetector-Row CT Syllabus, 2006. Palo Alto, CA: Stanford University School of Medicine, 2006:27–8.
8 Mori S, Endo M, Tsunoo T, et al. Physical performance evaluation of a 256-slice CT-scanner for four-dimensional imaging. Med Phys 2004; 31:1348–56.
9 Kalender WA, Seissler W, Klotz E, Vock P. Spiral volumetric CT with single-breath-hold technique, continuous transport, and continuous scanner rotation. Radiology 1990; 176:181–3.
10 Mahesh M, Scatarige JC, Cooper J, Fishman EK. Dose and pitch relationship for a particular multislice CT scanner. AJR Am J Roentgenol 2001; 177:1273–5.
11 Theocharopoulos N, Perisinakis K, Damilakis J, Karampekios S, Gourtsoyiannis N. Dosimetric characteristics of a 16-slice computed tomography scanner. Eur Radiol 2006; 16(11):2575–2585.
12 Fuchs T, Krause J, Schaller S, Flohr T, Kalender WA. Spiral interpolation algorithms for multislice spiral CTpart II: measurement and evaluation of slice sensitivity profiles and noise at a clinical multislice system. IEEE Trans Med Imaging 2000; 19:835–47.
13 Primak AN, McCollough CH, Bruesewitz MR, Zhang J, Fletcher JG. Relationship between noise, dose, and pitch in cardiac multi-detector row CT. Radiographics 2006; 26:1785–94.
14 Mettler FA, Jr., Wiest PW, Locken JA, Kelsey CA. CT scanning: patterns of use and dose. J Radiol Prot 2000; 20:353–9.
15 Gray JE. Safety (risk) of diagnostic radiology exposures. In: JanowerJL, LintonOW, eds. Radiation Risk: A Primer. Reston, VA: American College of Radiology, 1996:15–17.
16 Graser A, Wintersperger BJ, Suess C, Reiser MF, Becker CR. Dose reduction and image quality in MDCT colonography using tube current modulation. AJR Am J Roentgenol 2006; 187:695–701.
17 Kalra MK, Rizzo S, Maher MM, et al. Chest CT performed with *z*-axis modulation: scanning protocol and radiation dose. Radiology 2005; 237:303–8.
18 Iball GR, Brettle DS, Moore AC. Assessment of tube current modulation in pelvic CT. Br J Radiol 2006; 79:62–70.
19 Rydberg J, Sandrasegaran K, Tarver RD, Frank MS, Conces DJ, Choplin RH. Routine isotropic CT scanning of chest: value of coronal and sagittal reformations. Invest Radiol 2007; 42(1):23–28.
20 Remy-Jardin M, Campistron P, Amara A, et al. Usefulness of coronal reformations in the diagnostic evaluation of infiltrative lung disease. J Comput Assist Tomogr 2003; 27:266–73.
21 Chooi WK, Matthews S, Bull MJ, Morcos SK. Multislice computed tomography in staging lung cancer: the role of multiplanar image reconstruction. J Comput Assist Tomogr 2005; 29:357–60.
22 Lewis M, Keat N, Edyvean S. Report 06012. Sixteen slice CT scanner comparison report version 14. London, UK: ImPACT, 2006.
23 Lewis M, Keat N, Edyvean S. Report 06013. 32 to 64 slice CT scanner comparison report version 14. London, UK: ImPACT, 2006.

2

Dual PET-CT

Vikram Krishnasetty and Suzanne L. Aquino
Department of Radiology, Massachusetts General Hospital, Harvard Medical School, Boston, Massachusetts, U.S.A.

INTRODUCTION

In the past, the primary imaging technique for the diagnosis and evaluation of patients with thoracic disease, particularly lung cancer, has been CT. The basis of CT as the primary diagnostic modality in thoracic imaging is founded on its superior anatomic resolution as compared with other imaging modalities. A fundamental shortcoming of CT, however, is its dependence on change in morphology for diagnostic interpretation. The addition of FDG-PET technology has supplemented the radiologic staging and diagnosis of malignant disease with physiologic data (1). Research has shown that the added information regarding abnormal glucose metabolism within malignant cells in FDG-PET imaging has significantly impacted radiologic staging of patients with lung cancer by significantly and appropriately changing the management in a majority of affected patients. In a study by Hicks et al. (2), the addition of PET to conventional staging techniques identified patients with metastases to be converted to palliative therapy, sparing patients unnecessary surgery. An additional 10% of the patients in their study were downstaged based on PET results converting their therapy regimen from palliative to curative.

Recent advances in dual PET-CT imaging systems (3) as well as software-generated PET-CT image registration (4,5) have further improved lung cancer staging and management by combining the anatomically specific information of CT with the more sensitive metabolic findings of FDG-PET. This relatively new technology allows the fusion of anatomic and metabolic data into a comprehensive diagnostic tool. In this chapter, we review some of the technical aspects of dual PET-CT image acquisition, the role of combined PET-CT in the imaging of lung cancer, and some important pitfalls associated with dual PET-CT imaging.

TECHNICAL FEATURES

Historical Aspects

Historically, one of the first dual modality devices to combine functional and anatomic imaging was a combination of CT and single photon emission CT (SPECT) developed by Hasegawa et al. (6) and Lang et al. (7) in the early 1990s. The first dedicated PET-CT scanner, a prototype installed at the University of Pittsburgh Medical Center, did not become operational for patient studies until 1998 (8,9). Around the same time, PET emerged as an important imaging modality for diagnosis, staging, and therapeutic planning of cancer, and PET-CT technology, with its improved anatomic definition, is arising as an important oncologic imaging tool.

All of the modern dual PET-CT imaging systems are based on the hardware combination of modern multislice helical CT scanners and PET coincidence detection systems. The variations in the PET-CT hardware is primarily based on the relative level of performance of the PET and CT components, extent of hardware integration, and the level of software integration (9).

Clinical Protocols

Approximately 1 hour after injection of approximately 10 mCi (370 MBq) of FDG, the patient is positioned in a supine position on the gantry. From the acquired topogram, the range to be scanned by PET and CT is selected. The CT is then acquired after the patient is instructed to breathe quietly. A recent study by Gilman et al. demonstrated that misregistration in the thorax can be minimized with attenuation correction CT performed in expiration, mid suspended breath-hold, or quiet breathing; however, quiet breathing is most commonly used for patient comfort (Fig. 1) (10). Subsequently, PET images are also acquired with the patient in quiet breathing. Once the first bed position is completed, PET reconstruction commences (9). CT-based attenuation correction factors are calculated and three-dimension reconstructions are performed. Within a few minutes after the completion of the final PET bed position, reconstructed attenuation correction PET images coregistered to CT images are available for viewing.

Additional Technical Considerations

An additional advantage of dual PET-CT, beyond that of acquiring coregistered anatomic and functional data,

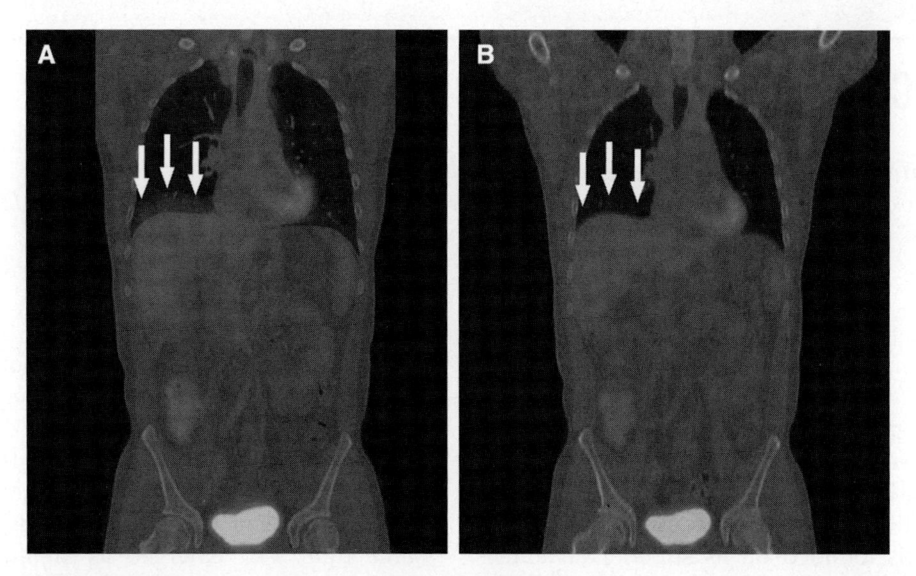

Figure 1 Dual PET-CT examinations of a 63-year-old male with history of non–small cell lung cancer. (**A**) Examination performed with breath-hold technique CT demonstrates misregistration of the right hemidiaphragm. (**B**) Examination performed with quiet breathing technique CT demonstrates excellent registration in the same area. (*See color insert.*)

is the potential to use CT images for attenuation correction of PET emission data. This eliminates the need for a separate, time-consuming PET transmission scan and allows for the reduction of whole-body scan times by at least 40% (9). CT attenuation correction also provides essentially noiseless attenuation correction factors as compared to transmission PET. However, the scaling of attenuation coefficients from CT energies to 511 keV is associated with certain problems (9). Because of the scaling algorithms used, there is the potential to create focal artifacts in PET imaging when pixels are incorrectly scaled to 511 keV, particularly in contrast-enhanced imaging. For this reason, most dual PET-CTs are acquired without the use of intravenous (or oral) contrast. Since standard-of-care CT scanning generally involves the use of contrast, one way to avoid these potential artifacts is to use a low-dose CT scan for attenuation correction and a separate contrast-enhanced scan (11).

Image Interpretation

Following image reconstruction, images are transferred to an off-line viewing station and the data can be archived. Images are best viewed on a workstation that can display the 3D reconstructed CT, PET, and coregistered fused data set in multiple planes. This alleviates the need of the interpreting radiologist to "visually fuse" the PET and CT data, thereby decreasing the potential for localization errors (12).

At this point, it should be noted that FDG uptake can be assessed by either qualitative means or semi-quantitative means [i.e., standard uptake value (SUV)]. In our clinical practice, we employ the qualitative assessment of FDG uptake because SUVs are subject to variations dependent on weight and circulating insulin levels (13). In addition, studies demonstrate a wide overlap of individual SUVs between malignant and benign lesions even though overall SUVs are higher in malignant lesions than benign lesions (14).

PRIMARY DIAGNOSIS OF LUNG CANCER

The detection and diagnosis of lung cancer is arguably the most important aspect of modern thoracic imaging. The goal is the detection of lung cancer in its earliest stage and the differentiation from benign disease. Although chest CT is useful for assessing the size and stability of a nodule over time, it lacks sufficient specificity to provide a definitive diagnosis. CT features of lung nodules that suggest malignancy or benignity are discussed in more detail in Chapter 9.

FDG-PET has been shown to be both highly sensitive and specific in the diagnosis of malignancy in pulmonary nodules (15,16). According to Patz et al. (17), the sensitivity and specificity of FDG-PET for detecting malignancy were 100% and 89%, respectively. A drawback of stand-alone FDG-PET imaging is the accurate localization of a focal FDG abnormality to the lesion in question.

The combination of PET-CT adds the potential to better localize an area of FDG uptake to a specific pulmonary nodule (Fig. 2). Additionally, by demonstrating an absence of FDG uptake within a pulmonary nodule, PET-CT has the potential to identify it as more likely benign. A study by Lowe et al. (18) demonstrated that, when FDG uptake within focal opacities was analyzed, a highly statistically significant difference was found between the PET SUV

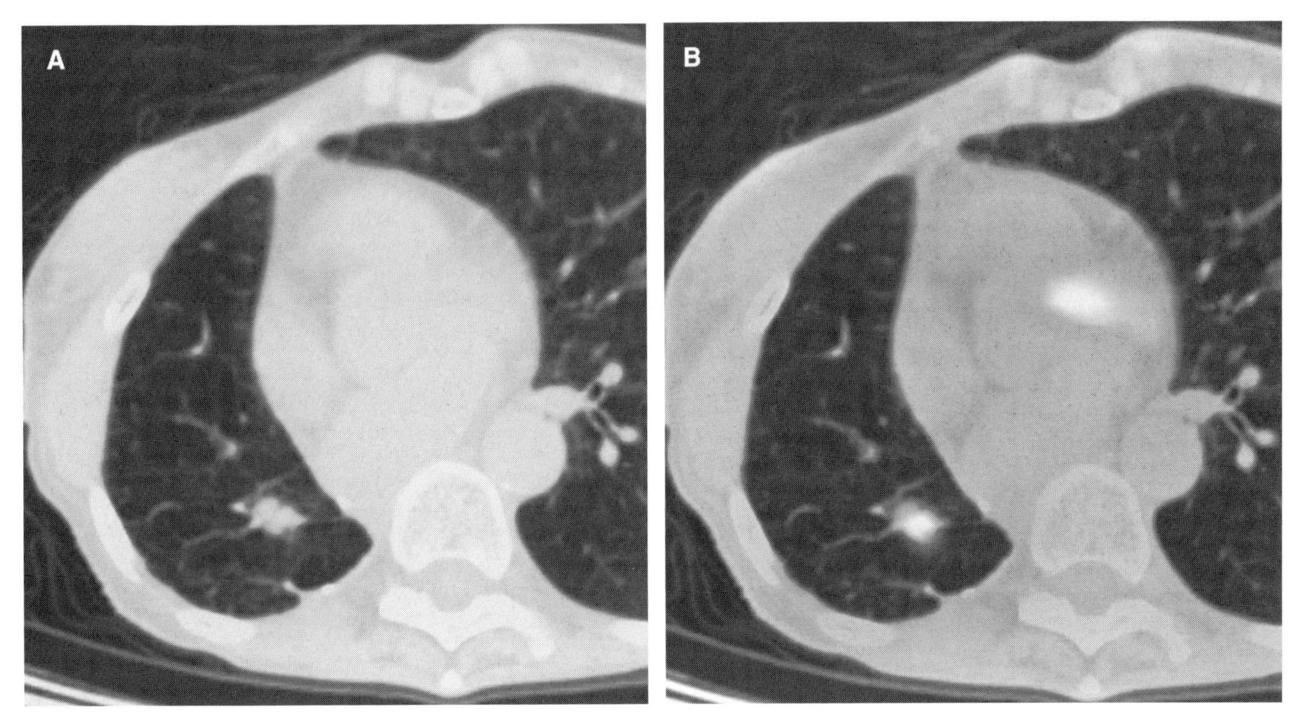

Figure 2 Evaluation of a pulmonary nodule in a 69-year-old woman. (**A**) CT image from a dual PET-CT examination demonstrates a nodule in the right upper lobe. (**B**) Fused image from a dual PET-CT examination clearly demonstrates focal intense FDG uptake, with the nodule indicative of malignancy. (*See color insert for* **B**.)

value of malignant and benign lesions (19). Combined PET-CT, however, is still limited for the evaluation of pulmonary nodules less than 8 mm since the limiting resolution of most commercially available PET-CT scanners is 7–8 mm (20).

In cases where the malignancy of a lesion needs to be confirmed by histologic sampling, localizing and targeting an area of FDG uptake within a lesion has the potential to provide a better positive diagnostic yield. Areas of low FDG uptake due to adjacent scar or necrosis could be avoided in favor of areas of increased FDG uptake that are more likely to have viable tumor (Fig. 3).

Studies have also revealed that certain malignancies in the thorax, e.g., bronchioloalveolar carcinoma (BAC) (21,22) and carcinoid tumor (23,24), demonstrate comparatively low FDG uptake. In these instances, CT characteristics of a lung nodule may

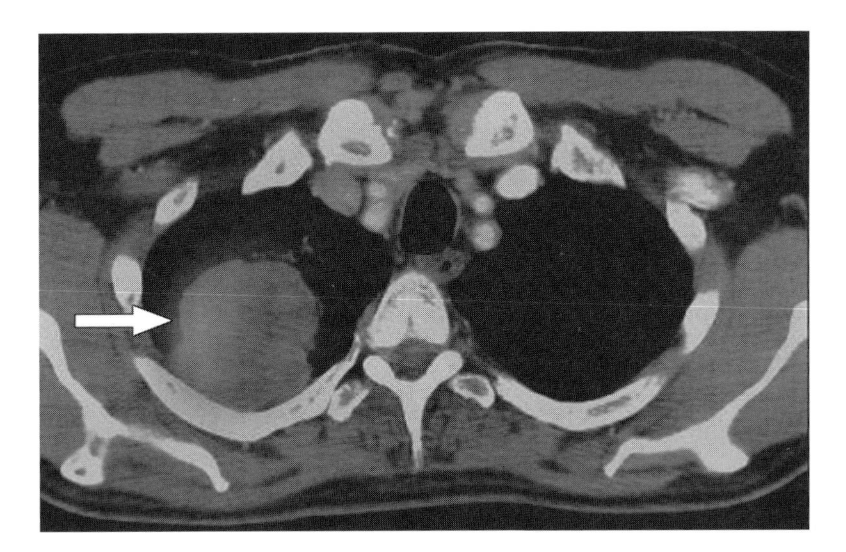

Figure 3 Dual PET-CT in a 61-year-old for initial staging of lung cancer. Large right apical mass demonstrates areas of intense FDG uptake corresponding to viable tumor and areas of lower FDG uptake corresponding to areas of necrosis confirmed on gross pathology. (*See color insert.*)

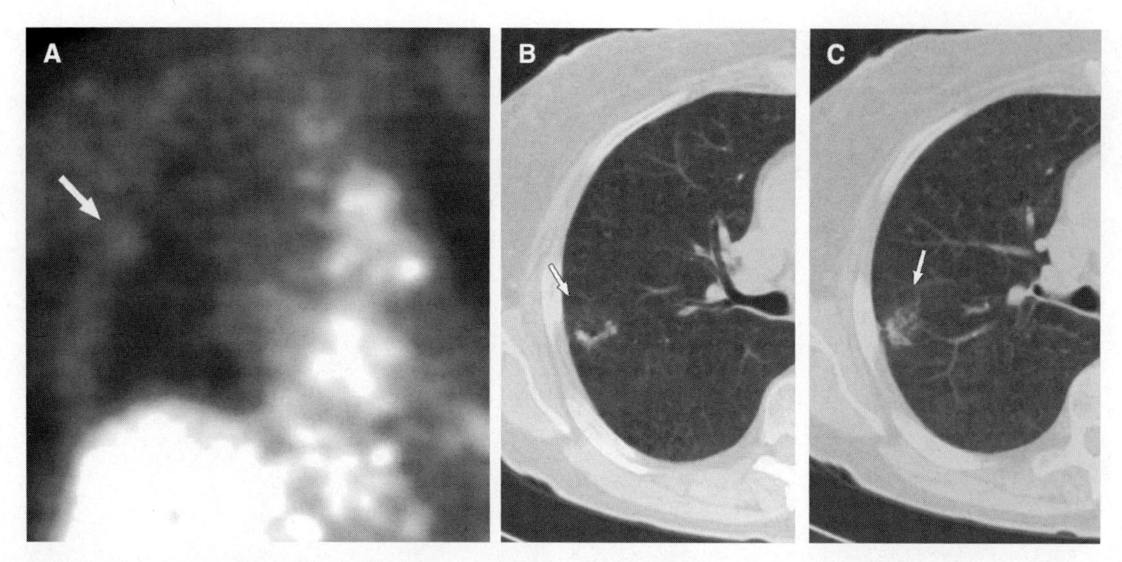

Figure 4 Bronchioloalveolar cell carcinoma in a 70-year-old woman. (**A**) FDG-PET image demonstrating a focus of low-level uptake that is equivalent to mediastinal uptake but slightly greater than surrounding lung parenchyma. (**B,C**) Ground glass nodule with a small area of cavitation corresponding to the focus of FDG-PET uptake.

need to be factored into the analysis of a nodule evaluated by PET. Nodules that have ground glass or mixed ground glass appearance on CT may need to be more aggressively approached since these patterns are more likely to be associated with BAC (25). For example, in Figure 4, a BAC demonstrates FDG uptake only slightly above background, however, its features on CT help distinguish it as a BAC. Carcinoid tumors are less distinct radiographically but may manifest as a discrete nodule associated with a bronchus (26). On the other hand, pulmonary diseases other than malignancy may create false-positive interpretations resulting from increased FDG activity that has been observed in a variety of benign conditions, such as granulomatous diseases and infection. This will be discussed in more detail in the following sections.

STAGING OF NON–SMALL CELL LUNG CANCER

Although imaging is useful for the initial detection of lung cancers, the most common role of radiological imaging in patients with lung cancer is initial staging. Recent studies evaluating combined PET-CT have shown significant improvement in lung cancer staging over both PET and CT (3,27). The current "International System for Staging Lung Cancer" published by Mountain in 1997 (28) is based on prognosis at time of presentation and is used to guide treatment planning.

Primary Tumor Staging

The high-spatial resolution of multidetector CT makes it an excellent modality for assessing the size and extent of the primary tumor (T). However, there are ways that combined PET-CT can improve the accuracy of primary tumor evaluation (3). For example, Lardinois et al. (3) found that combined PET-CT more accurately demonstrates chest wall and mediastinal invasion as compared to PET alone, CT alone, or visually correlated PET and CT. PET-CT has also been demonstrated to more precisely delineate the primary tumor, improving the detection of any involvement of the chest wall or pleura (29). For example, in Figure 5, CT demonstrates nonspecific pleural thickening, however PET-CT demonstrates focal areas of intense FDG uptake consistent with pleural involvement.

The improved delineation of primary tumor from postobstructive atelectasis by dual PET-CT allows for more accurate tumor measurement (Fig. 6) (30). As a result, radiation therapy targeting and portals can be planned more accurately. Nestle et al. demonstrated that 35% of radiation portals were changed (primarily reduced) after more accurate primary tumor staging was achieved with dual PET-CT imaging.

The combination of PET and CT imaging may also help distinguish benign from malignant pleural effusions, which can change the initial T stage. Malignant pleural effusions have been shown to demonstrate more intense uptake than the usual background FDG uptake seen in benign pleural effusions with accuracies approaching 91% (31).

Lymph Node Staging

Traditionally, CT has been used to detect and evaluate involved lymph nodes in patients with lung cancer. CT depends on morphologic criteria alone defining a mediastinal or hilar lymph node as pathologic if the short axis measurement is greater than 1 cm. However,

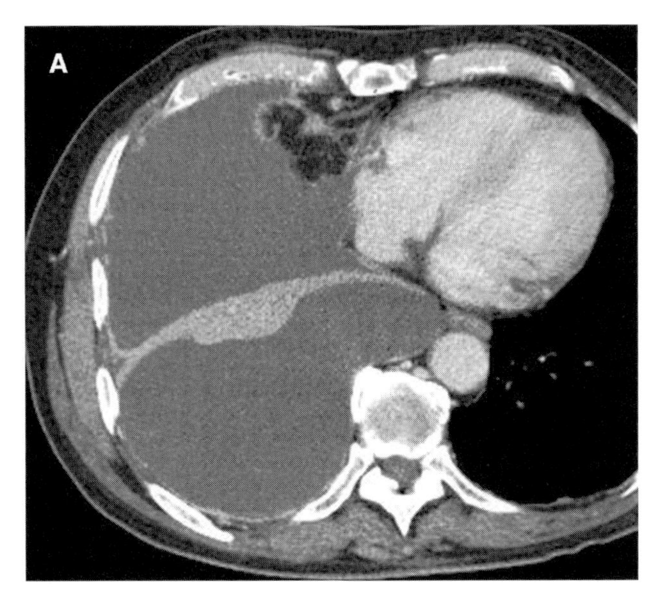

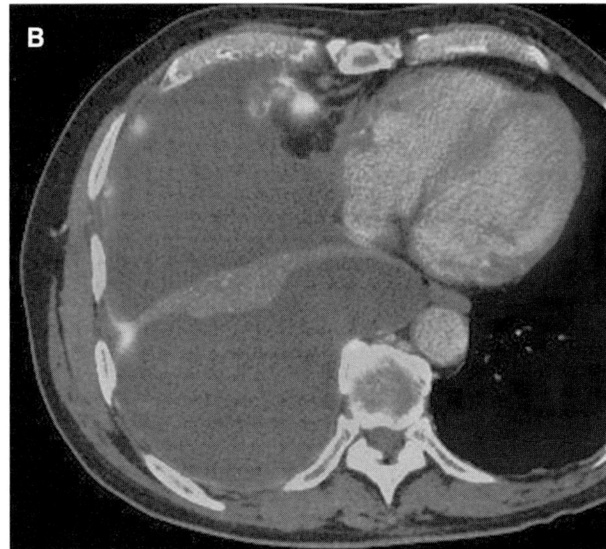

Figure 5 Dual PET-CT in a 79-year-old male with non–small cell lung cancer. (**A**) CT demonstrates nonspecific pleural thickening. (**B**) Fused dual PET-CT images demonstrate foci of intense pleural FDG uptake, confirming pleural involvement. (*See color insert for* **B**.)

in a study by McLoud et al. (32), 33% of enlarged lymph nodes on CT in patients with lung cancers were benign. In addition, Pieterman et al. (33) demonstrated that multiple small metastatic lymph nodes were missed on CT but were better detected by FDG-PET. In their study, PET was 91% sensitive and 86% specific compared to CT, which was 75% sensitive and 66% specific for the detection of mediastinal nodal metastases. Dual PET-CT further improves this sensitivity and specificity (33). Antoch et al. (34) reported sensitivity of 89% and specificity of 94% in regional nodal staging with dual PET-CT scan as compared to 89% sensitivity and 89% specificity with PET alone. Aquino et al. (5) reported improved sensitivities and specificities in detecting nodal metastases and overall staging among their readers when they compared staging of CT and PET images interpreted side-by-side with PET-CT data sets fused with registration software.

Detection of Metastases

Non–small cell lung cancer (NSCLC) can metastasize to a variety of sites throughout the body. Studies have found that whole-body PET has a 11–12% incidence of detecting metastases that were missed by

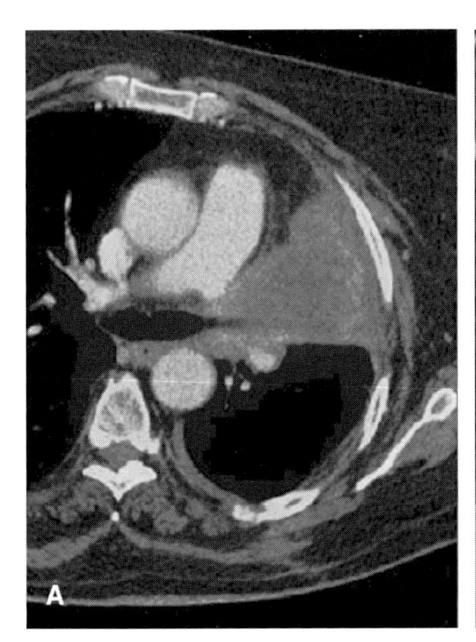

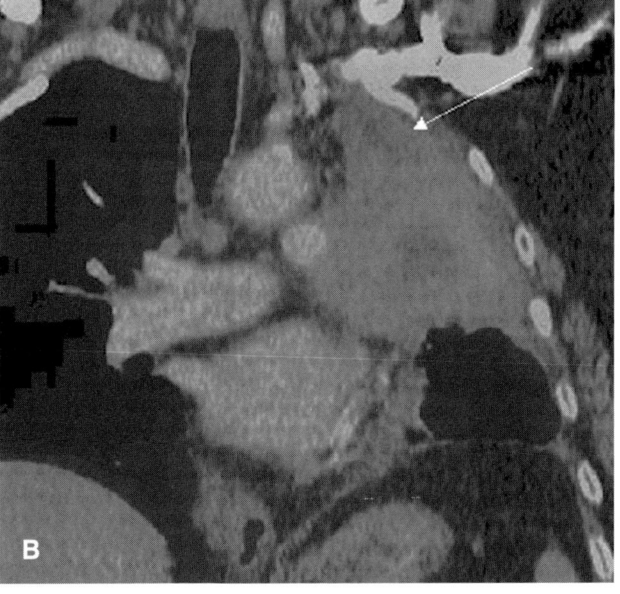

Figure 6 Dual PET-CT in a 64-year-old with non–small cell lung cancer. (**A**) Axial images demonstrate a necrotic mass in the left upper lobe with intense heterogeneous FDG uptake. (**B**) Coronal images demonstrate post-obstructive atelectasis distal to the large hilar mass that does not demonstrate intense FDG uptake. This allows more accurate measurement of the primary tumor mass. (*See color insert.*)

conventional staging methods (33,35). A study by Bury et al. has even demonstrated the usefulness of whole-body FDG-PET in the detection of bone metastases in patients with NSCLC (36). The exception is the use of FDG-PET in the evaluation of brain metastases (37). Rohren et al. theorized that the insensitivity (61% sensitivity) of FDG-PET in the detection of cerebral metastases may be secondary to the small size of the metastases as well as the inherent background FDG uptake of the gray matter. For these reasons, contrast-enhanced CT and MRI are still needed for the assessment of brain metastases.

The detection of metastases is further improved by dual PET-CT. Metastatic lesions that are not clearly evident or are missed on CT may be more easily identified on PET-CT. Prabhakar et al. (38) found that 8.4% of patients with cancer who received combined PET-CT scans had findings on combined image interpretation that were missed on CT alone. This number increased to 17.6% in patients with lung cancer.

SMALL CELL LUNG CANCER

The primary mode of treatment for small cell lung cancer (SCLC) is chemotherapy and/or radiation therapy, unlike NSCLC, which can be treated surgically. For this reason, the staging criteria used for NSCLC is not generally used for SCLC patients. Instead, clinical stage, which can be divided into limited disease (LD) and extensive disease (ED), is the most important factor affecting prognosis and treatment options for patients with SCLC (39). Although patients with LD are treated with a combination of chemotherapy and chest irradiation, those patients with ED are treated primarily with chemotherapy alone (40). LD is defined as disease confined to one hemithorax, mediastinum, and regional lymph nodes; in other words, disease that can be targeted with one radiation portal field (40). At initial presentation, two-thirds of the patients present with ED, which is defined as extrathoracic disease or malignant pleural effusion (39).

The primary role of diagnostic imaging is to accurately distinguish LD from ED for initial staging and treatment planning. Conventionally, CT, MRI, and bone scan have been the most commonly used diagnostic modalities for the staging of SCLC. However, recent studies, such as that by Kamel et al., have demonstrated that the addition of FDG-PET imaging was able to demonstrate otherwise occult metastatic sites that changed patients from a LD to ED category (40). They also demonstrated that PET excluded metastases in 12% of patients with suspicious lesions found on CT and MRI. Overall, Kamel and colleagues showed that the addition of FDG-PET affected staging and management in 29% of the 42 patients with SCLC in their study.

BRONCHIOLOALVEOLAR CARCINOMA

BAC accounts for 2–10% of all lung cancers but has increased in incidence over the past few years (41). This tumor is a well-differentiated adenocarcinoma, which frequently exhibits very slow growth. Studies prior to the reclassification of BAC suggested poor reliability of detection of BAC by FDG-PET (21,22). Kim et al. (22) theorize that the unique slow growth of BAC accounts for this lower peak SUV, thus decreasing the reliability of PET for the detection of BAC. However, a recent study by Yap et al. (41) demonstrated an 87% sensitivity for the detection of BAC by PET. In all of these studies, however, FDG-PET had the lowest sensitivity and specificity in the detection of pure BAC (100% BAC component) (22,41).

Although no study has yet examined combined PET-CT in the diagnosis of BAC, the addition of CT morphologic features and improved lesion localization may likely be as good or better than PET alone. Even though the peak SUV of pure BAC lesions may not be as high as other types of bronchogenic carcinoma, the combination of a ground glass CT appearance with slightly higher levels of uptake on FDG-PET may allow for better BAC detection by combined PET-CT. Figure 4 demonstrates a case of histologically proven BAC. Although the level of FDG uptake within the nodules is equivalent to mediastinal uptake and not as intense as seen in other types of NSCLC, the level of FDG uptake is still discernibly greater than that of the surrounding lung parenchyma.

LUNG CANCER RESTAGING

Regardless of the treatment, therapeutic response and potential for recurrence are monitored with imaging studies given that approximately 50% of patients with resected NSCLC will have recurrence (42). Before the advent of FDG-PET, imaging studies relied only on changes in anatomy to distinguish posttherapy changes from residual or recurrent tumor. However, due to the background of architectural distortion from surgery and radiation therapy, this differentiation based on morphologic CT features alone has proven to be difficult. Additionally, a negative biopsy result may actually be a false-negative secondary to sampling error.

Recurrence Following Surgical Therapy

Many patients will show increased FDG uptake at the surgical site secondary to postoperative inflammatory response. Although early postsurgical changes may be difficult to distinguish from recurrent disease, late postsurgical changes should be easier to distinguish from recurrent disease since postsurgical change should only demonstrate background low-level FDG

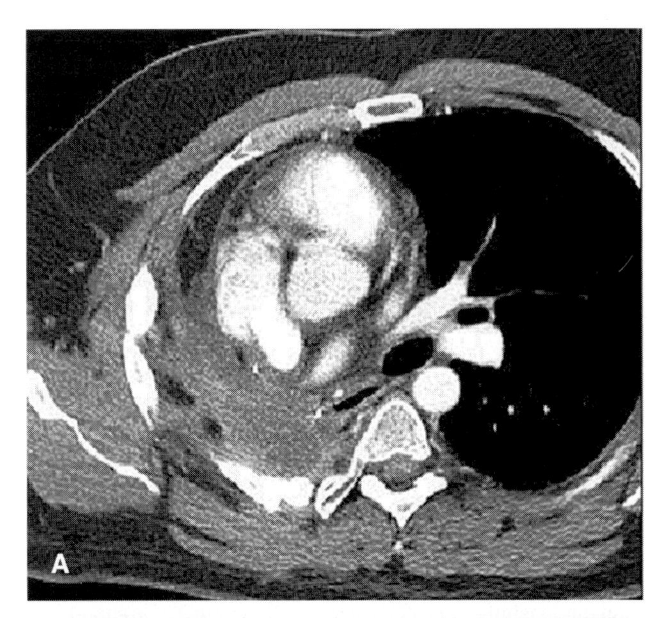

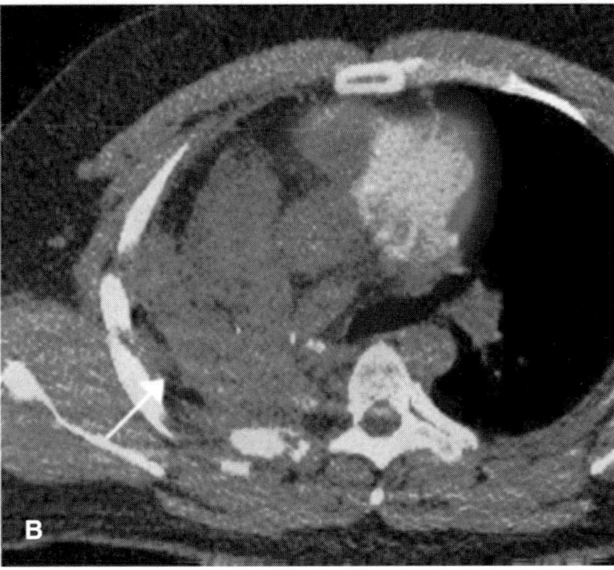

Figure 7 Dual PET-CT examination in a 43-year-old male, two years after a right pneumonectomy for non–small cell lung cancer. (**A**) Axial CT image demonstrates nonspecific post-operative findings status post pneumonectomy with a loculated pleural effusion and diffuse pleural thickening. (**B**) Dual PET-CT image demonstrates an area of pleural thickening with intense FDG uptake that likely represents recurrent disease. (*See color insert for* **B**.)

uptake (43). Areas of intense FDG uptake in the late postoperative should raise the suspicion of residual or recurrent disease. Recurrence should also be suspected if FDG uptake extends to locations that should not have been affected by the surgery. In the example shown in Figure 7, the postpneumonectomy changes on CT are difficult to distinguish from recurrent disease with CT imaging alone. Dual PET-CT imaging demonstrates intense nodular uptake within the post-pneumonectomy space, suggesting disease recurrence rather than just postsurgical changes.

Recurrence at the bronchial stump after pneumonectomy has traditionally been difficult to diagnose before disease progression beyond the stump (44). In a study by Verleden, 3.4% of patients followed after radical resection for NSCLC developed bronchial stump recurrence (45). They found a significant relationship between the time of recurrence and the distance of the primary tumor from the bronchial stump. Keidar et al. (43) reported a case where PET-CT was useful in excluding bronchial stump recurrence in a patient where CT findings were equivocal. Although studies have suggested that the appearance of soft tissue at the bronchial stump or change in the sharp appearance of the bronchial stump on CT can be used as signs of recurrence (46), the addition of PET imaging may be useful in the evaluation of such recurrence.

The administration of talc into the pleural space during thoracotomy may also create false-positive findings on FDG-PET. Talc causes a chronic granulomatous reaction in the pleural space that can mimic pleural tumor (47). The use of dual PET-CT imaging to localize the foci of increased FDG uptake to dense talc deposits in the pleura can be helpful to avoid such false-positives (Fig. 8). According to Kwek et al. pleural talc deposits will be abnormal on FDG-PET for an indefinite period of time. Therefore it is essential to carefully identify and track these areas on any follow-up FDG-PET scan in order to distinguish these area of posttreatment changes from any new foci of FDG uptake representing new tumor deposits.

Recurrence Following Radiation Therapy

Virtually all patients who receive therapeutic doses of radiation will have some degree of lung parenchymal reaction although not always radiographically detectable (48). Early radiation damage (1–4 months) results in radiation pneumonitis caused by cellular damage and subsequent repair (48). Some of the biochemical pathways involved in cellular repair depend on ATP as a source of energy (49), which may help explain the association of increased FDG uptake and radiation pneumonitis. The typical CT findings of acute radiation include indistinct pulmonary vasculature, airspace disease, and dense consolidation usually confined to the field of radiation. On FDG-PET these areas show moderate FDG uptake within the boundaries of the radiation port (48,50). Late radiation changes manifest as CT findings of fibrosis exclusively defined to the radiation portal (48). The typical CT findings of radiation fibrosis include well-defined areas of architectural distortion, fibrosis, traction bronchiectasis, and volume loss. On FDG-PET these areas of fibrosis will show relatively normalized levels of FDG uptake similar to background soft tissue uptake (48,50).

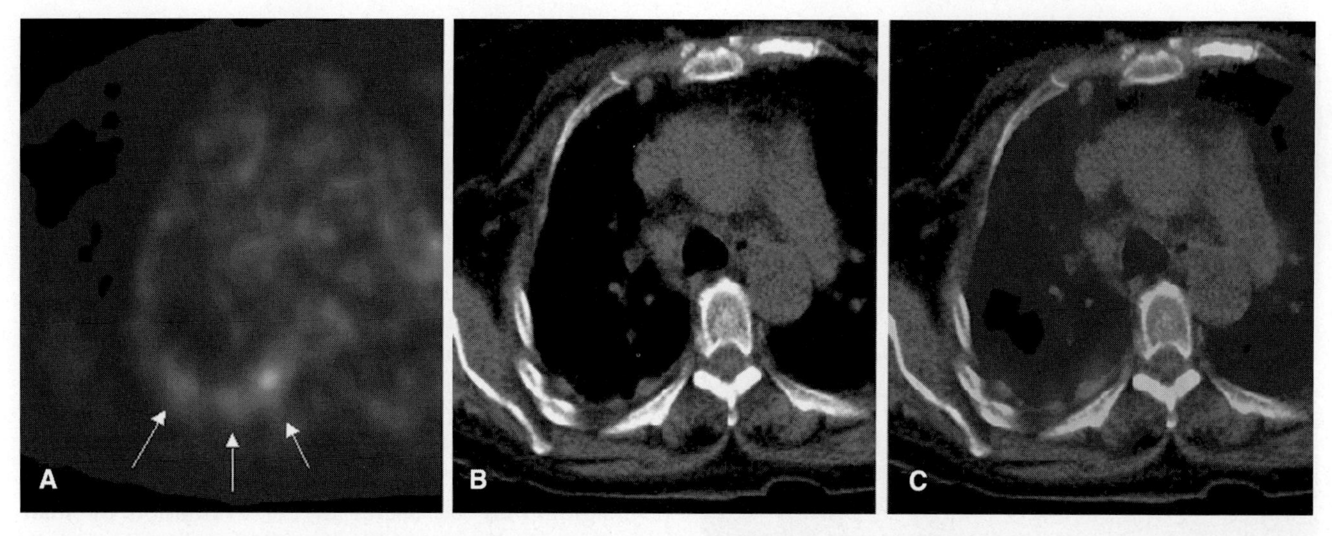

Figure 8 Images from a dual PET-CT on a 74-year-old woman with non–small cell lung cancer status post talc pleurodesis. (**A**) FDG-PET images demonstrate multiple foci of intense uptake in the right posterior pleura. (**B**) Corresponding axial CT image demonstrates high-density talc in the posterior right pleural space. (**C**) Fused dual PET-CT image demonstrates the foci of intense FDG uptake corresponding to the high-density talc. Finding is secondary to a granulomatous reaction to the talc rather than metastatic disease. (*See color insert for* **C**.)

The differentiation between posttreatment changes in the lungs from residual/recurrent tumor can be difficult during the period in which FDG uptake has not normalized. However, studies have demonstrated that FDG-PET imaging is useful for this purpose in the late posttreatment period (51). In a study by Patz et al. (51), persistent FDG uptake 2 months posttreatment was considered suspicious for malignancy since FDG uptake from posttreatment changes should have normalized in that time period. More recent studies, such as that by Keidar et al. (43) suggest that persistent FDG uptake can be seen in up to 6 months posttreatment. Although stand-alone PET is sensitive for the detection of recurrence, it lacks the anatomic detail to localize suspicious findings. Treatment-distorted anatomy along with posttherapeutic inflammation may hinder the diagnosis of recurrence. Keidar et al. (43) demonstrated that combined PET-CT scans improved the anatomic localization of suspicious lesions compared to PET or CT alone in patients with suspected NSCLC recurrence. Aquino et al. (5) found that fusion of PET and CT data sets of patients treated for lung cancer and other thoracic neoplasms improved the detection of recurrent or metastatic tumor. Patients who had undergone surgery or received radiation therapy often had areas of anatomic distortion. By fusing the PET and CT images, areas of increased FDG uptake were better localized to either areas of tumor or inflammation such as esophagitis or atherosclerosis. Figure 9 demonstrates the localization of abnormal mediastinal uptake to the esophagus, suggesting radiation-induced esophagitis rather than recurrence within a subcarinal lymph node.

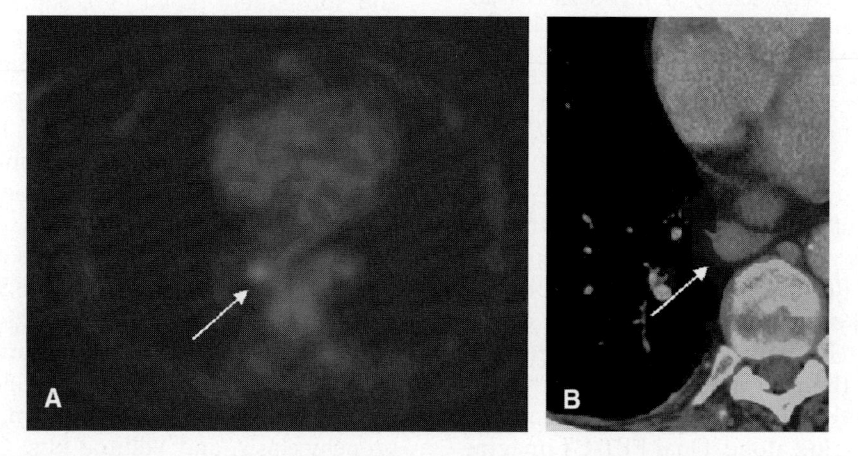

Figure 9 Dual PET-CT for restaging in patient with non–small cell lung cancer. (**A**) Focus of FDG uptake on PET images in the posterior mediastinum, which could be mistaken for uptake within a subcarinal lymph node. (**B**) Fused dual PET-CT image demonstrates that the focus of FDG uptake corresponds to the esophagus rather than an abnormal lymph node. In this patient who has had prior radiation treatment, this likely represents radiation induced esophagitis. (*See color insert for* **B**.)

Therapy Monitoring

PET-CT can determine changes in tumor metabolism and may be a valuable addition to CT and MRI alone in the monitoring of therapy in patients with lung cancer. Recent studies have described the usefulness of FDG-PET for monitoring response to therapy and determining prognosis after therapy for lung cancer (52–54). Because PET imaging evaluates the glycolytic metabolic rate of tumor cells, this technique should evaluate the effectiveness of various treatments earlier than anatomic imaging modalities (54). Normalization of FDG-PET uptake levels following therapy has been shown to be a good prognostic indicator in patients with NSCLC (55). Additionally, a case study presented by Erdi et al. (53) suggests that PET may predict outcome during the course of therapy. Monitoring response to therapy would require the acquisition of a PET-CT scan prior to the initiation of therapy, during therapy, and after the completion of therapy. Standardization of acquisition would be important for all follow-up scans since the biodistribution of FDG can be affected by various physiologic factors (54). Standard prescan fasting times, good hydration, and muscle relaxants may all be employed to ensure standardized acquisitions. Current data indicates that images can be obtained as early as after 1 to 2 cycles of chemotherapy (54).

FDG-PET imaging has also been shown to have prognostic value that correlates with survival rate in patients treated for lung cancer with radiation, surgery, and/or chemotherapy (52). Patz et al. demonstrated a relative risk ratio of 10:3 for patients with positive FDG-PET results. Although the therapeutic monitoring of lung cancer is still in relatively early stages of investigation, these early studies suggest that it should be a useful tool.

PITFALLS OF PET-CT IMAGING: FALSE-POSTIVES AND ARTIFACTS

Infection/Inflammation

The majority of the pitfalls of PET-CT imaging are related to false-positives. The most common cause of a false-positive result on FDG-PET imaging are foci of inflammation/infection that may be erroneously interpreted as malignant. In particular, active granulomatous disease, such as histoplasmosis, mycobacterial infection, or sarcoidosis, will show intense FDG uptake, mimicking malignant disease. For example, Figure 10 demonstrates a case of presumed malignancy on PET-CT that was histologically proven to be mycobacterium avium infection (MAI). False-positive uptake has also been reported in diseases such as Wegeners granulomatosis, acute and organizing pneumonias, and lipoid pneumonia (56). Lowe et al. (19) found that other acute infections, such as tuberculosis, coccidiomycosis, aspergillosis, and histoplasmosis, were sources of false-positive findings on FDG-PET. However, the authors also reported that some nongranulomatous pneumonias and viral infections displayed relatively lower levels of FDG uptake than malignancies and were less likely sources of false-positive results (19). Further complication of the issue arises when both an acute inflammatory process and malignancy coexist, such as in a postobstructive pneumonia. Although Nestle et al. (30) found PET useful in distinguishing primary tumor from postobstructive atelectasis, Strauss et al. (49) found inconclusive results in attempting to differentiate tumor from inflammation based on the intensity of FDG uptake. They found that visual interpretation and calculation of SUVs were not helpful in the differentiation of tumor when acute inflammation had to be excluded.

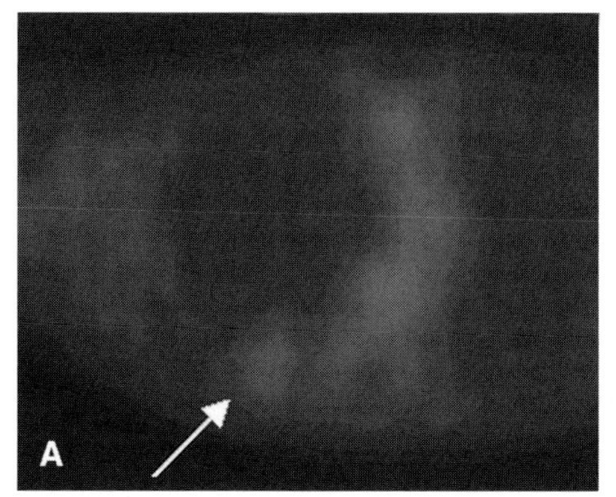

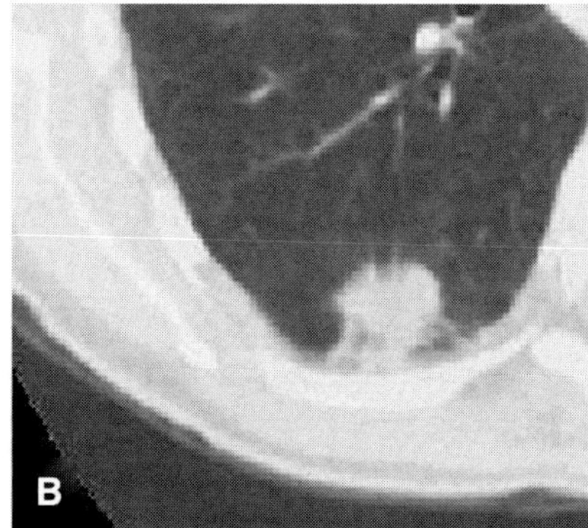

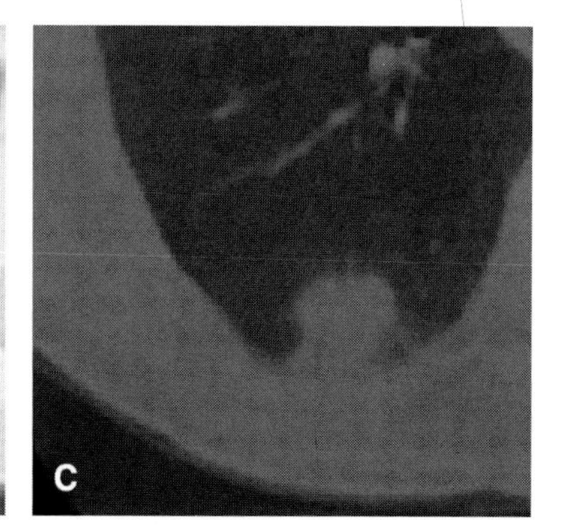

Figure 10 Dual PET-CT in a 63-year-old female with suspected lung cancer. (**A**) FDG-PET image demonstrates a focus of uptake in the posterior right lower lobe. (**B**) Corresponding CT image demonstrates a soft tissue nodule in the right lower lobe. (**C**) Fused images demonstrate FDG uptake corresponding to the right lower lobe nodule. A wedge resection was performed for suspected lung cancer and the nodule was proven to be an area of chronic inflammation secondary to mycobacterium avium infection (MAI). (*See color insert for* **C**.)

Brown Fat Uptake

The first description of brown adipose tissue (BAT) is generally attributed to Konrad Gessner who detected BAT in hibernating marmots more than 450 years ago, but only recently has it been identified as highly thermogenic tissue with a role in regulating body temperatures (57). BAT is a common potential source of false-positive results on FDG-PET (57). Recent studies have described increased FDG uptake in the supraclavicular and high-axillary fat region, as well as in the mediastinum, paraspinous fat, and upper abdominal fat. Hany et al. (58) showed that at least 2.5% of patients referred for PET had symmetrically increased uptake in the neck, shoulder regions, and thoracic spine. This pattern of uptake is more likely to be seen in women (1:6 male to female ratio) and children (59). People with low body mass index (BMI) are more prone to feel cold at normal room temperatures and, therefore, are more inclined to thermoregulation by activation of the sympathetic nervous system, which increases uptake in BAT (60). Prior to dual PET-CT imaging, these areas of increased FDG uptake were often interpreted erroneously as metastatic foci. Dual PET-CT imaging has been instrumental in solving the dilemma of distinguishing metabolic-active adipose tissue from soft tissue metastatic disease. Combined imaging successfully localizes areas of increased FDG uptake to regions of adipose tissue on CT (–190 to –30 HU) that clearly have no evidence for lymphadenopathy. For example, in Figure 11, FDG-PET demonstrates areas of supraclavicular FDG uptake that could be mistaken for abnormal uptake within lymph nodes. Dual PET-CT demonstrates that the bilateral FDG uptake localizes to areas of supraclavicular fat and confirms the absence of lymphadenopathy.

Skeletal Muscle Uptake

Physiologic uptake within muscles may also contribute to false-positive results on FDG-PET imaging. Focal FDG uptake within muscles, especially in the scalene muscles of the neck, may be falsely attributed to abnormal uptake within supraclavicular lymph nodes. However, with accurate image registration on dual PET-CT these areas of increased uptake can be localized to these specific muscle groups (Fig. 12). Cohade et al. (59) found dual PET-CT reliable in localizing muscle uptake. In their study evaluating potential supraclavicular FDG-PET false-positive results, all of the patients in whom supraclavicular uptake was assigned to muscle activity rather than nodal disease had no evidence of nodal disease in the neck on clinical follow-up.

Bone Uptake

Degenerative joint disease can be a source of foci of elevated FDG uptake on PET. Common areas of degenerative joint disease in the thorax are the sternoclavicular joints, acromioclavicular joints, glenohumeral joints, and the spine. Although some studies have demonstrated less intense uptake in areas of degenerative joint disease as compared to metastases (61), correlation with the CT portion of the dual PET-CT images as well as pattern of uptake on the PET are usually sufficient to distinguish the two.

False-positive results on FDG-PET can be due to the misinterpretation of focal uptake in healing bones as skeletal metastases. FDG uptake can be elevated in healing fractures for up to 6 months (62). The use of dual PET-CT to correlate areas of abnormal FDG uptake in the skeleton to CT findings of fracture can allow accurate differentiation between osseous metastases/pathologic fractures and benign fractures.

Heterogeneous bone marrow uptake on FDG-PET can also be mistaken for osseous metastatic disease. Correlation with the CT portion of a dual PET-CT examination may be helpful in distinguishing intraosseous metastases from normal heterogeneous bone marrow. If CT findings are equivocal, MRI may be helpful for further evaluation of the bone marrow. It

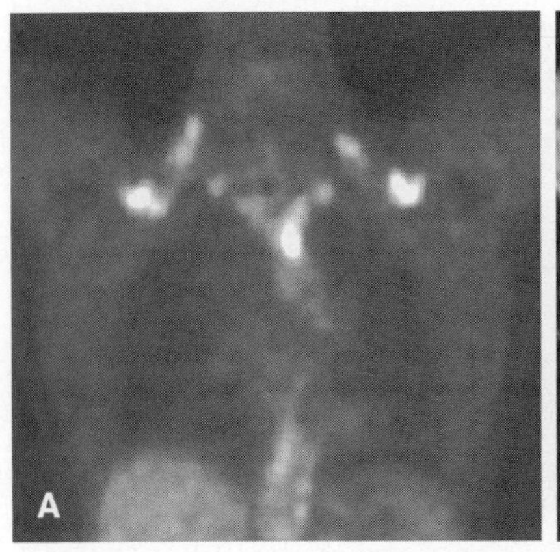

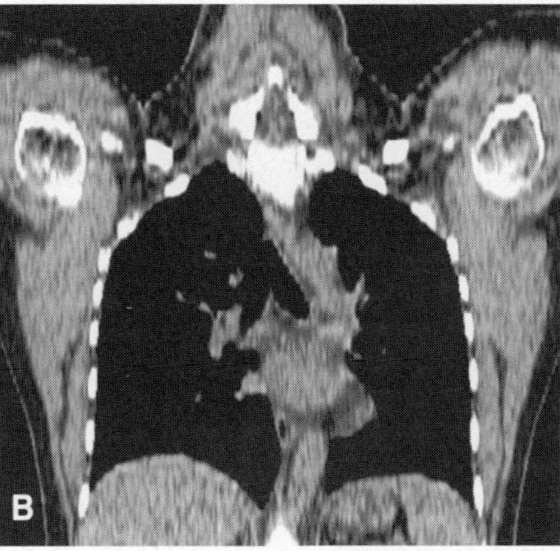

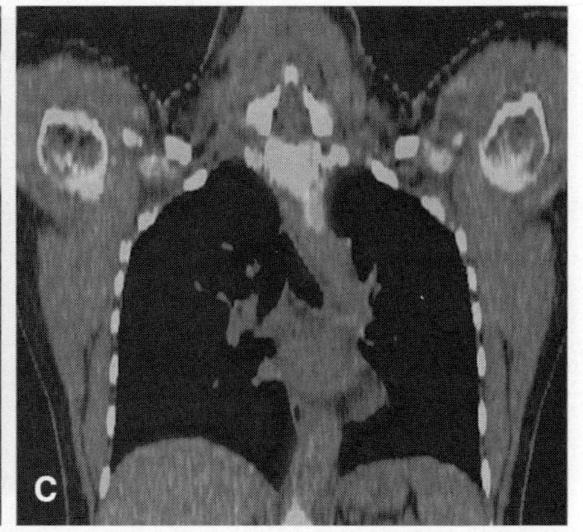

Figure 11 Dual PET-CT in a 32-year-old woman with thyroid cancer. (**A**) Intense symmetric uptake in the supraclavicular areas on PET. (**B**) CT demonstrates no evidence of supraclavicular lymphadenopathy. (**C**) Fused dual PET-CT image demonstrates localization of the intense supraclavicular uptake to regions of fat, consistent with uptake within brown adipose tissue. (*See color insert for* **C**.)

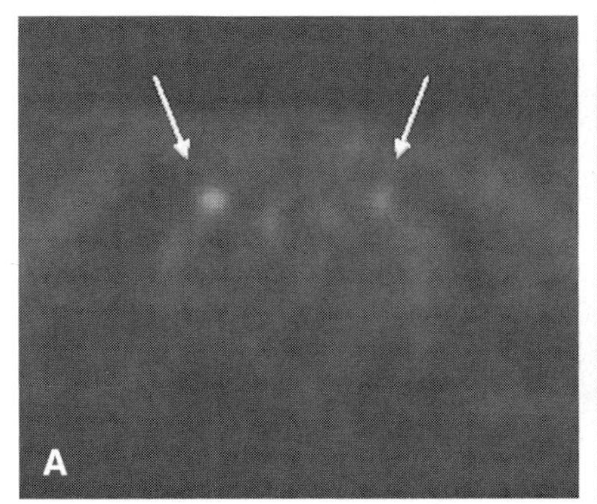

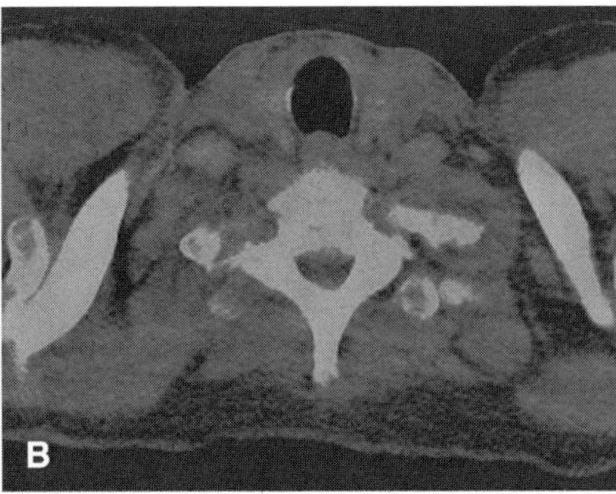

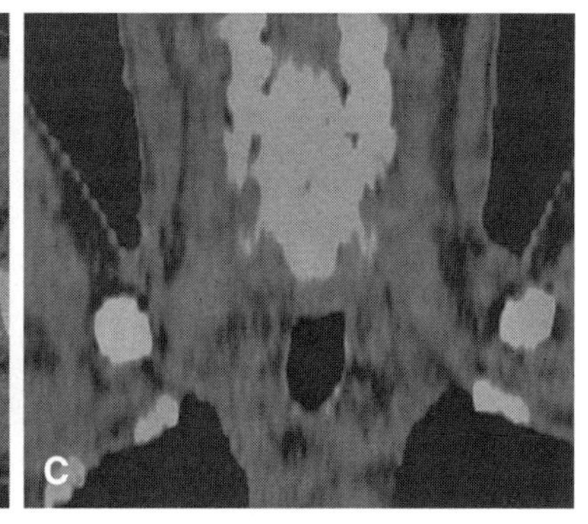

Figure 12 A 53-year-old male with a history of lymphoma. (**A**) PET portion of a dual PET-CT examination shows symmetric foci of uptake in the supraclavicular regions. (**B,C**) Axial and coronal fused images from the dual PET-CT demonstrate that the linear, symmetric, bilateral FDG uptake corresponds to the anterior scalene muscles bilaterally. No lymphadenopathy identified in the supraclavicular regions. (*See color insert for* **B** *and* **C**.)

should also be noted that intense FDG uptake secondary to activation from granulocyte colony stimulation factor (GCSF) treatment or chemotherapy should not be misinterpreted as diffuse metastatic disease (60).

Cardiac Uptake

Cardiac uptake is variable and can present as low background activity to intense FDG uptake, particularly in the left ventricle myocardium. Intense myocardial uptake can obscure mediastinal or pericardial lymph nodes on dual PET-CT imaging. Myocardial uptake is dependent on the fasting state of the patient. In a fasting state, myocardium preferentially utilizes free fatty acids for energy and, consequently, myocardial glucose and FDG uptake is low. In a nonfasting state or after a glucose load, glucose and FDG uptake of the myocardium can be three to five times that of uptake in the fasting state (60). For oncologic imaging of the thorax, cardiac activity can be minimized if the patient is fasting at least 4–6 h prior to FDG administration.

Brown fat is a known component of lipomatous hypertrophy of the interatrial septum (LHIS). This focus of increased fat deposit in the heart between the right and left atria may show very intense uptake on FDG-PET, which may mimic tumor spread in a patient with lung cancer (Fig. 13). According to Fan et al. (63), fusion imaging correctly localizes the area of intense uptake on FDG-PET to LHIS, thus preventing erroneous N staging in a patient with lung cancer.

Laryngeal Uptake

Talking during the injection of FDG and in the subsequent uptake period will cause symmetric

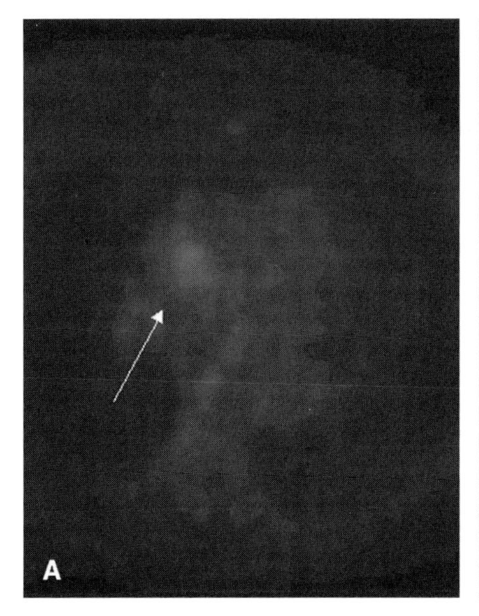

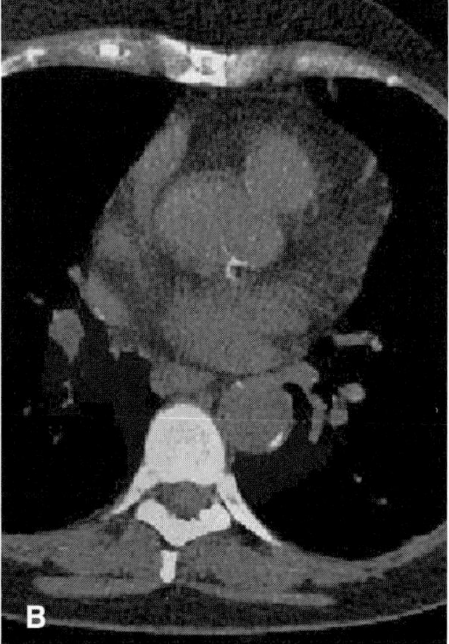

Figure 13 Dual PET-CT examination for staging in a 63-year-old man with a gastrointestinal stromal tumor. (**A**) PET portion of the examination demonstrates a focus of FDG uptake in the mediastinum. (**B**) Fused dual PET-CT images demonstrate the focus of FDG uptake corresponding to a focus of fat in the interatrial septum. Findings are consistent with lipomatous hypertrophy of the interatrial septum (LHIS). (*See color insert for* **B**.)

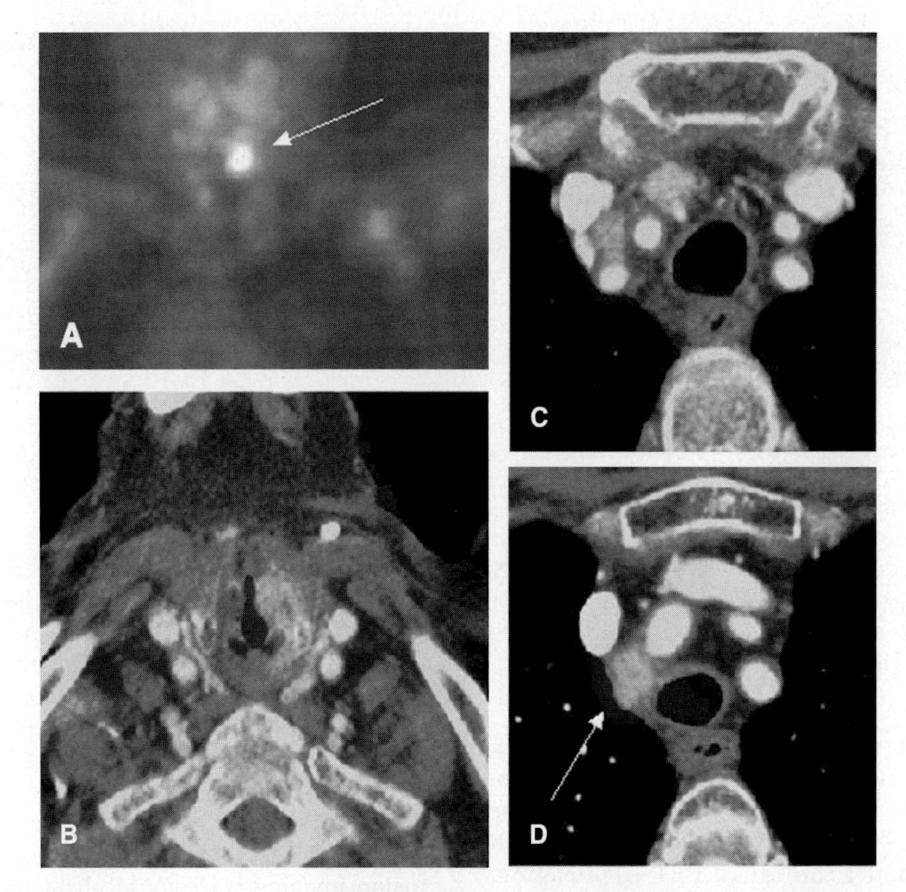

Figure 14 Restaging dual PET-CT in a 63-year-old female with non–small cell lung cancer. (**A**) FDG-PET image demonstrates a focus of uptake in the left neck. (**B**) Fused dual PET-CT images demonstrate intense FDG uptake in the region of the normal, nonparalyzed, left vocal cord. (**C,D**) Dual PET-CT images demonstrate FDG-avid, right, high, paratracheal lymphadenopathy in the region of the right recurrent laryngeal nerve. In this patient with right vocal cord paralysis from right recurrent laryngeal nerve impingement, there is compensatory increased uptake within the normal left vocal cord. (*See color insert for* **B**, **C**, *and* **D**.)

uptake in the vocal cords and laryngeal muscles (64). The extent of speaking is directly related to amount of uptake within the laryngeal muscles. On dual PET-CT imaging this symmetric uptake within the larynx can be localized to the vocal cords and laryngeal muscles, distinguishing it from laryngeal tumor. However, in cases of recurrent laryngeal nerve paralysis, which can be caused by a central bronchogenic carcinoma, there will be intense uptake in the contralateral normal larynx, which can mimic laryngeal carcinoma (60). An example of this is shown in Figure 14.

Thymus Uptake

Physiologic FDG uptake in the thymus in prepubescent children is a normal finding. However, FDG uptake in the adult thymus secondary to thymic hyperplasia after chemotherapy should not be mistaken for uptake within malignant mediastinal lymph nodes (65). Dual PET-CT can confirm the location of the mediastinal uptake within the typically triangular retrosternal bi-lobed thymic tissue avoiding false interpretation of mediastinal lymphadenopathy.

Attenuation Correction Errors

As noted above in the technical features section, iodinated contrast and metallic foreign objects can cause attenuation correction that present as areas of apparent FDG uptake on PET scan. Correlation with CT images will localize these foci of apparent FDG uptake to areas of concentrated iodinated contrast or to metallic foreign bodies.

CONCLUSION

In summary, dual PET-CT imaging has made a significant impact on the imaging of the thorax, particularly the staging and monitoring of lung cancer. By providing for more accurate anatomic localization of FDG uptake, dual PET-CT imaging allows for more accurate staging of patients with lung cancer. In addition, dual PET-CT may help resolve many of the pitfalls associated with conventional FDG-PET imaging alone. With a solid understanding of the normal physiologic distribution of FDG and the recognition of characteristic morphologic patterns of diseases on CT, radiologists have the ability to significantly contribute to the management of patients with thoracic diseases and malignancies with dual PET-CT imaging.

References

1 Eubank WB, Mankoff DA, Schmiedl UP, et al. Imaging of oncologic patients: benefit of combined CT and FDG-PET in the diagnosis of malignancy. AJR Am J Roentgenol 1998; 171:1103–10.
2 Hicks RJ, Kalff V, MacManus MP, et al. (18)F-FDG-PET provides high-impact and powerful prognostic stratification in staging newly diagnosed non-small cell lung cancer. J Nucl Med 2001; 42:1596–604.
3 Lardinois D, Weder W, Hany TF, et al. Staging of non-small-cell lung cancer with integrated positron-emission tomography and computed tomography. N Engl J Med 2003; 348:2500–7.
4 Krishnasetty V, Fischman AJ, Halpern EL, et al. Comparison of alignment of computer-registered data sets: combined PET/CT versus independent PET and CT of the thorax. Radiology 2005; 237:635–9.
5 Aquino SL, Asmuth JC, Moore RH, et al. Improved image interpretation with registered thoracic CT and positron emission tomography data sets. AJR Am J Roentgenol 2002; 178:939–44.
6 Hasegawa BH, Stebler B, Rutt BK, et al. A prototype high-purity germanium detector system with fast photon-counting circuitry for medical imaging. Med Phys 1991; 18:900–9.
7 Lang TF, Hasegawa BH, Liew SC, et al. Description of a prototype emission-transmission computed tomography imaging system. J Nucl Med 1992; 33:1881–7.
8 Beyer T, Townsend DW, Brun T, et al. A combined PET/CT scanner for clinical oncology. J Nucl Med 2000; 41:1369–79.
9 Townsend DW, Beyer T, Blodgett TM. PET/CT scanners: a hardware approach to image fusion. Semin Nucl Med 2003; 33:193–204.
10 Gilman MD, Fischman AJ, Krishnasetty V, et al. Optimal CT breathing protocol for combined thoracic PET/CT. AJR Am J Roentgenol 2006; 187:1357–60.
11 Antoch G, Freudenberg LS, Beyer T, et al. To enhance or not to enhance? ^{18}F-FDG and CT contrast agents in dual-modality 18F-FDG PET/CT. J Nucl Med 2004; 45 (Suppl 1):56S–65S.
12 Wahl RL. Why nearly all PET of abdominal and pelvic cancers will be performed as PET/CT. J Nucl Med 2004; 45 (Suppl 1):82S–95S.
13 Sugawara Y, Zasadny KR, Neuhoff AW, et al. Reevaluation of the standardized uptake value for FDG: variations with body weight and methods for correction. Radiology 1999; 213:521–5.
14 Lapela M, Eigtved A, Jyrkkio S, et al. Experience in qualitative and quantitative FDG-PET in follow-up of patients with suspected recurrence from head and neck cancer. Eur J Cancer 2000; 36:858–67.
15 Dewan NA, Shehan CJ, Reeb SD, et al. Likelihood of malignancy in a solitary pulmonary nodule: comparison of Bayesian analysis and results of FDG-PET scan. Chest 1997; 112:416–22.
16 Duhaylongsod FG, Lowe VJ, Patz EF, Jr., et al. Detection of primary and recurrent lung cancer by means of F-18 fluorodeoxyglucose positron emission tomography (FDG-PET). J Thorac Cardiovasc Surg 1995; 110:130–9; discussion 139–40.
17 Patz EF, Jr., Lowe VJ, Hoffman JM, et al. Focal pulmonary abnormalities: evaluation with F-18 fluorodeoxyglucose PET scanning. Radiology 1993; 188:487–90.
18 Lowe VJ, Naunheim KS. Current role of positron emission tomography in thoracic oncology. Thorax 1998; 53:703–12.
19 Lowe VJ, Hoffman JM, DeLong DM, et al. Semi-quantitative and visual analysis of FDG-PET images in pulmonary abnormalities. J Nucl Med 1994; 35: 1771–6.
20 Gould MK, Maclean CC, Kuschner WG, et al. Accuracy of positron emission tomography for diagnosis of pulmonary nodules and mass lesions: a meta-analysis. Jama 2001; 285:914–24.
21 Higashi K, Ueda Y, Seki H, et al. Fluorine-18-FDG-PET imaging is negative in bronchioloalveolar lung carcinoma. J Nucl Med 1998; 39:1016–20.
22 Kim BT, Kim Y, Lee KS, et al. Localized form of bronchioloalveolar carcinoma: FDG-PET findings. AJR Am J Roentgenol 1998; 170:935–9.
23 Jadvar H, Segall GM. False-negative fluorine-18-FDG PET in metastatic carcinoid. J Nucl Med 1997; 38: 1382–3.
24 Erasmus JJ, McAdams HP, Patz EF, Jr., et al. Evaluation of primary pulmonary carcinoid tumors using FDG-PET. AJR Am J Roentgenol 1998; 170:1369–73.
25 Henschke CI, Shaham D, Farooqi A, et al. Computerized tomography screening for lung cancer: new findings and diagnostic work-up. Semin Thorac Cardiovasc Surg 2003; 15:397–404.
26 Fink G, Krelbaum T, Yellin A, et al. Pulmonary carcinoid: presentation, diagnosis, and outcome in 142 cases in Israel and review of 640 cases from the literature. Chest 2001; 119:1647–51.
27 Aquino SL, Asmuth JC, Alpert NM, et al. Improved radiologic staging of lung cancer with 2-[^{18}F]-fluoro-2-deoxy-D-glucose-positron emission tomography and computed tomography registration. J Comput Assist Tomogr 2003; 27:479–84.
28 Mountain CF. Revisions in the international system for staging lung cancer. Chest 1997; 111:1710–7.
29 Goerres GW, von Schulthess GK, Steinert HC. Why most PET of lung and head-and-neck cancer will be PET/CT. J Nucl Med 2004; 45(Suppl. 1):66S–71.
30 Nestle U, Walter K, Schmidt S, et al. 18F-deoxyglucose positron emission tomography (FDG-PET) for the planning of radiotherapy in lung cancer: high impact in patients with atelectasis. Int J Radiat Oncol Biol Phys 1999; 44:593–7.
31 Gupta NC, Rogers JS, Graeber GM, et al. Clinical role of F-18 fluorodeoxyglucose positron emission tomography imaging in patients with lung cancer and suspected malignant pleural effusion. Chest 2002; 122:1918–24.

32 McLoud TC, Bourgouin PM, Greenberg RW, et al. Bronchogenic carcinoma: analysis of staging in the mediastinum with CT by correlative lymph node mapping and sampling. Radiology 1992; 182:319–23.
33 Pieterman RM, van Putten JW, Meuzelaar JJ, et al. Preoperative staging of non-small-cell lung cancer with positron-emission tomography. N Engl J Med 2000; 343:254–61.
34 Antoch G, Stattaus J, Nemat AT, et al. Non-small-cell lung cancer: dual-modality PET/CT in preoperative staging. Radiology 2003; 229:526–33.
35 Reske SN, Kotzerke J. FDG-PET for clinical use. Results of the 3rd German Interdisciplinary Consensus Conference, "Onko-PET" III, 21 July and 19 September 2000. Eur J Nucl Med 2001; 28:1707–23.
36 Bury T, Barreto A, Daenen F, et al. Fluorine-18 deoxyglucose positron emission tomography for the detection of bone metastases in patients with non-small cell lung cancer. Eur J Nucl Med 1998; 25:1244–7.
37 Rohren EM, Provenzale JM, Barboriak DP, et al. Screening for cerebral metastases with FDG-PET in patients undergoing whole-body staging of non-central nervous system malignancy. Radiology 2003; 226:181–7.
38 Prabhakar H, Aquino SL, Sharma A, et al. Impact of dual PET/CT findings on the interpretation of thoracic CT in patients with malignancy, RSNA Abstract, Chicago, IL, 2004.
39 Tas F, Aydiner A, Topuz E, et al. Factors influencing the distribution of metastases and survival in extensive disease small cell lung cancer. Acta Oncol 1999; 38:1011–5.
40 Kamel EM, Zwahlen D, Wyss MT, et al. Whole-body (18)F-FDG PET improves the management of patients with small cell lung cancer. J Nucl Med 2003; 44: 1911–7.
41 Yap CS, Schiepers C, Fishbein MC, et al. FDG-PET imaging in lung cancer: how sensitive is it for bronchioloalveolar carcinoma? Eur J Nucl Med Mol Imaging 2002; 29:1166–73.
42 Martini N, Bains MS, Burt ME, et al. Incidence of local recurrence and second primary tumors in resected stage I lung cancer. J Thorac Cardiovasc Surg 1995; 109:120–9.
43 Keidar Z, Haim N, Guralnik L, et al. PET/CT using 18F-FDG in suspected lung cancer recurrence: diagnostic value and impact on patient management. J Nucl Med 2004; 45:1640–6.
44 Miura H, Konaka C, Kato H, et al. Recurrence at the bronchial stump after resection of lung cancer. Ann Surg 1994; 219:306–9.
45 Verleden G, Deneffe G, Demedts M. Bronchial stump recurrence after surgery for bronchial carcinoma. Eur Respir J 1990; 3:97–100.
46 Gruden JF, Campagna G, McGuinness G. The normal CT appearances of the second carina and bronchial stump after left upper lobectomy. J Thorac Imaging 2000; 15:138–43.
47 Kwek BH, Aquino SL, Fischman AJ. Fluorodeoxyglucose positron emission tomography and CT after talc pleurodesis. Chest 2004; 125:2356–60.
48 Logan PM. Thoracic manifestations of external beam radiotherapy. AJR Am J Roentgenol 1998; 171:569–77.
49 Strauss LG. Fluorine-18 deoxyglucose and false-positive results: a major problem in the diagnostics of oncological patients. Eur J Nucl Med 1996; 23: 1409–15.
50 Lin P, Delaney G, Chu J, et al. Fluorine-18 FDG dual-head gamma camera coincidence imaging of radiation pneumonitis. Clin Nucl Med 2000; 25:866–9.
51 Patz EF, Jr., Lowe VJ, Hoffman JM, et al. Persistent or recurrent bronchogenic carcinoma: detection with PET and 2-[F-18]-2-deoxy-D-glucose. Radiology 1994; 191:379–82.
52 Patz EF, Jr., Connolly J, Herndon J. Prognostic value of thoracic FDG-PET imaging after treatment for non-small cell lung cancer. AJR Am J Roentgenol 2000; 174:769–74.
53 Erdi YE, Macapinlac H, Rosenzweig KE, et al. Use of PET to monitor the response of lung cancer to radiation treatment. Eur J Nucl Med 2000; 27:861–6.
54 Kostakoglu L, Goldsmith SJ. PET in the assessment of therapy response in patients with carcinoma of the head and neck and of the esophagus. J Nucl Med 2004; 45:56–68.
55 Hebert ME, Lowe VJ, Hoffman JM, et al. Positron emission tomography in the pretreatment evaluation and follow-up of non-small cell lung cancer patients treated with radiotherapy: preliminary findings. Am J Clin Oncol 1996; 19:416–21.
56 Asad S, Aquino SL, Piyavisetpat N, et al. False-positive FDG positron emission tomography uptake in non-malignant chest abnormalities. AJR Am J Roentgenol 2004; 182:983–9.
57 Weber WA. Brown adipose tissue and nuclear medicine imaging. J Nucl Med 2004; 45:1101–3.
58 Hany TF, Gharehpapagh E, Kamel EM, et al. Brown adipose tissue: a factor to consider in symmetrical tracer uptake in the neck and upper chest region. Eur J Nucl Med Mol Imaging 2002; 29:1393–8.
59 Cohade C, Osman M, Pannu HK, et al. Uptake in supraclavicular area fat ("USA-Fat"): description on ^{18}F-FDG PET/CT. J Nucl Med 2003; 44:170–6.
60 Rosenbaum SJ, Lind T, Antoch G, et al. False-positive FDG-PET uptake the role of PET/CT. Eur Radiol 2006; 16:1054–65.
61 Dehdashti F, Siegel BA, Griffeth LK, et al. Benign versus malignant intraosseous lesions: discrimination by means of PET with 2-[F-18]fluoro-2-deoxy-D-glucose. Radiology 1996; 200:243–7.
62 Shon IH, Fogelman I. F-18 FDG positron emission tomography and benign fractures. Clin Nucl Med 2003; 28:171–5.
63 Fan CM, Fischman AJ, Kwek BH, et al. Lipomatous hypertrophy of the interatrial septum: increased uptake on FDG PETAJR Am J Roentgenol 2005; 184: 339–42.
64 Kostakoglu L, Wong JC, Barrington SF, et al. Speech-related visualization of laryngeal muscles with fluorine-18-FDG. J Nucl Med 1996; 37:1771–3.
65 Brink I, Reinhardt MJ, Hoegerle S, et al. Increased metabolic activity in the thymus gland studied with ^{18}F-FDG PET: age dependency and frequency after chemotherapy. J Nucl Med 2001; 42:591–5.

3

Functional MR Imaging

David L. Levin
Department of Radiology, Mayo Clinic, Rochester, Minnesota, U.S.A.

Talissa A. Altes
Department of Radiology, Children's Hospital of Philadelphia, Philadelphia, Pennsylvania, U.S.A.

INTRODUCTION

Radiologists traditionally rely on the correlation between changes in structure, as identified on radiological studies, and pathology to aid them in the diagnosis of disease. For example, a spiculated mass arising from the lung parenchyma suggests a primary carcinoma. Changes in structure may also be used to infer a change in pulmonary function. For example, tracheal collapse during expiration is associated with tracheomalacia and obstructive physiology. Newer imaging methods now allow for the direct evaluation of pulmonary function. The primary function of the lung is gas exchange, and the two primary determinants of gas exchange are blood flow and ventilation. Novel MR imaging techniques have the ability to directly evaluate pulmonary blood flow and ventilation. While these methods are not widely used in clinical practice, they have already had a significant impact on our understanding of lung function in a research setting. In this chapter, we will examine MR techniques for the evaluation of pulmonary blood flow and ventilation, and discuss current research and potential clinical applications.

Pulmonary Physiology

The matching of pulmonary blood flow with ventilation is crucial to the function of the lung as an efficient gas exchanger. As such, changes in regional pulmonary blood flow and ventilation may have major effects on pulmonary function. Alterations in pulmonary blood flow are a common feature in cardiopulmonary disease and changes in blood flow are also seen in healthy subjects in response to exercise, hypoxia, and other physiological stresses. Alterations in regional ventilation are commonly seen with emphysema and reactive airway disease.

MR Imaging of the Lung

MR imaging is a widely available and accepted clinical imaging technique. Conventional proton MR imaging relies on the differences in the magnetic properties of tissues to produce contrast in the images. However, the lung is inherently difficult to image with conventional techniques because of a low proton density and substantial magnetic susceptibility artifacts that are created by the many air–soft tissue interfaces. An additional difficulty in the evaluation of the lung with MR imaging techniques is the need to image within a breath-hold. Many of the imaging methods that will be described use sequences and hardware modifications to overcome many of these limitations.

MR IMAGING OF BLOOD FLOW

Two general types of MR sequences can be used to evaluate pulmonary blood flow. The first approach to the evaluation of blood flow with MR uses multiple images obtained rapidly during the first pass of intravascular contrast through the pulmonary circulation (1). The second approach uses sequences that do not require intravenous contrast material, and instead magnetically label inflowing blood. Collectively, these are known as arterial spin labeling (ASL) sequences (see Ref. 2 for a review). Each of these techniques has its advantages and disadvantages.

Contrast-Enhanced MR Imaging Techniques

Of the two approaches, contrast-enhanced techniques are the most straightforward. Multiple images are acquired rapidly during a bolus administration of an intravenous contrast agent, such as gadopentetate dimeglumine. The images can be acquired either using a two-dimensional (2D) or three-dimensional (3D) imaging scheme (3,4). An increase in the signal intensity of the lung parenchyma is seen as the contrast passes through the pulmonary vasculature. The pulmonary vasculature and systemic vessels demonstrate significant enhancement using these sequences. There is also a generalized increase in signal throughout the lung parenchyma from enhancement of capillary beds (Fig. 1) Regions of decreased

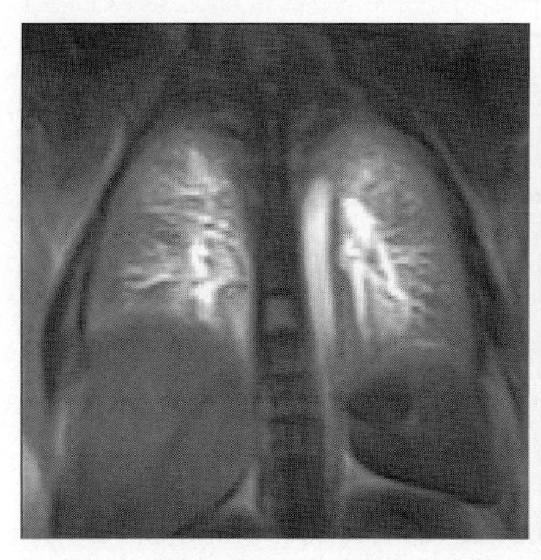
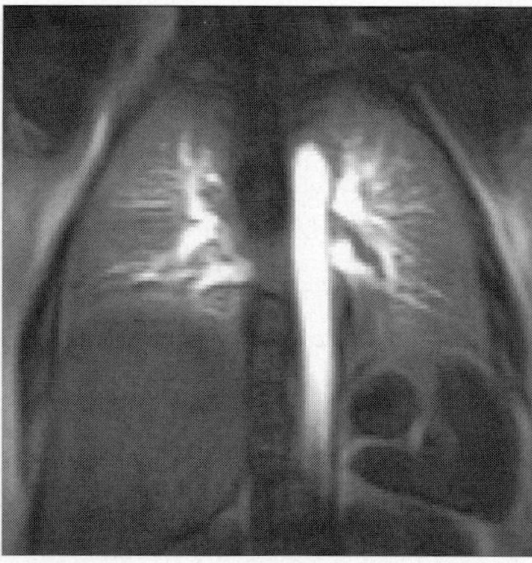
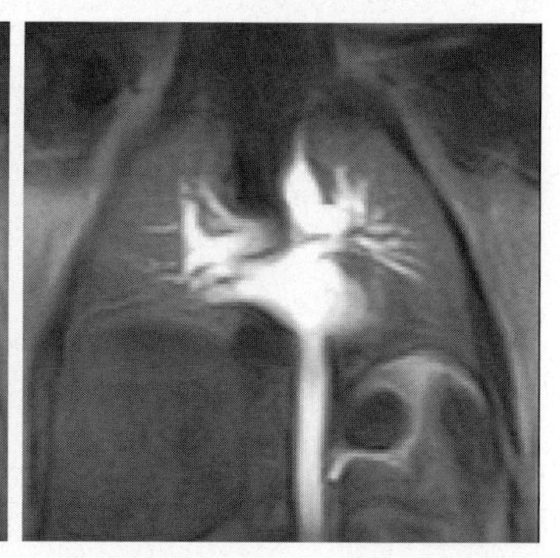

Figure 1 Contrast-enhanced MR images in healthy subject. There is uniform enhancement throughout the lungs. Both large and small vessels are identified along with a diffuse "blush" from the capillaries.

parenchymal blood flow will be identified qualitatively as areas of poor regional contrast enhancement (Fig. 2). Contrast-enhanced sequences have several advantages over noncontrast techniques. They are typically easier to implement and have greater spatial resolution and signal-to-noise ratio. However, the use of exogenous contrast substantially limits repeated measurements over shorter time frames.

Quantitative values for pulmonary perfusion can be obtained by applying the principles of indicator dilution techniques. An example of the change in signal intensity seen within a region of lung parenchyma using a 2D ultrafast imaging scheme is shown for a healthy volunteer in Figure 3. The signal intensity (open circles) is plotted as a function of time following the injection of contrast. Following a brief transit delay to the region of interest, a sharp rise in signal intensity is seen with the arrival of contrast to the region of interest. The signal intensity will decline as the contrast bolus washes out from the region of interest. In this example, a second peak due to recirculation of the contrast is present. The first-pass portion of the curve can be fit to a gamma-variate function (solid line). From this curve, quantitative values for blood volume, blood flow, and mean transit time (MTT) can be obtained (5,6). Regional blood volume is determined directly by calculating the area under the observed tissue concentration curve (7). The calculation of regional blood flow and MTT, however, is less straightforward and may be subject to substantial error (8). Additionally, the relationship between gadolinium contrast concentration and signal intensity is nonlinear. Thus, either a small dose of contrast must be used, to stay within a linear range, or an inherent inaccuracy must be accepted.

Initial studies to validate these methods were performed in a pig model of pulmonary embolism (9). Pulmonary emboli were produced by the injection of autologous clot into the systemic venous system. Regional pulmonary blood flow within the lung parenchyma was assessed simultaneously using both bolus tracking MR and colored microspheres. A strong correlation was seen between regional blood

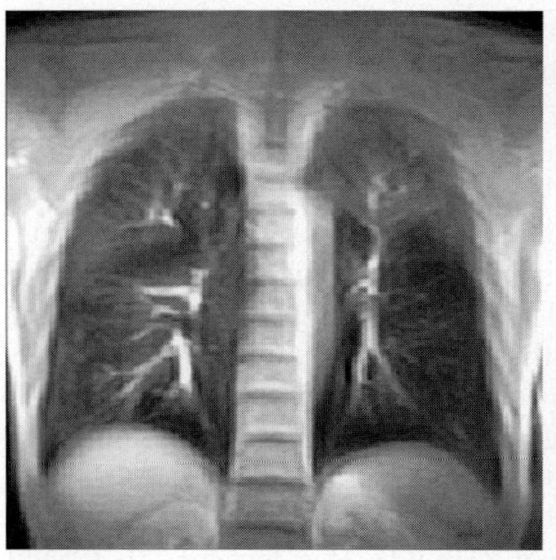
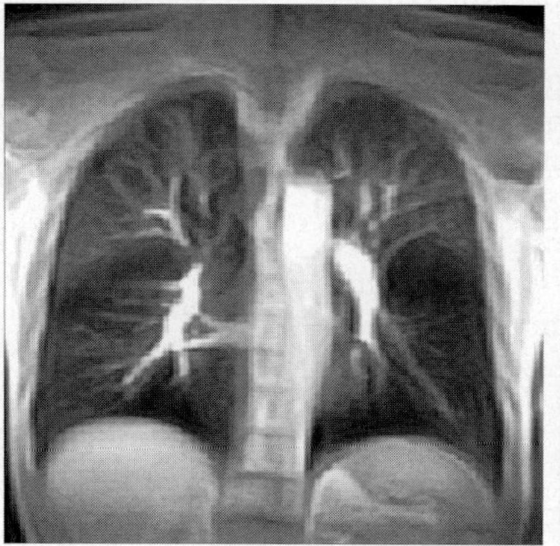
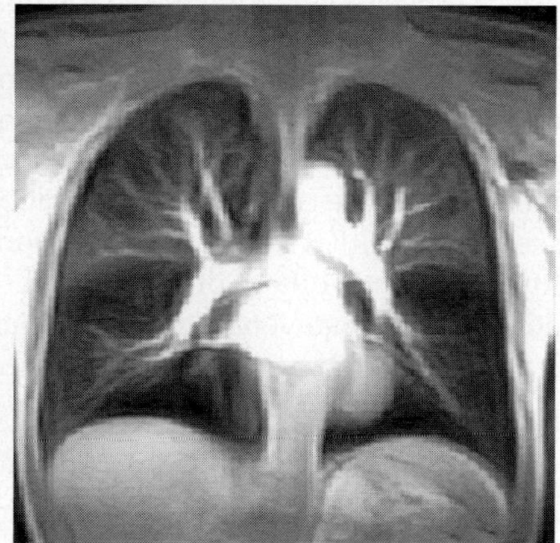

Figure 2 Contrast-enhanced MR images from a patient with severe emphysema. Regions of absent or severely diminished enhancement are present bilaterally, suggesting a reduction in blood flow.

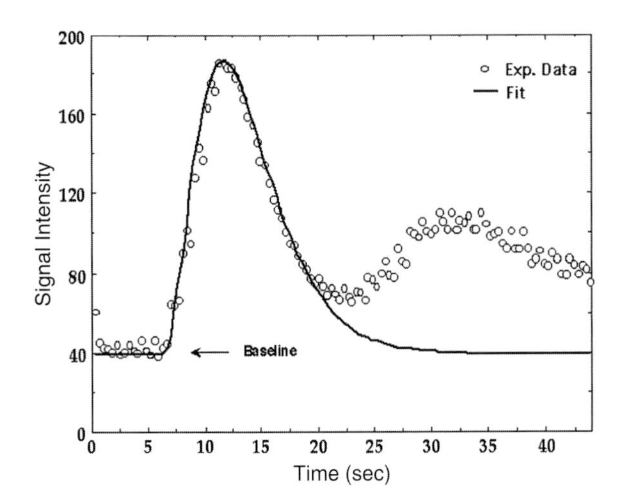

Figure 3 Changes in the signal intensity for a region of lung parenchyma during bolus administration of intravenous contrast. Following a brief transit delay, there is a sharp rise in signal intensity during the first pass of contrast. A small peak is noted from recirculation.

flow measured using MR and blood flow measured using colored microspheres. Subsequently, this technique was used to investigate regional pulmonary perfusion in healthy human subjects (3). Regional pulmonary blood flow, blood volume, and MTT were calculated for each voxel within the lung parenchyma. Parametric image maps were then created to display regional variations in these variables (Fig. 4). In these images, variation in color is used to represent blood flow, blood volume, or transit time.

Noncontrast MR Imaging Techniques

The basic principle for noncontrast techniques is that MR signal from stationary lung tissue is eliminated and signal from flowing blood produces an image. Typically, this is done by producing two images: one where both flowing blood and stationary tissues contribute to signal and one where only stationary tissues contribute to MR signal. When these two images are subtracted from each other, the signal from the stationary tissues is eliminated, and only signal from flowing blood is left. This produces a perfusion-weighted image map (Fig. 5). In this image, the brightness, or the signal intensity, of each part of the image directly reflects the amount of blood delivered to that region. Absolute, or relative quantification, blood flow can be obtained from this image. There are two primary advantages of ASL sequences: regional blood flow is determined directly from the signal intensity of the perfusion image, and no intravenous contrast is needed. This allows for repeated measurements within the same subject over very short intervals. They have several disadvantages, however, when compared to contrast-enhanced techniques: they are more difficult to develop and use, and they usually have poorer spatial resolution and signal-to-noise. While ASL techniques are typically used to produce qualitative images of blood flow, they can be adapted to provide quantitative measures (10).

In the simplest terms, the quantification of regional perfusion requires a knowledge of the volume of protons (blood) delivered to a region of interest, and the duration of time needed to deliver that particular volume. This principle has been applied to healthy human subjects (11). The data obtained using ASL suggested an average pulmonary blood flow of 2.0 mL/min-mL of tissue, which compared well to an estimate of average perfusion of 1.7–2.5 mL/min-mL based on cardiac output and lung tissue volume. A similar analysis has been performed using a different ASL technique, which also yielded similar values for average pulmonary blood flow (12).

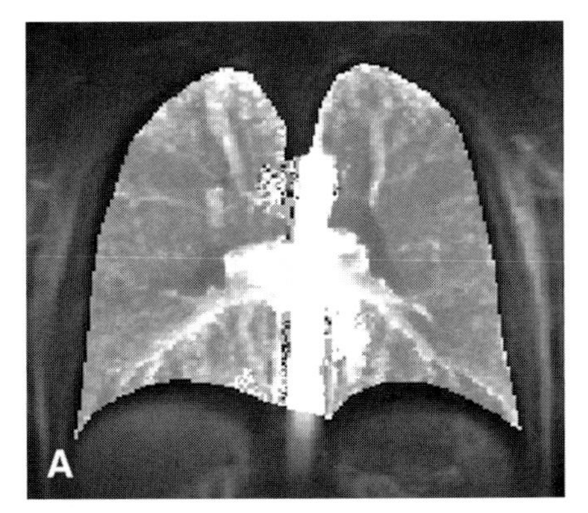

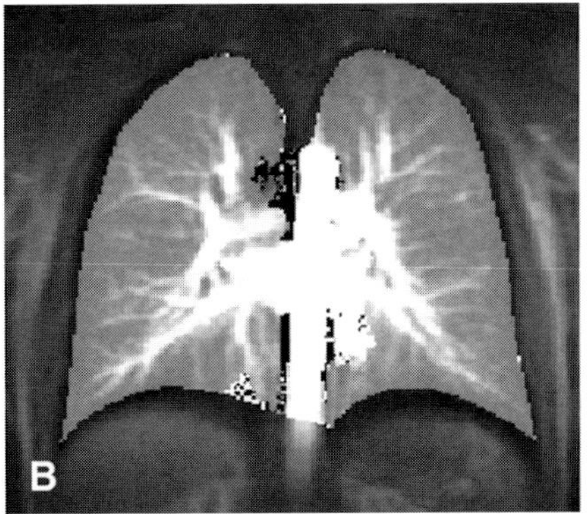

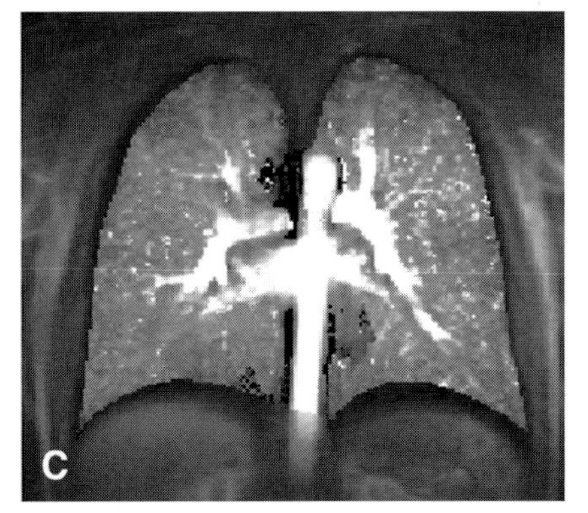

Figure 4 Parametric maps of transit time (**A**), blood volume (**B**), and blood flow (**C**). The value for each of these parameters is converted to a color scale to allow for better visualization of data. Regions with faster transit times are represented by areas of red or orange, while greater blood volumes or flows are represented by areas of white or yellow. In this healthy subject, faster transit times are seen in the apex compared to the lung base. There is relatively uniform blood flow throughout the lungs with slight decrease at the lung periphery. *Source*: Modified from Ref. 3. (*See color insert.*)

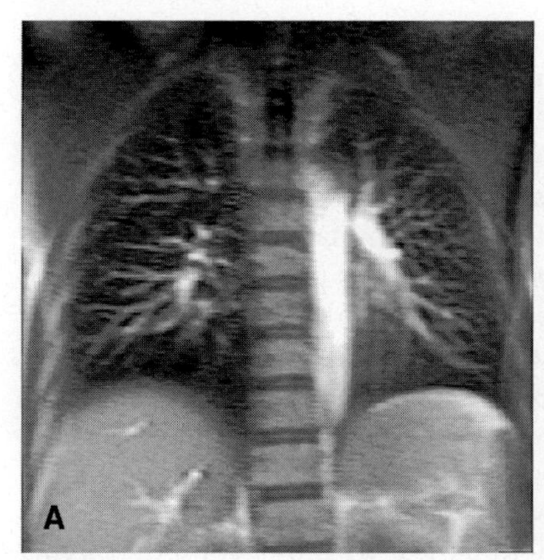

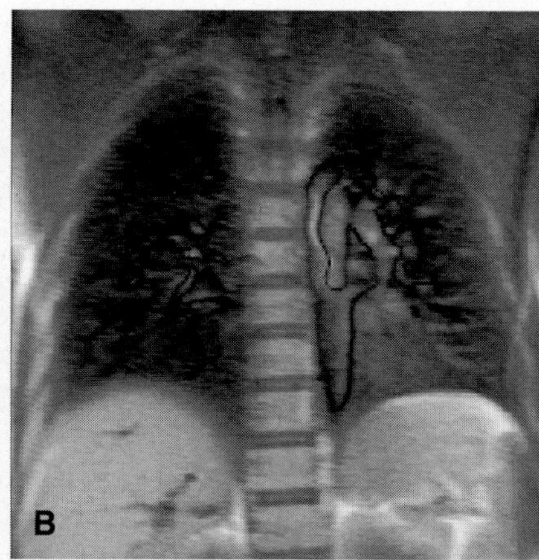

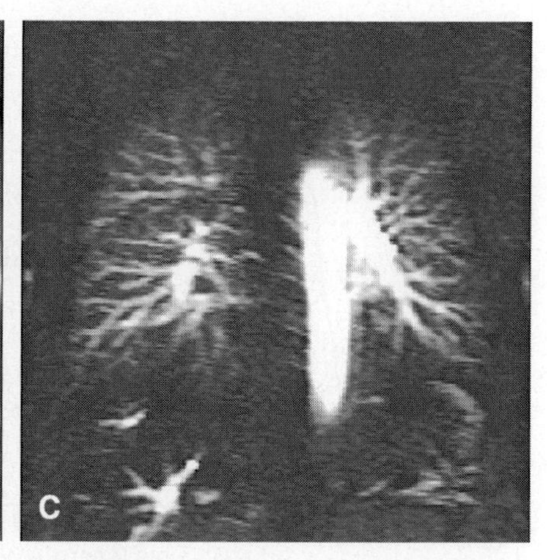

Figure 5 Coronal MR images showing the creation of a perfusion-weighted image map using ASL-FAIRER. Two images are obtained during a single breath-hold: a control image (**A**) and a tag image (**B**). Subtraction of these two images generates the perfusion-weighted image map (**C**).The images are presented with standard radiographic conventions—the subject's left is to the right on the image. The descending aorta is seen as a bright tubular structure immediately to the left of midline.

MR IMAGING OF PULMONARY VENTILATION

The airspaces of the lung produce a very low MR signal because of the low physical density and thus low proton density of inspired gas. Two approaches have been developed to permit MR imaging of lung ventilation and both require the use of an inhaled contrast agent: either molecular oxygen (13) or hyperpolarized gas (14).

Oxygen-Enhanced MR Ventilation Imaging

Oxygen is a paramagnetic substance, like gadolinium, although oxygen's paramagnetic properties are much weaker. However, like gadolinium, oxygen can be used to alter the spin-lattice relaxation time (T1) of adjacent tissues. If MR images of the lung are obtained with the subject breathing room air (21% oxygen) and again following the inhalation of gas containing a high concentration of oxygen, the comparative signal change can be used to assess lung ventilation (13). Regions that are well-ventilated receive a large amount of inspired gas and thus have a large signal change following the inhalation of gas with a high oxygen concentration. Conversely, poorly ventilated regions receive little of the inspired oxygen so the signal change following the inhalation is small. Oxygen is soluble in blood, so the oxygen-enhanced MR images likely reflect a combination of both ventilation and perfusion (15). One of the difficulties with this method is that the difference in signal from the lung parenchyma with 21% and high oxygen concentrations is relatively small. This results in a rather low signal-to-noise level in the resulting MR oxygen-enhanced images. Furthermore, the subtraction of the images obtained at different oxygen concentrations results in significant artifacts if the subjects moves even slightly between breath-holds or if the breath-hold volumes are not identical. However, oxygen-enhanced MRI requires no special equipment and can be performed using common MR sequences. Furthermore, medical-grade molecular oxygen is inexpensive, so, despite the limitations with regard to image quality, this is a promising technique. To date, few clinical studies have been performed with oxygen-enhanced MR ventilation imaging.

Hyperpolarized Gas MR Ventilation Imaging

Hyperpolarized gases are new type of MR contrast agent in which a high degree of nuclear polarization is achieved outside of the MR scanner using a variety of techniques (16–18). This high degree of nuclear polarization, several orders of magnitude greater than the nuclear polarization of protons in a 3 T scanner, provides a large MR signal despite the low physical density of the gas. The two commonly polarized isotopes of noble gases are helium-3 and xenon-129, both nonradioactive isotopes. Xenon is soluble in biological tissues and has anesthetic properties. Until recently the polarizations achievable with xenon were lower than with helium. Thus, most clinical studies with hyperpolarized gas MR have been done with helium-3.

The basis of contrast enhancement with a paramagnetic agent, such as gadolinium or oxygen, is a reduction in T1 of the water molecules nearby the contrast agent. Hyperpolarized gases are fundamentally different, in that the hyperpolarized gas atoms themselves are directly imaged. This has several important implications. First, the MR scanner must be equipped to image at the precession frequency of the hyperpolarized gas atoms, which for helium-3 is approximately 48 MHz at 1.5 T. The gas is polarized outside of the MR scanner so the MR signal generated by the hyperpolarized gas atoms is, to first order, independent of the field strength of the MR scanner

(19). Since susceptibility effects increase with increasing field strength, lower field strengths are thought to be better for hyperpolarized gas MR. Finally, the nuclear polarization is not renewable, which has important implications for the MR sequence design.

A variety of mechanisms of contrast have been exploited for hyperpolarized gas MRI. The most straightforward is spin density imaging, in which the subject inhales the hyperpolarized gas and images are acquired during the subsequent breath-hold. The MR signal received is proportional to the spin density of the hyperpolarized gas atoms. Regions of the lung that are well ventilated receive a large amount of the hyperpolarized gas and thus appear bright on the spin density images. Poorly ventilated regions receive little hyperpolarized gas and thus appear dark. Thus, this type of imaging is often called ventilation imaging (20–22). This technique depicts the homogeneity of lung ventilation, but does not provide a quantitative assessment of regional ventilation as defined by lung physiologists. Since the MR scanner is tuned to the hyperpolarized gas frequency, no signal is obtained from structures that do not contain the hyperpolarized gas, such as the chest wall, mediastinum, and pulmonary vasculature (Fig. 6).

Other mechanisms of contrast include dynamic ventilation imaging (23,24), oxygen-sensitive imaging (25,26), and diffusion imaging (27–29). With dynamic ventilation imaging, images are collected very rapidly during inspiration or expiration, typically at a single-slice position, to prove information about the dynamics of gas flow within the lungs (Fig. 7). Oxygen-sensitive imaging takes advantage of one of the properties of hyperpolarized gases to provide regional maps of the partial pressure of oxygen within the airspaces of the lung. Diffusion imaging provides information about the size of the distal airspaces of the lung.

APPLICATION TO PULMONARY DISEASE AND PHYSIOLOGY

Pulmonary Perfusion

Pulmonary Embolism

The diagnosis of pulmonary embolism remains a significant clinical challenge. As scanner technology improves, CT has become increasingly relied upon for the evaluation of suspected embolism. MR imaging techniques have also been used for the detection of pulmonary embolism and may play a clinical role in selected patients, such as those with contrast allergies or renal insufficiency. Qualitative MR perfusion imaging methods using both contrast and noncontrast techniques have been used to identify regional changes in pulmonary blood flow associated with pulmonary embolism.

Chen et al. (30) used bolus tracking techniques to identify altered perfusion in a pig model of pulmonary embolism. Blood clots were created ex vivo and injected into the inferior vena cava. Following this, images were rapidly acquired during the first pass of contrast through the pulmonary circulation. Regions of reduced or absent perfusion were seen in regions distal to nonocclusive or occlusive thrombus (Fig. 8). These findings were confirmed with conventional angiography and pathological examination.

Keilholz et al. (31) compared bolus tracking methods with an ASL technique for the detection of local perfusion abnormalities. A balloon occlusion catheter was used to occlude the left pulmonary artery in a rabbit. Pulmonary blood flow was evaluated using both a FAIRER perfusion-weighted sequence and a turbo FLASH bolus tracking sequence. While perfusion defects were noted with both techniques, a greater difference in enhancement between normally perfused

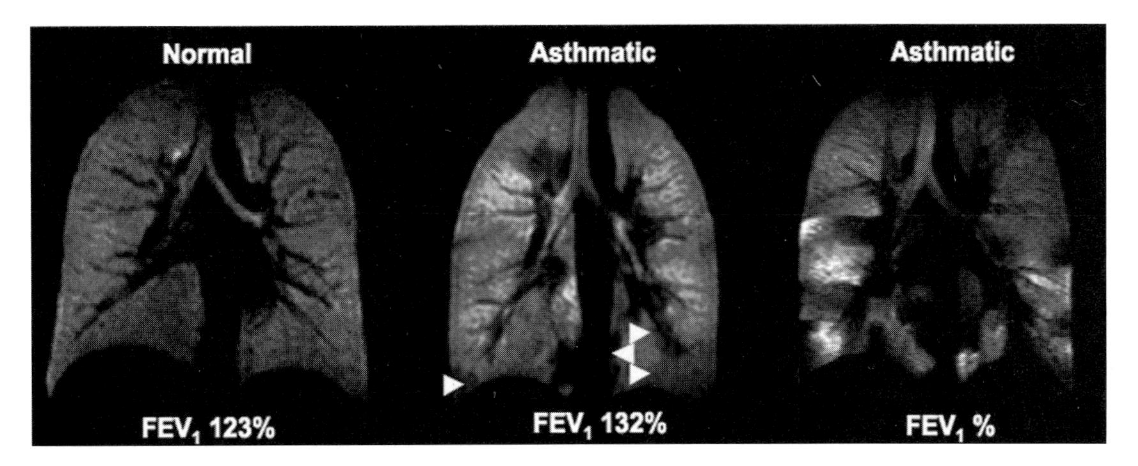

Figure 6 Coronal hyperpolarized helium MR ventilation images of a normal subject, and two subjects with asthma. The normal subject has homogeneous ventilation through their lung. The asthmatics have ventilation defects (*arrows*) with more ventilation defects in the subject with a lower FEV_1 % predicted.

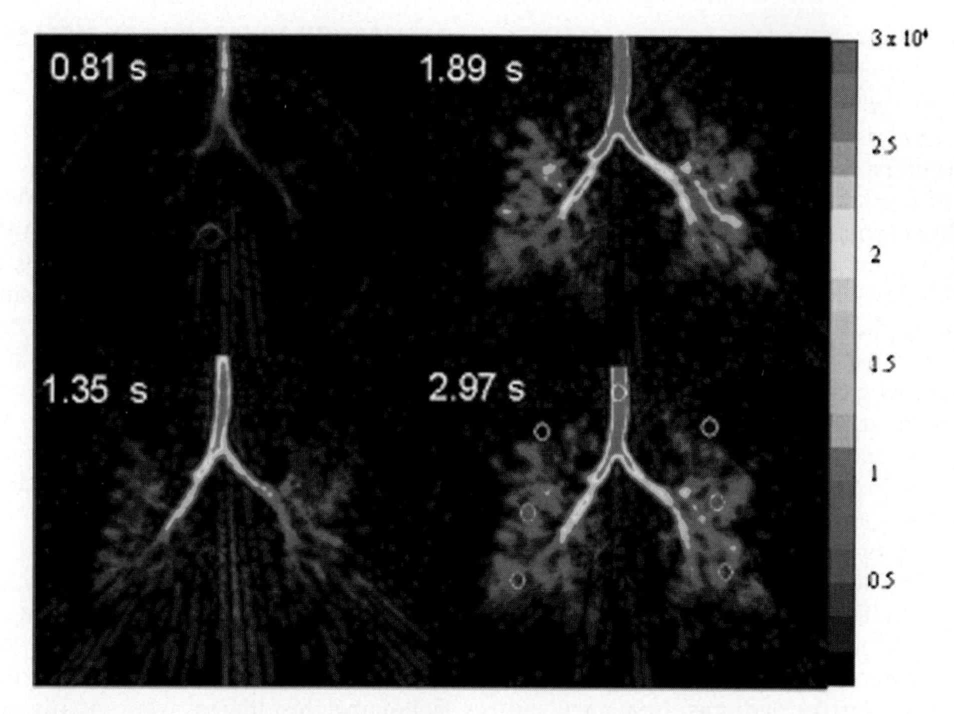

Figure 7 Dynamic coronal hyperpolarized helium MR ventilation images from a patient with cystic fibrosis showing inhomogeneity of ventilation. *Source*: Courtesy of James Wild, from Ref. 39. (*See color insert.*)

lung and occluded lung was seen with the bolus tracking technique.

MR has also been used to qualitatively evaluate pulmonary perfusion in the setting of suspected pulmonary embolism in select groups of patients. These patients typically have a contraindication to CT angiography, such as renal failure, contrast allergy, or pregnancy. Most frequently, MR angiography has been used (32). However, combined MR protocols using MR angiography as well as perfusion imaging demonstrate excellent sensitivity for the detection of pulmonary embolism when compared to CT (33).

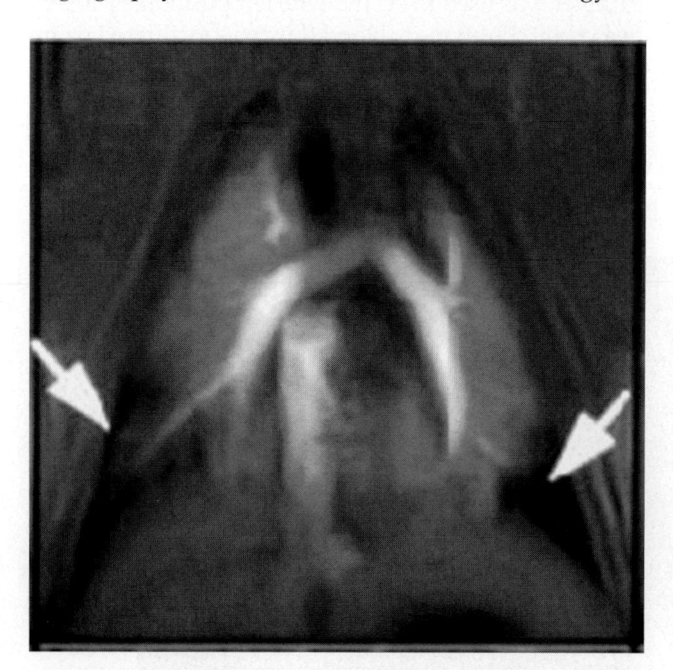

Figure 8 Perfusion MR images using a contrast-enhanced technique showing multiple regions of absent perfusion (*arrows*) in a swine experimental model of pulmonary embolism. *Source*: Modified from Ref. 25.

Pulmonary Hypertension

While a variety of pathologies can lead to pulmonary arterial hypertension, one of three histological patterns is typically identified: plexogenic arteriopathy, thrombotic arteriopathy, or veno-occlusive disease. The distinction between these causes is important, as different therapies and outcomes are expected for each pattern of disease. It is difficult to distinguish among these causes clinically. However, different patterns of pulmonary perfusion may be identified with each of these causes. Patients with thrombotic hypertension frequently have a patchy distribution of blood flow, while patients with plexogenic angiopathy may have a more uniform distribution of flow (34,35). MR evaluation of pulmonary blood flow may be able to distinguish between these two etiologies. An ASL image from a patient with chronic thromboembolic pulmonary hypertension is shown in Figure 9. A nonuniform decrease in pulmonary perfusion is present with multiple regions of markedly decreased signal intensity. While MR perfusion techniques are able to document changes in blood flow with pulmonary hypertension, the importance of these techniques in the diagnosis and management of these diseases is not known.

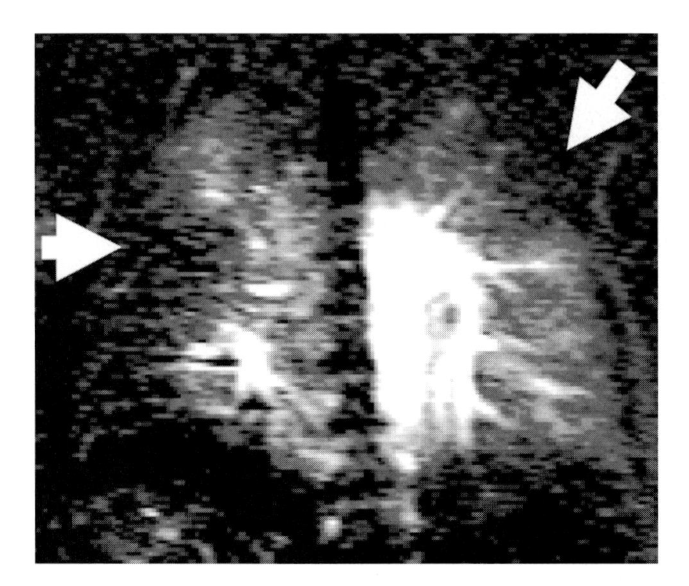

Figure 9 Perfusion-weighted image map in a patient with chronic thrombotic pulmonary hypertension obtained using ASL-FAIRER imaging. Decreased signal intensity is present bilaterally (*arrows*) corresponding to absent flow distal to chronic emboli.

Pulmonary Ventilation

Hyperpolarized gas MRI has been used to evaluate a variety of obstructive lung diseases including asthma (36,37), smoking-related lung disease (28,29), and cystic fibrosis (CF) (38,39). The majority of the studies in asthmatics and patients with CF have used ventilation imaging. Both ventilation and diffusion imaging have been assessed in smoking-related lung disease.

Asthma

A number of studies using hyperpolarized gas MRI have been reported in asthmatics. It has been shown that asthmatics have more areas of the lung that are poorly ventilated (ventilation defects) than age-matched normal subjects, and that these defects increase in number with increasing asthma severity or with provocation, such as exercise or methacholine (Fig. 6) (36,37,40). Thus, the ventilation defects on hyperpolarized gas MRI appear to be depicting the reversible airway obstruction that was known to occur in asthmatics but that was previously difficult to visualize. Recently, it has been shown that the locations of the ventilation defects are remarkably persistent, or recur in the same location, over time, suggesting that the underlying processes that cause airway obstruction are not homogeneously or randomly distributed throughout the lung, but are heterogeneous and relatively stable with time (41).

Smoking-Related Lung Disease

Patients with chronic obstructive pulmonary disease (COPD) have been shown to have more extensive helium MRI ventilation defects than subjects who never smoked. Healthy smokers were found to have more ventilation defects than never smokers but had fewer defects than the patients with COPD, demonstrating the expected dose response characteristics of cigarette smoke exposure on pulmonary ventilation (42). Diffusion helium MRI has been used to investigate emphysematous change in the lung. When inhaled, the diffusion of the helium atoms is restricted by the walls of the alveoli and airways. Measuring the apparent diffusion coefficient (ADC) of the helium gas within the lung provides information about the degree to which the lung structure restricts the diffusion of the helium atoms, and thus provides information about the size and connection of the lung microstructure. In animal models of emphysema, the helium ADC has been shown to be correlated with histological measures of alveolar size with elevated ADC values corresponding to alveolar enlargement and destruction (43–45). In humans with COPD, the helium ADC has been demonstrated to elevated relative to healthy controls, suggesting the helium ADC is able to noninvasively evaluate the structural changes that characterize emphysema (28). Furthermore, elevations of the helium ADC were found in some healthy smokers suggesting that diffusion helium MRI may be a sensitive method for detecting early or subclinical emphysematous change in the lung (Fig. 10) (46).

Cystic Fibrosis

As with asthma and COPD, helium MRI ventilation defects are increased in patients with CF, including the subset of CF subjects with an FEV1% predicted in the normal range, as compared to age-matched normal control subjects (25). Further, changes in the ventilation defects were detected following standard airway mucus clearance techniques in CF patients. However, only weak to moderate correlations were found between helium MRI ventilation defects and spirometry or chest X-ray in 18 children with CF (47). The authors postulated that the weak correlations were the result of a greater sensitivity of hyperpolarized helium MRI to ventilatory abnormalities. In 8 adults with CF, helium MRI ventilation defects were strongly correlated with abnormalities of structure on CT on a regional basis (Fig. 11) (48). Thus, hyperpolarized helium MRI appears to detect airway obstruction in CF, even in mild CF, and may represent a safe alternative to CT for the evaluation of CF lung disease.

SUMMARY

Functional MR imaging of the lung, by providing regional information about the ventilation and

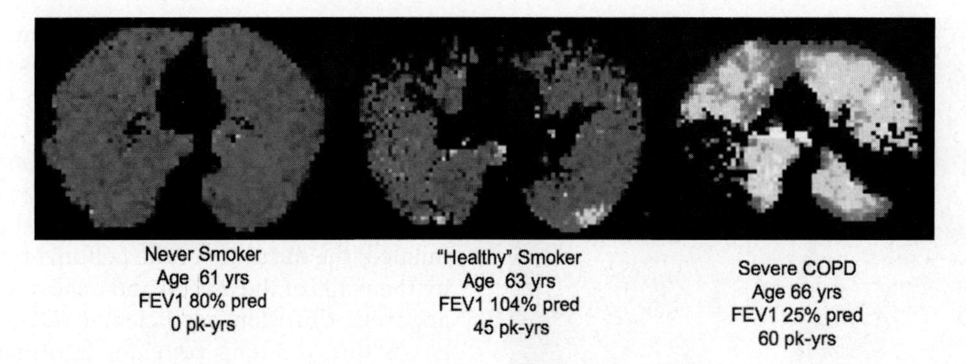

Figure 10 Axial hyperpolarized helium MR apparent diffusion coefficient (ADC) maps in a subject who never smoked, a healthy smoker, and a patient with chronic obstructive pulmonary disease (COPD). The never smoker has homogeneously low ADC values (*red pixels*) indicating small homogeneously sized alveoli. The healthy smoker has two small areas of ADC elevation (*yellow pixels*) suggesting there are focal areas of lung structural damage. The patient with COPD has markedly elevated ADC values (*yellow to white pixels*) throughout the lung suggesting widespread structural damage to the lung. (*See color insert.*)

perfusion, allows us to noninvasively explore aspects of lung physiology and pathophysiology that previously were accessible only by invasive means. These new MR imaging techniques have already provided new information about diseases such as asthma and high altitude pulmonary edema and will facilitate new lines of inquiry into pulmonary disease. The combination of perfusion and ventilation imaging may be particularly powerful. Initially, these techniques may be most useful for the pharmaceutical industry in the drug discovery and development process since they may be more sensitive outcome measures than standard outcome measures, such as pulmonary function tests. However, as new treatments are developed for pulmonary diseases, these techniques may play a crucial role clinically in the identification of patients who may respond to treatment and in the assessment of the response to treatment.

REFERENCES

1 Hatabu H, Gaa J, Kim D, Li W, Prasad PV, Edelman RR. Pulmonary perfusion: qualitative assessment with dynamic contrast-enhanced MRI using ultra-short TE and inversion recovery turbo FLASH. Magn Reson Med 1996; 36:503–8.

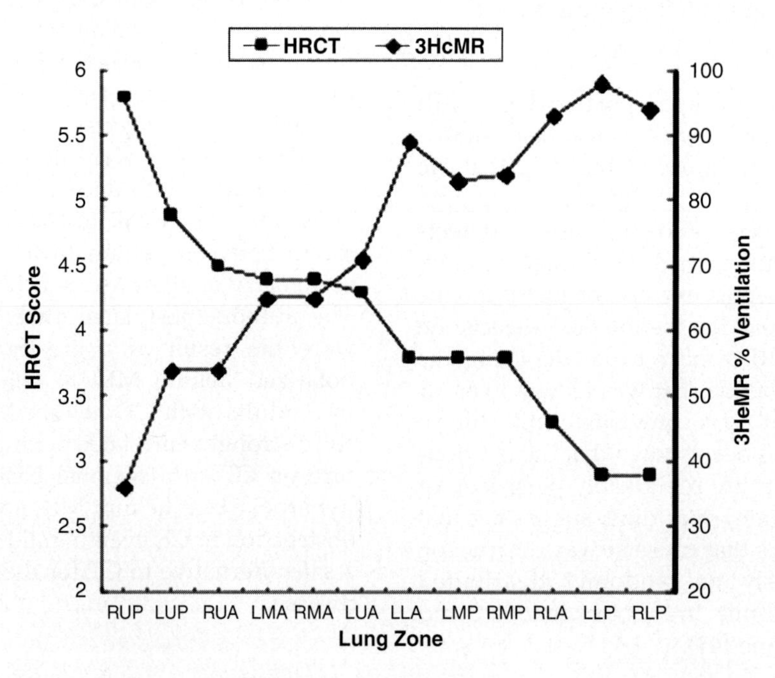

Figure 11 Regional hyperpolarized helium ventilation MRI and CT scores from a patient with CF. Areas with poor hyperpolarized helium ventilation tend to have a high (worse) score on CT and vice versa demonstrating the regional concordance of the information obtained on CT and helium MR. *Abbreviations*: RUP, right upper posterior; LUP, left upper posterior; RUA, right upper anterior; LMA, left middle anterior; RMA, right middle anterior; LUA, left upper anterior; LLA, left lower anterior; LMP, left middle posterior, RMP, right middle posterior; RLA, right lower anterior; LLP, left lower posterior; RLP, right lower posterior. *Source*: Courtesy of Jim Wild, from Ref. 48.

2 Buxton RB. Arterial spin labeling techniques. In: Introduction to Functional Magnetic Resonance Imaging. Cambridge, UK: Cambridge University Press, 2002: 351–87.
3 Levin DL, Chen Q, Zhang M, Edelman RR, Hatabu H. Evaluation of regional pulmonary perfusion using ultrafast magnetic resonance imaging. Magn Reson Med 2001;46:166–71.
4 Ohno Y, Hatabu H, Murase K, et al. Quantitative assessment of regional pulmonary perfusion in the entire lung using three-dimensional ultrafast dynamic contrast-enhanced magnetic resonance imaging: preliminary experience in 40 subjects. J Magn Reson Imag 2004; 20: 353–65.
5 Wilke N, Jerosch-Herold M, Stillman AE, et al. Concepts of myocardial perfusion imaging in magnetic resonance imaging. Magn Reson Q 1994; 10:249–86.
6 Thompson HK, Starmer CF, Whalen RE, McIntosh HD. Indicator transit time considered as a gamma variate. Circ Res 1964; 14:502–15.
7 Axel L. Methods using blood pool tracers. In: Binha DL, ed. Magnetic Resonance Perfusion and Diffusion Imaging. New York: Raven Press, 1995:205–11.
8 Weisskoff RM, Chesler F, Boxerman JL, Rosen BR. Pitfalls in MR measurement of tissue blood flow with intravascular tracers: which mean transit time? Magn Reson Med 1993; 29:553–58.
9 Hatabu H, Tadamura E, Levin DL, et al. Quantitative assessment of pulmonary perfusion with dynamic contrast-enhanced MRI. Magn Reson Med 1999; 42:1033–8.
10 Buxton RB, Frank LR, Wong EC, Siewert B, Warach S, Edelman RR. A general kinetic model for quantitative perfusion imaging with arterial spin labeling. Magn Reson Med 1998; 40(3):383–96.
11 Hatabu H, Tadamura E, Prasad PV, Chen Q, Buxton R, Edelman RR. Noninvasive pulmonary perfusion imaging by STAR–HASTE sequence. Magn Reson Med 2000; 44(5):808–12.
12 Bolar DS, Levin DL, Hopkins SR, et al. Quantification of regional pulmonary blood flow using ASL-FAIRER. Magn Reson Med 2006; 55(6):1308–17.
13 Edelman RR, HatabuH, Tadamura E, Li W, Prasad PV. Noninvasive assessment of regional ventilation in the human lung using oxygen-enhanced magnetic resonance imaging. Nat Med 1996; 2:1236–9.
14 Middleton H, BlackRD, Saam B, et al. MR imaging with hyperpolarized ^{3}He gas. Magn Reson Med 1995; 33:271–5.
15 Keilholz S, Knight-Scott J, Mata J, et al. The contribution of ventilation and perfusion in O2-enhanced MRI: results from rabbit models of pulmonary embolism and bronchial obstruction. In: Tenth Annual Scientific Meeting of International Society of Magnetic Resonance in Medicine (ISMRM), Hawaii, May 2002.
16 Kauczor H, Surkau R, Roberts T. MRI using hyperpolarized noble gases. Eur Radiol 1998; 8(5):820–7.
17 van Beek EJ, Wild JM, Kauczor HU, Schreiber W, Mugler JP III, de Lange EE. Functional MRI of the lung using hyperpolarized 3-helium gas. J Magn Reson Imag 2004; 20(4):540–54.
18 Moller HE, Chen XJ, Saam B, et al. MRI of the lungs using hyperpolarized noble gases. Magn Reson Med 2002; 47:1029–51.
19 Parra-Robles J, Cross AR, Santyr GE. Theoretical signal-to-noise ratio and spatial resolution dependence on the magnetic field strength for hyperpolarized noble gas magnetic resonance imaging of human lungs. Med Phys 2005; 32:221–9.
20 Altes TA, Rehm PK, Harrell F, Salerno M, Daniel TM, de Lange EE. Ventilation imaging of the lung: comparison of hyperpolarized helium-3 MR imaging with Xe-133 scintigraphy. Acad Radiol 2004; 11:729–34.
21 de Lange EE, Mugler JP III, Brookeman JR, et al. Lung air spaces: MR imaging evaluation with hyperpolarized ^{3}He gas. Radiology 1999; 210:851–7.
22 Kauczor HU, Hofmann D, Kreitner KF, et al. Normal and abnormal pulmonary ventilation: visualization at hyperpolarized He-3 MR imaging. Radiology 1996; 201:564–8.
23 Saam B, Yablonskiy DA, Gierada DS, Conradi MS. Rapid imaging of hyperpolarized gas using EPI. Magn Reson Med 1999; 42:507–14.
24 Salerno M, Altes TA, Brookeman JR, de Lange EE, Mugler JP III. Dynamic spiral MRI of pulmonary gas flow using hyperpolarized (3)He: preliminary studies in healthy and diseased lungs. Magn Reson Med 2001; 46:667–77.
25 Deninger AJ, Eberle B, Ebert M, et al. Quantification of regional intrapulmonary oxygen partial pressure evolution during apnea by (3)He MRI. J Magn Reson 1999; 141:207–16.
26 Eberle B, Weiler N, Markstaller K, et al. Analysis of intrapulmonary O(2) concentration by MR imaging of inhaled hyperpolarized helium-3. J Appl Physiol 1999; 87:2043–52.
27 Mugler JP III, Brookeman JR, Knight-Scott J, Maier T, de Lange EE, Bogorad PL. Regional measurement of the ^{3}He diffusion coefficient in the human lung. In: Proceedings of the International Society for Magnetic Resonance in Medicine (ISMRM), 1998, Sydney, Australia.
28 Salerno M, de Lange EE, Altes TA, Truwit JD, Brookeman JR, Mugler JP III Emphysema: hyperpolarized helium 3 diffusion MR imaging of the lungs compared with spirometric indexes—initial experience. Radiology 2002; 222:252–60.
29 Saam BT, Yablonskiy DA, Kodibagkar VD, et al. MR imaging of diffusion of (3)He gas in healthy and diseased lungs. Magn Reson Med 2000; 44:174–9.
30 Chen Q, LevinDL, Kim D, et al. Pulmonary disorders: ventilation-perfusion MR imaging with animal models. Radiology 1999; 213:871–9.
31 Keilholz SD, Mai VM, Berr SS, Fujiwara N, Hagspiel KD. Comparison of first-pass Gd-DOTA and FAIRER perfusion imaging in a rabbit model of pulmonary embolism. J Magn Reson Imag 2002; 16:168–71.
32 Meaney JFM, Weg JG, Chenevert TL, Stafford-Johnson D, Hamilton BH, Prince MR. Diagnosis of pulmonary embolism with magnetic resonance angiography. N Engl J Med 1997; 336:1322–427.
33 Kluge A, Luboldt W, Bachmann G. Acute pulmonary embolism to the subsegmental level: diagnostic

accuracy of three MRI techniques compared with 16-MDCT. Am J Roentgenol 2006; 187:W7–14.

34 WollmerP, Rozkoven A, Rhodes CG, Allan RM, Maseri A. Regional pulmonary blood volume in patients with abnormal blood pressure or flow in the pulmonary circulation. Eur Heart J 1984; 5:924–31.

35 Fraser RG, Pare JA, Pare PD: Pulmonary hypertension and edema. In: Pare PD, ed. Diagnosis of Diseases of the Chest. Philadelphia, PA: W.B. Saunders, 1999:1879–945.

36 Altes TA, Powers PL, Knight-Scott J, et al. Hyperpolarized ^{3}He MR lung ventilation imaging in asthmatics: preliminary findings. J Magn Reson Imag 2001; 13:378–84.

37 Samee S, Altes T, Powers P, et al. Imaging the lungs in asthmatic patients by using hyperpolarized helium-3 magnetic resonance: assessment of response to methacholine and exercise challenge. J Allergy Clin Immunol 2003; 111:1205–11.

38 Mentore K, FrohDK, de Lange EE, Brookeman JR, Paget-Brown AO, Altes TA. Hyperpolarized He 3 MRI of the lung in cystic fibrosis: assessment at baseline and after bronchodilator and airway clearance treatment. Acad Radiol 2005; 12:1423–9.

39 Koumellis P, van Beek EJ, Woodhouse N, et al. Quantitative analysis of regional airways obstruction using dynamic hyperpolarized ^{3}He MRI-preliminary results in children with cystic fibrosis. J Magn Reson Imag 2005; 22:420–6.

40 de Lange EE, Altes TA, Patrie JT, et al. Evaluation of asthma with hyperpolarized helium-3 MRI: correlation with clinical severity and spirometry. Chest 2006; 130:1055–62.

41 de Lange EE, Altes TA, Patrie JT, et al. Assessing the regional variability of airflow obstruction with hyperpolarized helium-3 MR imaging. J Allergy Clin Immunol (in press).

42 Woodhouse N, WildJM, Paley MN, et al. Combined helium-3/proton magnetic resonance imaging measurement of ventilated lung volumes in smokers compared to never-smokers. J Magn Reson Imag 2005; 21:365–9.

43 Chen XJ, HedlundLW, Moller HE, Chawla MS, Maronpot RR, Johnson GA. Detection of emphysema in rat lungs by using magnetic resonance measurements of ^{3}He diffusion. Proc Natl Acad Sci USA 2000; 97:11478–81.

44 Mata J, Altes T, Cai J, et al. Evaluation of emphysema severity and progression in a rabbit model: a comparison of hyperpolarized He-3 and Xe-129 diffusion MRI with lung morphometry. J Appl Physiol 2007; 102(3): 1273–1280.

45 Woods JC, ChoongCK, Yablonskiy DA, et al. Hyperpolarized (3)He diffusion MRI and histology in pulmonary emphysema. Magn Reson Med 2006; 56(6): 1293–300.

46 Fain SB, Panth SR, Evans MD, et al. Early emphysematous changes in asymptomatic smokers: detection with ^{3}He MR imaging. Radiology 2006; 239:875–83.

47 van Beek EJ, Hill C, Woodhouse N, et al. Assessment of lung disease in children with cystic fibrosis using hyperpolarized 3-Helium MRI: comparison with Shwachman score, Chrispin–Norman score and spirometry. Eur Radiol (in press).

48 McMahon CJ, DoddJD, Hill C, et al. Hyperpolarized (3) helium magnetic resonance ventilation imaging of the lung in cystic fibrosis: comparison with high resolution CT and spirometry. Eur Radiol 2006; 16:2483–90.

4

Digital Chest Radiography

Matthew Freedman
Department of Oncology, Lombardi Comprehensive Cancer Center, Georgetown University, Washington, D.C., U.S.A.

THE IDEAL CHEST IMAGE

The chest radiograph is a complex image containing information on many structures in the thorax. In this image, one can see the lungs and their diseases; the pulmonary vessels and their diseases; the heart; the mediastinum; the bony thorax; the chest wall; and portions of the neck, abdomen, and arms. Because of the great differences in the absorption and inherent tissue contrast in these regions, the ideal chest radiograph has conflicting requirements. All current chest radiographs, both analog and digital, represent compromises to accommodate these conflicting optimal requirements. Digital radiography currently comes closer to meeting these requirements than analog radiography, but current systems are still not able to produce the ideal image and further developments are needed.

In the ideal chest image, one would want to be able to assess each structure in the chest with sufficient contrast to detect disease and sufficient resolution to define the structural features of what is seen. The fundamental problem in chest radiography is that the absorption of different parts of the chest varies widely and the inherent contrast of different structures—the inherent differences in absorption of different tissues—varies widely. To "create" an ideal chest radiograph, one must consider both general regional differences in absorption and the local differences in the absorption of the tissues within the region. One needs an image that accommodates the large differences in regional absorption within the mediastinum and the local differences in absorption, such as visualization of the structures within the lung. For the bedside chest examination, we need one that either has some method for automatic exposure control (AEC) or that uses some method of post-processing of the image to correct for exposure differences among images that are very difficult to control in standard chest radiography where both under- and overexposure are common.

Digital radiography helps to overcome this problem of varying exposures in bedside radiography (1,2). In one study, bedside screen-film radiographs had a mean lung optical density of 2.43 with a standard deviation of 0.31. High lung optical density was used to provide adequate mediastinal density to visualize the tubes within the mediastinum, an important part of the evaluation of postcardiac-surgery patients. Digital radiographs had an average lung density of 1.44, standard deviation of 0.13 (2). Digital chest radiographs were closer to the optimum optical density recommended by the International Labor Organization (hilar regions at a minimum of 0.2 optical density units above fog; parenchymal regions at a maximum of 1.8 units of optical density above fog) (3) and showed less variation film to film and patient to patient, allowing easier comparison.

Image processing of digital chest radiographs allows one to adjust partially for the regional differences in absorption and to enhance the contrast of specific structures within the lung. While such corrections can improve the image, they are only a partial solution to the problems in projection chest radiography. There are three main substances that absorb and scatter X-ray photons: air, water, and calcium. The variable absorption and scattering encode the original X-ray beam with information. Only those X-ray photons that reach the detector are used to form the image, so if the photons are absorbed or scattered sufficiently, they do not reach the detector. Air absorbs and scatters the least, calcium the most. The thickness of each of these substances also affects absorption; the more there is of any of these substances in the path of the X-ray beam, the more it absorbs and scatters. For each portion of the chest, the proportion of the X rays reaching the image recording system will depend on the types of substances in the X ray beam and their combined thickness for each location in the projected image. The chest has a wide range of absorption differences. If one attempts to display the entire range of absorption differences, two things can happen: either the image is of low contrast, or some areas are of high contrast and others of low contrast. The standard screen-film chest radiograph is generally presented as an image where the contrast in the lungs is moderately high and that in the mediastinum and projected over the upper abdomen is relatively low. The areas of lower contrast, however, may contain important details in the image. Digital chest radiography can be adjusted so that these areas of lower contrast are altered to become regions of higher contrast, while leaving the contrast of the lungs nearly unchanged. When using a soft copy viewing workstation, the brightness and contrast of the image can be adjusted to correct or partially correct for the differences in absorption and image contrast; the image can then be viewed twice, once for the lungs and a second version for the mediastinum.

Correct positioning and instruction of the patient also helps create a better image. If the patient fails to take a deep breath, the lung bases will show crowded markings and disease may be simulated by the lung markings or obscured by them. If the scapulae overlie the lungs, small peripheral lung nodules and infiltrates may be obscured or densities appearing like nodules and infiltrates may be produced. Rotation will affect the apparent symmetry of lung size and lung radiodensity simulating disease.

Requirements for the Lungs

In the region of the image where the lungs are projected, there is far less water density material to absorb and scatter the X rays than there is in the mediastinum and lateral chest wall. For this reason, the lung regions need less X-ray exposure than the mediastinum to produce an image of appropriate optical density (for an analog system) or appropriate signal-to-noise (for a digital system). Ideally, the maximum contrast between the vessels, interstitium, and the air in the lungs is desired. Current analog and digital images must compromise on this because of the differences in the thickness and absorbing characteristics of different parts of the chest. In general, because there is less air and more water and calcium absorption in the lateral and apical portions of the lung, the region projected behind the heart, and in the lung area projected behind the diaphragm, these areas require more exposure. Unfortunately, the exposure level necessary for these regions to have an ideal exposure is excessive for the lungs and would make them very dark, sufficient to obscure disease. With digital chest images, different display settings can be used to adjust the density range of the image, allowing one to gain optimum settings for each of these regions, but at a cost of the time required to make these separate adjustments.

Special Requirements for the Lung Apices

The clavicles and the upper ribs (which are more closely spaced than the lower ribs) overlie the lung apices. The presence of these bony structures can obscure underlying lung disease (4). In addition, the apical lung is relatively small, so that processes are more likely to reach a pleural surface. When a process reaches a pleural surface, it tends to extend along the surface, thus losing its sharp edge, making it harder to identify. In the ideal image, one would want to decrease the degree to which the bony structures obscure the apical lung. There are two current and one future method that can help accomplish this. The first is to obtain the chest radiograph at the highest kilovolt peak possible since the absorption differences between calcium and water decrease with increasing kilovolts. With a higher kilovolt peak, any lung process becomes more equal in density to the bone projected over it. The second method is to use energy subtraction. With this method (described below), special image acquisition and image processing can form an image in which the bone is largely subtracted away. Special equipment and image processing are necessary for this technique. Third, experimentally, several groups are developing temporal subtraction chest radiography. If one has two chest radiographs that are similar in their positioning, it is possible to process them so that they are nearly superimposed. Once superimposed, the computer can subtract one image from the other. The bony structures are unlikely to change, while the lung can develop pneumonias, cancers, and so on. Thus, the subtraction image provides a potentially better view for the detection of change in the apical lung. This technique is demonstrated below.

Processes in the lung apices may not have sharp margins, so that the major sign of disease may be a difference in the absorption of the X rays when the two apices are compared. The detection of this difference in absorption can be mimicked or obscured by mild degrees of rotation of the patient or by a different degree of elevation of the two arms. When the lungs are well inflated, the apical bones (ribs and clavicles) separate more and make it possible to better see the regions of lung between the bony structures. Proper positioning of the patient aids in the detection of otherwise subtle and poorly defined abnormalities in the lung apices.

Special Requirements for Lateral Margin of the Chest

Because of the generally ovoid shape of the lungs, there is less lung and there are more chest wall structures, both bone and soft tissue, near the edges of the chest. This increase in soft tissue and bony structures results in the lungs appearing more opaque (whiter) peripherally than centrally. This factor, combined with the shadows from female or male breast tissue, makes it harder to show lung detail with maximum contrast. If one chooses maximum contrast centrally, the lung periphery may be underexposed. Equalizing these lung densities across the chest should enhance the ability to use higher contrast imaging of the lungs. A common problem in detecting subtle disease in the lateral margins of the chest is the presence of the scapulae when they overlie the chest. The differential density caused by the scapulae may hide or simulate disease (especially small lung nodules). Proper positioning of the patient will help alleviate this problem. The density of the breasts on a chest radiograph can often be decreased if the patient is positioned with the lower portion of the chest tight against the cassette thereby flattening the breasts and pushing them down and to the side, decreasing their superimposition on the lungs. Sometimes, if an area of concern is at the lung bases in a woman, having the patient lift up her breasts with her hands may allow one to decide if an image radiodensity is due to lung disease or normal soft tissues, potentially avoiding the use of fluoroscopy or CT.

Special Requirements for the Region Projected Behind the Heart and Diaphragm

Portions of the lungs project behind the heart and behind the diaphragm. These areas are difficult to visualize on screen-film chest radiographs because of the larger amount of water density absorbers there than over the central portions of the lungs and because there is less lung tissue. A lateral view of the chest partially compensates for this, but not completely. Moreover, with bedside chest radiographs, a lateral view is often not feasible. Image processing of digital radiographs can partially correct this density difference. One method is to increase the optical density of the entire image when one looks at these regions and then use a different processing setting to look at the central portions of the lungs (Fig. 1A and B). A second technique is to use regional density equalization methods to enhance these regions (Fig. 2A and B). Because the blackness of a film can be adjusted by image processing, it can be more difficult to assess whether there is disease behind the heart or whether this region is simply underexposed (since image processing can make it as black as one could desire). A useful guide is that the region is adequately exposed for lung disease if one can see the ribs projected through the heart. If the ribs cannot be seen, despite image processing, the image is underexposed and the failure to see normal lung vessels is not a sign of disease (Fig. 3). The same rule applies for the assessment of mediastinal tubes. If the spine can be seen, the exposure should be adequate for the detection of tubes and lines. Be aware, however, that some noise-suppression algorithms can obscure tubes while maintaining some degree of visibility of larger structures, such as the spine. In general, noise-suppression image processing can hide or partially hide the sharp edges of structures lowering their conspicuity. In digital chest imaging, lack of visible noise in the mediastinum should alert the radiologist that the edges of tubes and lines may be obscured, too much noise indicates underexposure.

Special Requirements for Specific Disease Processes

Pneumothorax

On both screen-film and digital chest radiographs, pneumothoraces may be difficult to detect. Detection of a pneumothorax depends on the detection of two findings: the first is the radiolucency of the lung zone outside of the edge of the lung; the second is the detection of the lung edge. Because digital image processing can change the density of regions of the image, density equalization programs may make the radiolucency harder to detect. The pleural edge can be very thin and can be superimposed on the ribs. Detection of

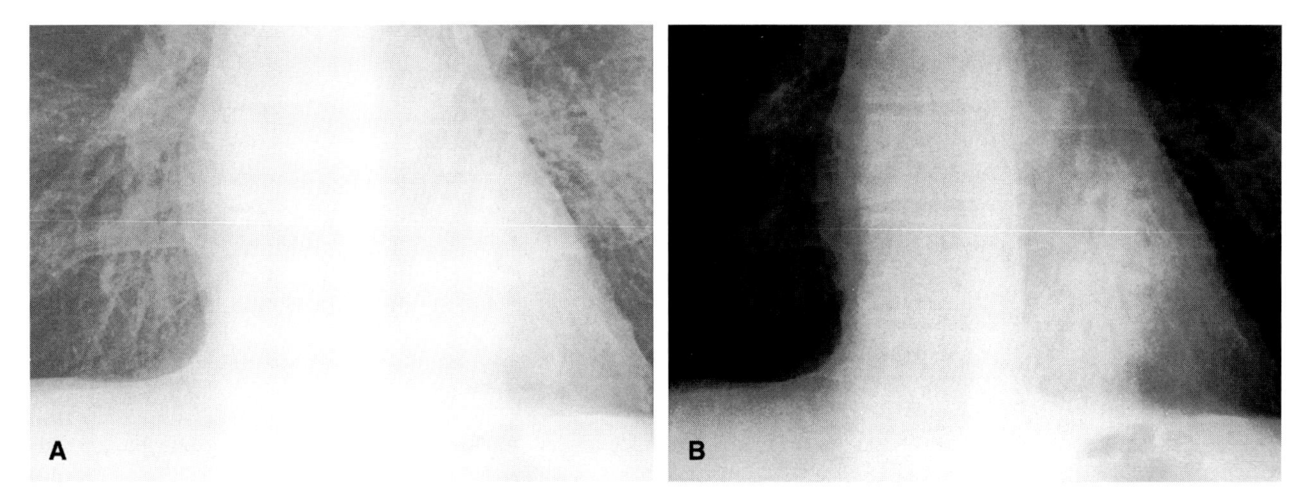

Figure 1 (**A** and **B**) Improved detection of retrocardiac pneumonia using image processing. A small area of pneumonia behind the heart can be seen on both images, but is more conspicuous on the image that has been processed to be darker (**B**).

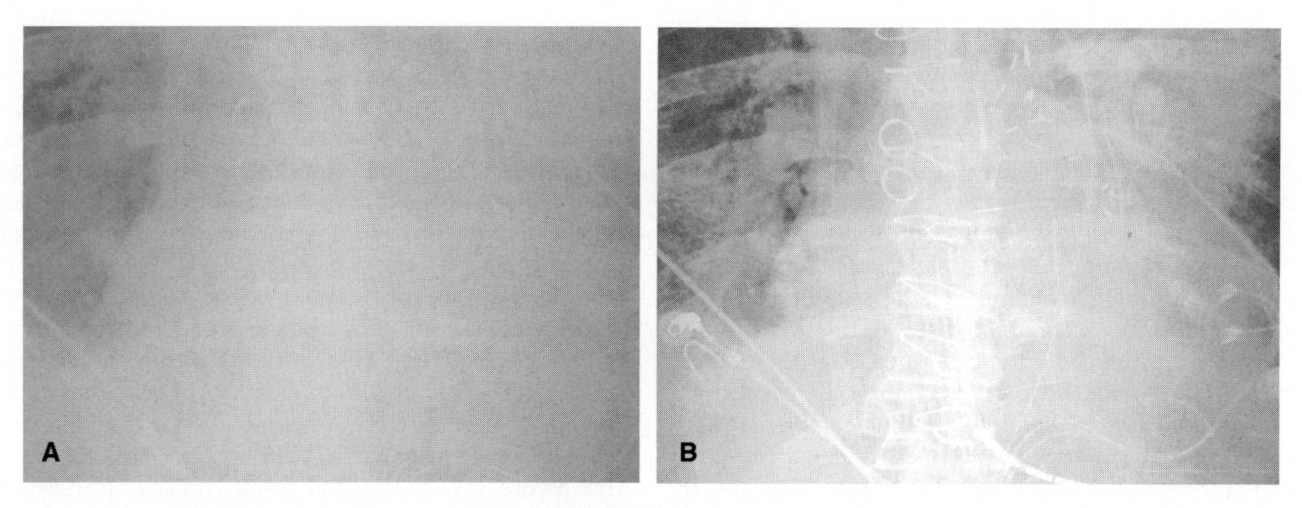

Figure 2 (**A** and **B**) Improved visualization of retrocardiac tubes and lines by using optical density equalization algorithm. The tubes and lines are better visualized on (**B**), in which optical density equalization has been applied.

the edge of the lung depends somewhat on the thickness of that edge, which varies among individuals. Using a slight degree of image processing to enhance edges increases the conspicuity of the lung edge and makes it easier to see a pneumothorax (Fig. 4). When the edge of the lung is superimposed on a rib, a low-kilovolt-peak chest X-ray technique may make it harder to see the lung edge because the relative radiodensity of the ribs is increased; therefore a high-kilovolt-peak technique is preferred. The outer 2 cm of the lungs are more radiolucent than the more central portion since there is less lung, fewer blood vessels, and therefore less tissue density. If the image is too dark, it may become quite difficult to see detail in this region. If you are using a workstation to look at the image, making the image lighter can enhance the conspicuity of a pneumothorax. In carefully controlled settings, the detection of pneumothoraces on screen-film and digital images has been shown to be equivalent (5–7).

Bedside chest radiographs may be obtained with the patient upright, semi-upright, or supine. When the patient is supine, the air will collect in the anterior pleural space and small amounts of air may be undetectable. Sometimes this air can be detected because the pleural edge can be seen in the cardiophrenic or costophrenic angles. Sometimes, the only evidence is a difference in the radiolucency of one hemithorax, an appearance that is sometimes mimicked by histogram equalization digital image processing. When the patient is semi-upright, the technologist will often obtain the bedside radiograph with the X-ray beam perpendicular to the patient, rather than horizontal. This may hide the pneumothorax. Since the pneumothorax air will usually rise to the pleural apex, when there is a question, a

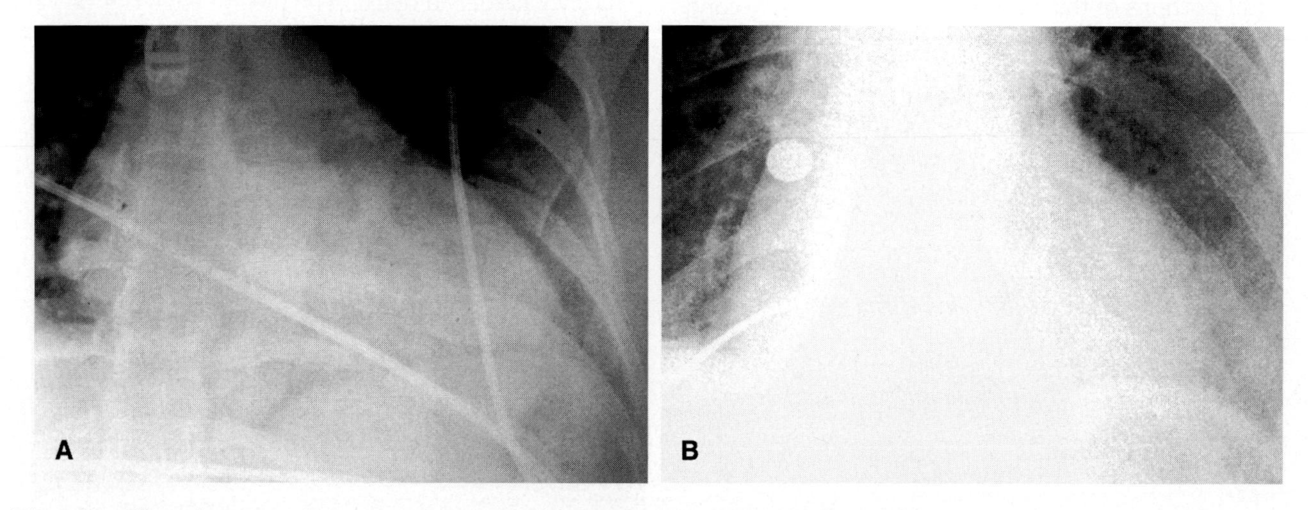

Figure 3 Effect of exposure factors on assessment of the retrocardiac region. (**A**) Retrocardiac atelectasis is visible; the ribs can be seen. (**B**) Retrocardiac area cannot be evaluated; the ribs cannot be seen. Underexposed Fuji film (Fuji Photo Film Corp., Tokyo, Japan) with an "S" of 8955 (the "S" number of a properly exposed chest radiograph is approximately 200–400). Due to underexposure, one cannot tell whether there is retrocardiac airspace disease or effusion. The system has, however, permitted overcorrection of the density of the lungs to be blacker than those of a properly exposed bedside chest radiograph.

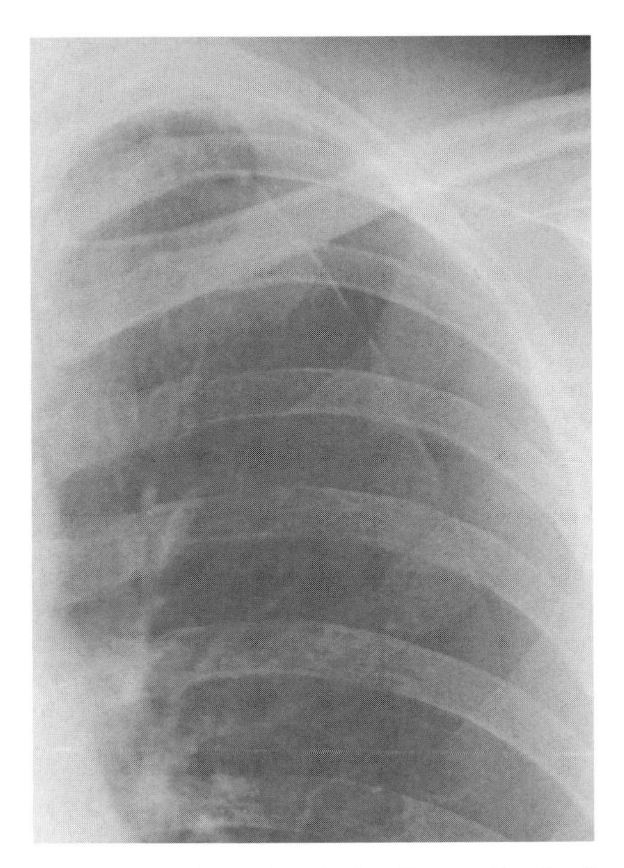

Figure 4 Pneumothorax detection in a 22-year-old male with a spontaneous pneumothorax. The pneumothorax is visible laterally. A few very small blebs are minimally visible at the apex of the lung.

repeat film with the X-ray beam horizontal may reveal a small pneumothorax; with a semiupright patient, however, a horizontal beam X-ray image may project less of the lungs between the top of the diaphragm and the lung apex, thereby hiding disease at the lung bases. Digital image processing can be used to enhance the visibility of structures projected through the diaphragm.

Emphysema

The edges of emphysematous bullae and blebs are often very fine-curved lines. Such lines can be blurred by the penumbra resulting from the X-ray tube focal spot. Small degrees of edge enhancement can enhance the conspicuity of these structures. For this reason, it can be easier to detect small amounts of emphysema on digital images (Fig. 4).

Interstitial Disease

Edge enhancement will increase the conspicuity of normal lung structures and interstitial lung disease. With edge enhancement, several reports document no difference in detection of interstitial lung disease (5,8,9). Without edge enhancement, one study (10) showed that interstitial disease is less conspicuous (Fig. 5A–C).

Interstitial disease is composed of fine and coarse lines and nodules. The conspicuity of these can be increased by a small amount of edge enhancement. The interstitial disease seen on digital chest radiographs, when minimal, may be quite difficult to see on conventional screen-film chest radiographs.

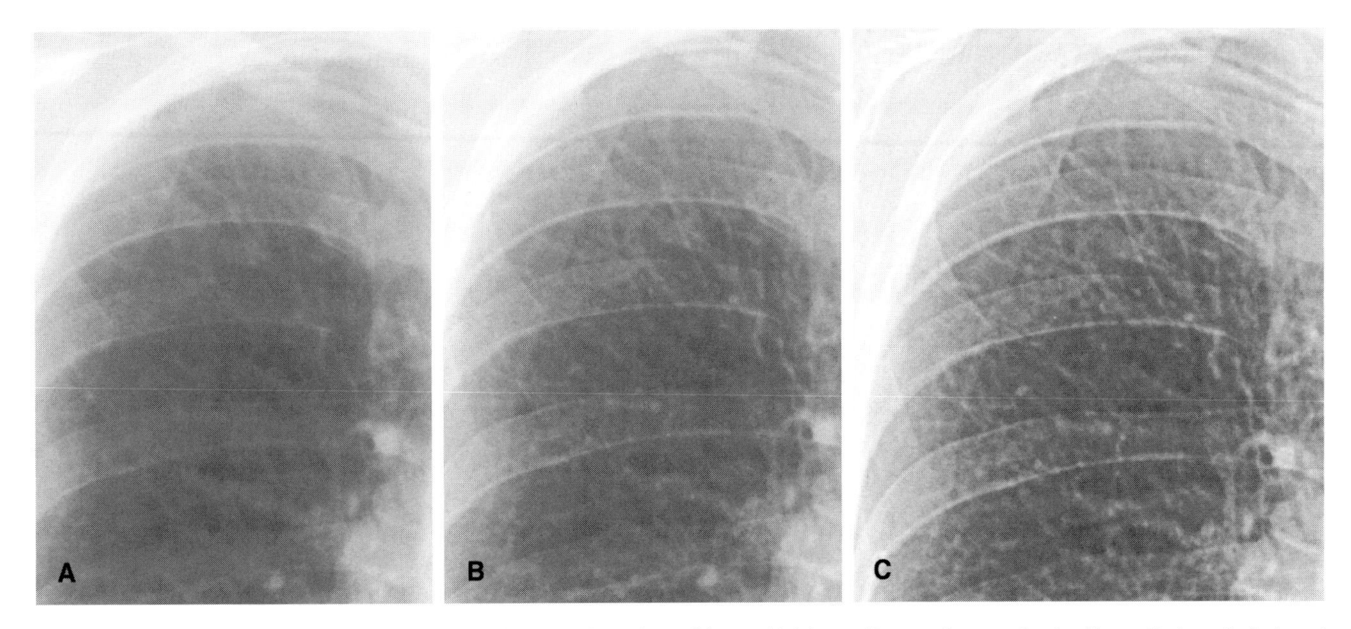

Figure 5 Effect of edge enhancement algorithm on detection of interstitial lung disease in a patient with methotrexate-induced interstitial lung disease. Interstitial disease shown with no edge enhancement (**A**), standard edge enhancement (**B**), and exaggerated edge enhancement (**C**). Increasing enhancement accentuates the fine-curved fibrotic lines. However, the small nodules are better seen in the less enhanced images. A small degree of edge enhancement (**B**) shows the pattern of interstitial disease best.

Thus, one is likely to detect minimal interstitial disease more often on the digital images. At the same time, the vessels may be more conspicuous on digital chest radiographs, so it is important to carefully assess visible lines. In general, if the lines branch, they are vessels; if they fail to branch, they are likely interstitial lines. On underexposed images, the noise can become visible and may simulate very small, miliary-like nodules. Figure 3B shows the nodular appearance of noise on a severely underexposed film. Conversely, the use of a blurring algorithm to decrease the visibility of noise may also blur fine interstitial lines and nodules decreasing their conspicuity, particularly if they are in lighter (less well exposed) areas of the image.

Masses and Nodules

Digital chest radiography has not resulted in problems in the detection of small lung nodules (5,8,9,11,12). A group of studies show radiologists have equivalent to slightly better ability to detect lung nodules on digital chest radiographs when compared to standard screen-film chest radiographs (13–18). Digital radiographs have been shown likely superior to screen-film radiographs in detecting nodules superimposed on the mediastinum (11,19). Because the contrast scale on digital chest radiographs can be changed, it may be more difficult to tell if a nodule is calcified. However, when techniques of image processing are standardized, this problem does not occur. The detection equivalence of lung nodules is seen when appropriate image processing is used (19). Inappropriate image processing of digital chest radiographs, however, can decrease the visibility of lung nodules. The conspicuity of lung nodules is equivalent with high-kilovolt-peak, high-contrast images. On the other hand, if the image processing produces a low-contrast image or if a low-kilovolt-peak image results in increased conspicuity of the ribs, nodules may be less visible (Fig. 6).

The detection of large lung masses and large areas of pneumonia may appear different on digital images when regional density equalization algorithms are used. These density equalization algorithms may partially equalize their density so they may not appear as dense for their size as they would on screen-film images.

Detection of Calcium in Lung Nodules

Digital image processing allows one to change the contrast of the chest image. Calcium in lung nodules is detected by two findings: first, the identification of the irregular shape of the calcifications and second by the greater density of a nodule for its size than would be expected for a noncalcified nodule. While the first sign remains unchanged with digital images, image processing can change the contrast of a nodule compared to its background, making it appear more radiodense or less radiodense. If techniques for image processing are standardized, there is usually no problem, but if one varies the image-processing technique for different patients, it may be confusing to the radiologist. A newer method, energy subtraction (also called dual-energy subtraction) imaging produces soft tissue and calcium emphasis images of the chest enhancing the ability of radiologists to separate calcified and noncalcified nodules. This method is discussed below.

Requirements for the Mediastinum

In the mediastinum and chest wall, there is much more water density material to absorb and scatter the X rays. The absorption difference between normal

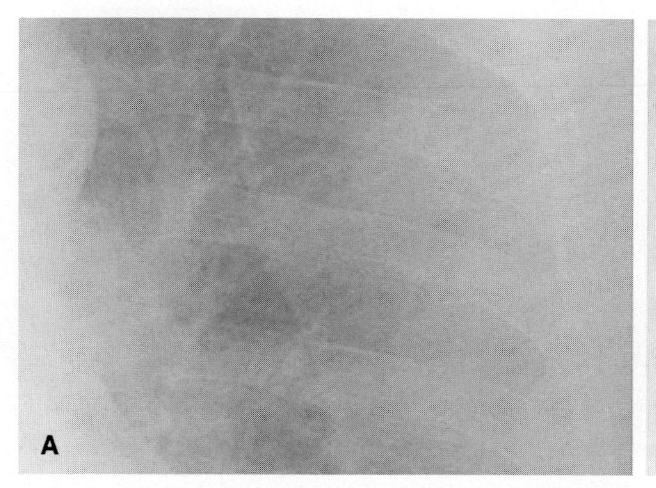

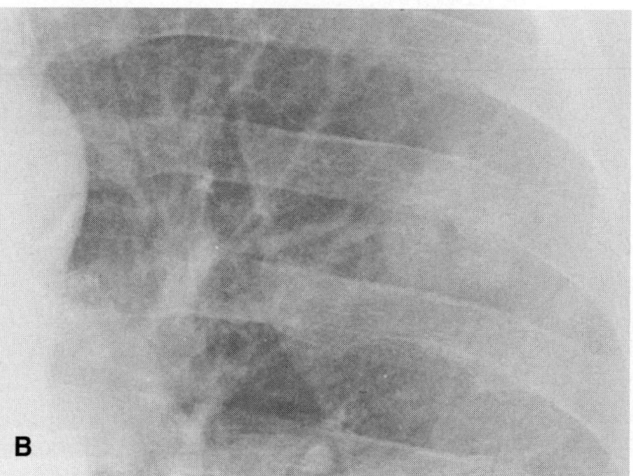

Figure 6 Effect of edge and contrast enhancement on lung nodule detection. Non–small cell primary lung cancer in the periphery of the left upper lobe shown (**A**) without and (**B**) with minimal edge and contrast enhancement. The mass is more easily seen with the edge and contrast enhancement.

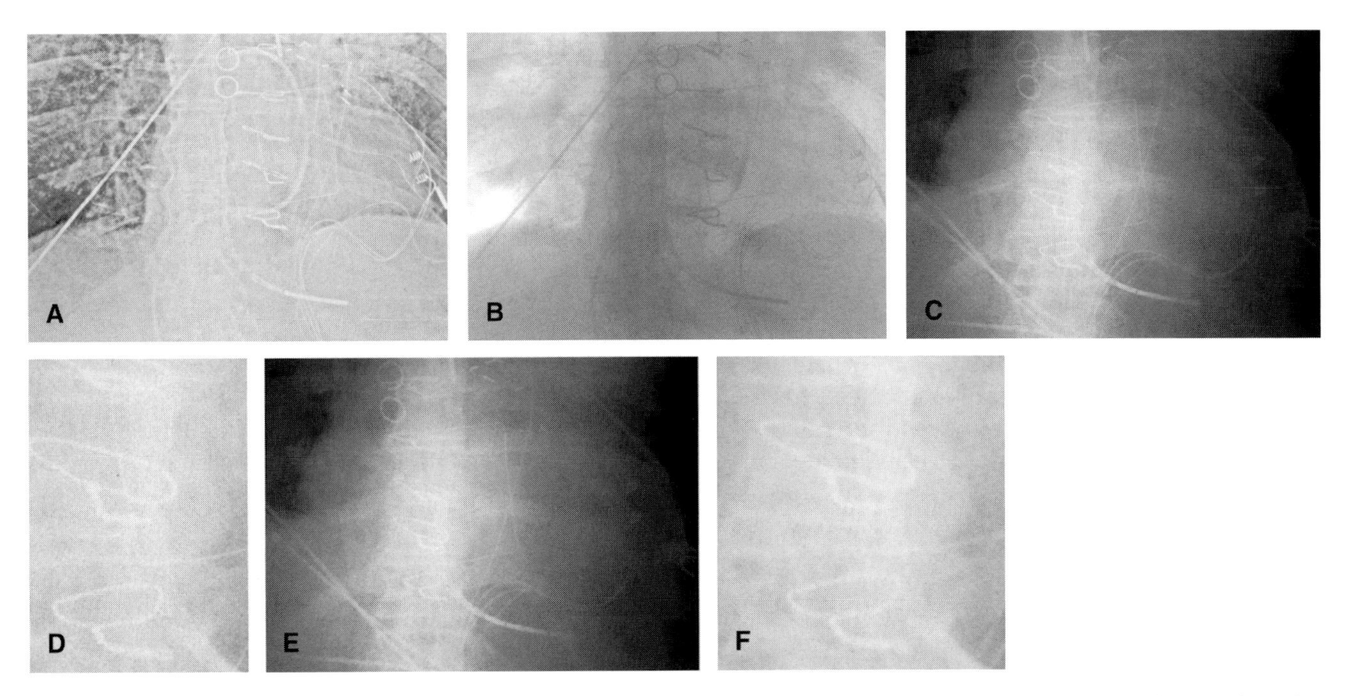

Figure 7 Assessment of lines and tubes using digital radiography. Retrocardiac tubes shown with histogram equalization plus edge enhancement (**A**) and black/white inversion (**B**). (**C**) Same patient, different day. Film is underexposed. Noise is more visible on local view shown in (**D**). (**D**) Same image as (**C**), but a local view. The noise is visible, but the edges of the lines can be seen. (**E**) Image blurring has been used to decrease visible noise. (**F**) Same image as (**E**), but a local view. Lines blurred by image smoothing, and less noise is visible. The edges of the lines are harder to see as compared to those in (**D**).

structures and the findings of mediastinal disease (such as lymph nodes) is relatively low. For this reason, one would ideally want to have high contrast to see the anatomic changes in the mediastinum and a higher exposure than we need to see the lungs. Digital chest radiographs have been shown to enhance the visibility of mediastinal structures (11,20).

Special Requirements for Seeing Tubes and Devices in the Mediastinum

Especially in bedside examinations, it is of great importance to identify the location of tubes and lines within the mediastinum since a misdirected line may have serious consequences for the patient. Digital chest radiography allows one to enhance the identification of the locations of these tubes and lines using three different methods (Fig. 7A–C). The first is to increase the optical density of the image so that the mediastinum is projected in the maximum contrast density of the film or monitor one is using. The second is to black/white invert the image. The third is to use density equalization algorithms. If the film is properly exposed, any of these techniques will usually suffice. If the image is underexposed, the necessary information may not have been captured.

Digital radiography software allows one to smooth the image to make the noise that occurs in regions of low exposure less visible. This smoothing may also smooth the edges of tubes and lines making them less visible (Fig. 7C–F). For this reason, we prefer to have a somewhat noisy-appearing mediastinum on our images since that increases the chance that we will be able to identify the edges of the tubes and lines.

DIGITAL RADIOGRAPHY VS. ANALOG RADIOGRAPHY

Analog Chest Radiography

Analog chest radiography is the commonly used method of acquiring chest radiographs using an X-ray machine, a phosphorescent screen that generates light when exposed to X rays, and film that is exposed by the light generated by the screen. The film is then processed in chemicals and is viewed on a viewbox or lightbox.

Relationship of Intensity of X-Ray Exposure to Degree of Blackness on Film

In the standard form of chest radiography, the degree of blackness in each part of the film is related to the exposure of the phosphorescent screen to X-ray photons. The response of the film is determined by its characteristic curve of response, a curve that is usually S-shaped. This characteristic curve is usually divided into three parts: the bottom (or toe), the midportion, and the top (or shoulder). Exposure of the film in the midpoint results in a near-linear relationship of exposure to film blackening. Exposures in the bottom (or toe) region and the top (or shoulder) region have nonlinear responses. Most importantly, in these regions, the degree of darkening for any set amount of increase or decrease in exposure results in less change in blackening than the same exposure change in the midportion. This means that the contrast in the bottom and top of the curve is less than that in the midportion so that it becomes harder to identify small nodules and infiltrates in regions that are relatively light or dark. Since the characteristic curve differs for different types of film, the optical density in regions where lower contrast occurs vary. In general, if you need to use a bright light to see through the image to see the details, that region will be of low contrast. The bright light may correct for the darkness of the image, but does not correct the loss of contrast in the dark region.

Factors Affecting Contrast

The phosphorescent screens used in analog chest radiography vary in the amount of light they produce for each unit of X-ray exposure and in their resolution. Films vary in their contrast scale (how steep the midportion of the characteristic curve is) and in the shape of that curve. They also vary in resolution, but it is the screen rather than the film that has the greatest effect on resolution.

Contrast in analog radiography depends on the contrast inherent in the film used, in the screen used, on the kilovolt peak used to form the image, and on the methods used for film processing. One can choose a specific level of contrast for the entire image by selecting an appropriate screen-film combination and a specific set of film development parameters. One can change the contrast on a specific film by adjusting the kilovolt peak. A higher kilovolt peak range produces a lower contrast image. These traditional methods, however, affect the entire image and do not allow one to specifically alter the contrast in a specific region of the image.

Asymmetric Screen-Film Analog Methods

Special asymmetric screen-film combinations have been developed that have different characteristics on their front and back surfaces. In these special combinations, the back screen and the backside of the film emulsion have been made to provide increase blackening predominately in regions of low intrinsic exposure, such as in the mediastinum and behind the heart. These regions are enhanced by the special systems, but with lower contrast than the remainder of the image. They provide at least some of the advantages of digital optical density equalization algorithms (21).

Size of Analog Images

Depending on the analog methods used, the image can be close to life size, enlarged, or decreased in size.

Digital Methods

Digital chest radiography is a method by which a chest radiograph is obtained as or converted into computer-readable form. There are three basic forms: (1) digitization of an analog chest radiograph (sometimes called digitized radiography); (2) storage devices that capture the exposure with delayed extraction of image data, computed radiography (CR), or storage phosphor radiography are common names for one type; digital selenium radiography is a competing type; and (3) exposure capture systems that in near real-time convert the analog exposure information to digital data these are sometimes called direct radiography (DR) or direct digital radiography (DDR) systems. Each of these three methods for obtaining digital images provides generally similar advantages, but they are not equivalent.

The main advantage of digital methods is that they allow the separation and separate optimization of four different parts that are included in an analog system: acquisition of image data representing different amounts of X-ray exposure, image processing (or enhancement), image storage, and image display. Image processing and enhancement by a computer provides the main disease detection and diagnostic advantage of digital methods. Image storage and retrieval provides the main economic argument for its benefit.

Film Digitization

Film digitization was the first method applied to obtain digital chest data and still has specific indications. It is by far the cheapest in equipment costs, but because of film handling, it has the highest labor costs.

In film digitization, the film is placed in a special machine that shines light through the film. The light may be broad spectrum, narrow spectrum, or laser light. In regions of the film radiograph where the image is more transparent, more light is transmitted, and in regions where the image is more opaque (blacker areas), less light is transmitted. Because the signal-to-noise ratio varies with the amount of light transmitted, there is more noise in dark areas of the original image. In general, in chest radiography, this is not a problem if the original image was of high quality, since there should be no very dark regions of the image. If the lungs are too dark, however, information may be lost. In the areas of lung projected through the heart and diaphragm, the image is usually lightly exposed. Digitizers may not capture all of the information in these low contrast areas.

Application of Film Digitization

Film digitization provides an important economic advantage in providing teleradiology from low-volume sites. If one starts with high-quality radiographs, the transmitted images can be interpreted with accuracy similar to that for the original film. A high-quality original image is a necessity.

Chest films, once digitized, can also be used for digital storage and for use in computer-aided diagnosis systems.

Techniques to Enhance the Quality of Digitized Film Chest Radiography

Analog chest radiographs have regions of high contrast and low contrast, high optical density and low optical density. Film digitizers will produce the best digital data for teleradiology in regions of high contrast and medium optical density. The best way to achieve an optimal analog image for teleradiology is to acquire the image with a lower contrast scale than would normally be used for nonteleradiology purposes. One can do this by using a screen-film system with relatively low contrast. If one acquires relatively low-contrast data, one can use image processing to recreate a high-contrast image and can process it for both the mediastinum and lungs. If one starts with a high-contrast image, the region behind the heart and in the mediastinum may be underexposed and image processing may not provide sufficient enhancement. Film digitizers are designed to capture information from a specified range of film optical densities. If one exceeds the optimal range, the digitizer may not capture all of the information. Different digitizers have different optimal ranges. In general, less expensive digitizers have a more limited optimum range. The type of film digitizer selected should be based on the optical density of the films to be digitized.

Digital Systems That Capture the Image Data for Delayed Data Extraction: Computed Radiography and Digital Selenium Radiography

In this second type of digital chest radiography system, the X rays produce a change in the charge in a flat plate of material that can then be moved to a reader that extracts the image. Currently, most available commercial systems use special phosphor imaging plates to store the data. The X rays are encoded with information as they pass through the patients body and interact with a special phosphor material that both produces some light, but also stores an electron charge in its molecules. When this plate with stored data is exposed to a laser, the electron charges are released, producing a new flash of light that can be detected, amplified, and used to create an image. To produce the image, the laser is scanned over the imaging plate and the light emitted at each point is recorded along with its location. The initial flash of light is measured using analog methods but is then converted to digital format through a device called an analog-to-digital converter. From that point on, it is handled as digital data. Systems are available from several sources and some of these systems are called CR. Newer systems show a clear improvement in image quality compared to older systems.

The Imaging Plates Are Usually Placed in a Cassette

The advantages of this type of system are that it uses cassettes that are the same size as standard screen-film cassettes and these cassettes can be transported from many radiographic rooms to one plate reader. The use of cassettes also allows use of the system for bedside chest radiographs. Because one system can serve as the imaging plate reader for multiple rooms, this technique is, for equipment costs, the most cost-effective current method for digital chest radiography. Once the equipment is purchased, it may have a small cost advantage compared to screen-film systems in that the number of repeat films for incorrect exposure decreases. The system records a wider range of exposures than the analog screen-film systems normally used for chest radiography. It therefore provides a better set of data than digitized screen-film radiographs for image processing.

The disadvantages of this system compared to standard screen-film radiography are its equipment costs. Its disadvantage compared to "direct" digital systems is that it can have higher labor costs than direct digital systems.

There are also digital storage systems that do not use cassettes. These cassetteless systems use an imaging plate or imaging cylinder. Once this plate or cylinder is exposed, it is moved to a different position in the same device where the stored data is extracted. The cylinder system uses a thin layer of selenium on a drum to temporarily store the encoded X-ray information (12).

Data Capture Devices with Near Real-Time Analog-to-Digital Conversion: "Direct" Digital Radiography

The third general type of digital chest radiography system is designed to provide for more immediate output of the digital data. This type is designed so that the X-ray-encoded data is detected by a system into which is embedded the method for extracting the data and converting it to digital format. In this type of system, there is no need for the technologist to move a cassette from the site of acquisition to a separate image plate reader. These devices are based either on selenium or silicon. The silicon methods resemble transistors in their structure. Some use a layer of phosphor to convert the X-ray photons into light that is then detected by the device, and others directly capture the X-ray photon and then extract the stored data. These systems are composed of a tightly packed array of smaller cells. Each of these has a charge produced in it either from direct X-ray photon interaction or from the light produced by the X-ray photon interaction with a phosphor. The charge is extracted as an analog signal and then converted within the device into a digital signal by an analog-to-digital converter.

These devices provide an important advantage in that they provide digital data in near real-time. This allows the technologist to rapidly survey the image to see if it needs to be repeated. Because of this time-saving aspect for the technologist, productivity can be increased. In theory, the efficiency of the detection of X rays can be greater than that of the phosphor storage systems.

The main disadvantage of these systems is that each X-ray room must has its own detector system, thus increasing costs. Currently, these systems are not suitable for bedside examinations, but this is likely to change in the near future.

These systems are relatively new and the quality of images produced by them is still improving. Current image quality is more than satisfactory and shows substantial improvement from systems previously available.

Advantages and Disadvantages of the Various Digital Methods

Briefly, each method for digital chest radiography has advantages and disadvantages. Digitized film is the lowest costs method. It is suitable for low-volume sites. High-quality films are necessary for good-quality results. In particular, exposure factors must be carefully controlled. This method is moderately labor-intensive. The resulting imaging quality can be good to very good.

The image storage systems are of intermediate cost and are suitable for moderate to high volume. It can accept images obtained under less optimal conditions and is therefore very well suited for bedside chest radiography. It provides images of very high quality when used for either in-department or bedside examinations. There is a low– to moderate-improvement in technologist productivity compared to standard screen-film chest radiography.

Near-real-time digital radiography systems ("direct" digital radiography) require that the image recording system is duplicated for each room in which it is used. It is therefore of higher initial cost if several rooms are to be equipped. It provides a greater improvement in technologist productivity that may in some settings justify its cost. It is not currently suitable for bedside chest radiography, but likely will be in the future. Images are of very high quality.

Special Methods of Image Acquisition Using Digital Systems: Dual-Energy Methods

Digital techniques make it possible to obtain two separate images with different energy spectra. Calcium shows more of a decrease in X-ray photon absorption than water as the energy of the X-ray photons increases. Because of this difference, if one obtains radiographs with two different X-ray photon energy spectra, it is possible to produce a bone-emphasis or a soft-tissue-emphasis image. Digital acquisition, because of the linear response of the data to X-ray exposure, makes it easier to create these emphasis images. Devices have been built for the storage phosphor systems and for the near-real-time digital systems. These images have their main advantage in the apices where the lungs are extensively covered by bone, but also have advantages elsewhere by removing the clutter of the ribs and thereby improving the conspicuity of lung lesions. Dual-energy methods are further discussed and examples are shown below.

X-Ray System Effects on Acquired Data

The X-ray system used to produce the X-ray photons for chest radiographs has a major effect on the quality of the resulting analog or digital chest radiograph. Three effects are of greatest importance: kilovolt peak, penumbra based on focal spot size, and patient motion (related to exposure time). Because image processing can make images look better, one could be misled to think that these postprocessing methods of contrast and edge enhancement available on digital images can correct for technical flaws in image acquisition. Image processing only partially corrects for image acquisition errors; thus, high-quality X-ray technique remains very important.

Kilovoltage Peak

In analog systems, high-kilovolt-peak technique is often used to decrease the conspicuity of the ribs based on the relatively lower absorption of X-ray photons by calcium at high compared to low photon energies. For digital chest radiography with storage phosphor methods, lower kilovolt peaks are often recommended since these enhance the absorption of X-ray photons by the imaging plate. One can then reduce the conspicuity of the ribs by image processing. Unfortunately, this method can also decrease the contrast of lung disease and normal lung structures. For this reason, I have chosen to use 125 kVp for my chest radiographs. Three-phase systems produce a better energy spectrum for chest radiography. There does not appear to be a diagnostic accuracy study such as a receiver operating characteristic (ROC) study to determine the benefit of a higher versus a lower kilovolt peak for digital radiographs.

X-Ray Focal Spot

The X-ray focal spot size and patient motion are the main factors in image blurring. To detect disease, the sharpest image is desired. The focal spot size affects the penumbra along the margins of lung structures. A larger focal spot size will decrease the edge sharpness of lung objects. When these objects are thin interstitial lines, these lines will become less distinct. Digital image processing using edge enhancement methods will restore some of this edge sharpness, but high-quality initial acquisition is more important. For both analog and digital images, one should use the smallest focal spot size that provides sufficient output for a properly exposed image. A maximum focal spot size of 1.2 mm is preferred (22).

Stopping Patient Motion

The second major effect resulting in edge blurring is patient motion. Not all patients can completely stop lung motion when asked to take in a deep breath and hold it. Vessel pulsation is always present and some patients have slight tremors or unsteadiness. The shorter the exposure time, the less likely these factors are to have an effect on the image. For this reason, one should use the highest kilovolt peak, highest milliamperage (mA), and shortest time (s) possible for both analog and digital chest radiography systems. In an individual patient who has difficulty holding very still, the best radiograph may result from the use of a larger focal spot with a shorter exposure rather than from the use of the smallest available focal spot.

X-Ray Exposure

One of the great advantages of digital chest radiography is the ability to correct for underexposure and overexposure through digital image processing. The digital receptors have a wider range of acceptable exposure than the screen-film systems used for chest radiography. Importantly, this factor allows them to accommodate variations in exposure to a greater degree than conventional systems. This accommodation, image processing to correct the optical density of the final image, is acceptable for a single image, but careful control of exposure is still important since image processing may not restore the full information content of an underexposed image or, conversely, systematically overexposed images will result in patients receiving higher than necessary X-ray exposures.

The Risk from Overexposure

Overexposure on a digital chest radiograph contains three potential problems. First, the patient is not receiving a dose meeting the "as low as reasonably achievable (ALARA)" recommendation. Second, at sufficiently high exposures, the digital detectors become nonlinear and image quality deteriorates. Third, digital imaging systems are very sensitive to low exposures of radiation. Scatter and backscatter increase as exposure increases. This scattering may produce detectable artifactual images from the back of the cassette or from the back of the digital detector with high exposures. Scatter and backscatter on a collimated image may be sufficiently intense to confuse the part of the computer algorithm that determines the edge of the collimated field. This can result in the computer algorithm overestimating image size, underestimating exposure, and thereby adjusting the image to one in which the lungs are too dark. When using screen-film systems, technologists adjust their exposure settings according to the blackening seen on the resulting films. In digital radiography, the digital system adjusts the resulting image to correct for under- and overexposure. This could result in a risk of systematic overexposure. We have not found this to happen in our facility, but intermittent monitoring of this parameter is recommended (23).

The Decrease in Image Quality from Underexposure

Underexposure increases the noise in the image by decreasing the signal. The digital system provides image processing with smoothing parameters to make the noise less visible. It does this by decreasing the high-spatial-frequency component of the image in regions with low exposure. The problem with this method is that the edges of catheters are of high-spatial frequency and this image smoothing may cause them to have low conspicuity or even disappear. When there are very high levels of noise, the noise may start to resemble high-spatial-frequency information in the lungs, either concealing fine interstitial disease or causing the radiologist to report interstitial disease when it is not present.

The Proper Exposure for Digital Systems

The proper level for digital chest radiographic exposures has been established by testing for the Fuji CR® FCR 9000 system (Fuji Photo Film Corp., Tokyo, Japan) to be in the range of a 200- to 400-speed screen-film radiographic system. At lower exposure levels, noise in the mediastinum can obscure the edges of catheters. Systems with improved X-ray photon capture including newer Fuji systems may be usable at lower exposures, but the appropriate exposure range would have to be established for each of these systems through observational or experimental clinical trials.

Automatic Exposure Control and Digital Chest Radiography Systems

The storage phosphor digital systems rely on the Automatic Exposure Control (AEC) device built into the chest cassette holder. Some cassettes used for digital radiography are lead backed. This can result in an increase in patient exposure compared to a standard screen-film system because the lead will absorb some of the radiation so that the AEC senses less of the exposure that the patient received and does not stop the exposure at the same low level used for conventional screen-film radiographs. When changing to a storage phosphor digital system, the exposure levels used should be checked. On the Fuji system, the average "s" number for each technologist should be in the 200–400 range. If it is outside of this range and an AEC device is used, then the AEC device needs to be reset. Intermittent monitoring of technologists as they use the system is recommended to avoid exposure drift. A method for this has been proposed (23).

For the near-real-time systems, it is possible for the system to monitor online the exposure reaching each cell and to stop exposure once a certain minimum exposure has reached each cell or once an average preset exposure has been reached. Thus, a near-real-time digital detector can serve as its own AEC device. In theory, the near-real-time devices could be designed to select exposure measurements from any group of cells, potentially enhancing the image quality by better compensating for unusual patient anatomy or extensive disease affecting only one lung (like a severe unilateral pneumonia).

IMAGE PROCESSING

Image processing is the computer manipulation of digital image data done with the goal of enhancing image quality. Sometimes the image processing is done to enhance the attractiveness of the image, sometimes it is done to enhance disease conspicuity, and sometimes both attractiveness and improved conspicuity result at the same time. Image processing is discussed in three different parts: standard commercial methods, special commercial methods, and experimental methods that may potentially provide additional benefits.

Currently Available Commercial Image-Processing Methods

Currently available image-processing methods produce six different effects on image appearance. They define the "window of clinically useful exposure data," they affect the degree of image blackness and image contrast, they equalize image blackness in different parts of the image, and they provide edge enhancement or provide blurring of noise in parts of the image. The steps described below have been written in a logical progression, but may or may not be actually carried out in this way or in this sequence. More detail on these methods is available (24–26).

Defining the "Window of Clinically Useful Exposure Data"

Digital acquisition systems are designed to record data from a wide range of X-ray exposures in a relatively linear relationship of exposure to pixel value. This wide range of recorded exposure is desirable because it can correct for X-ray exposure errors and for patients with different body builds. If one used this "raw" data to create the images, they would be of very low contrast. By design, the width of the window of pixel values set for accepting this information is set very wide.

The raw data that has been received by the imaging device contains both useful and non-useful exposure data. Non-useful data, for example, include the exposure that occurs from X-ray photons that passed through the area outside of the patient and areas outside of the collimated field. Because the imaging device received unimportant exposure data, the digital data will contain unimportant exposure data. To cope with this, the first step in image processing is to define what data is likely to represent the data encoded as the X-ray photons pass through the body.

At least two different methods are involved in this analysis. One defines the edge of the collimated field and excludes the data outside of the collimated field from further analysis. Different companies use different proprietary methods for this purpose and these methods are moderately effective.

The second method uses information from the exposure histogram. The exposure histogram is a map of the different intensity values of the picture elements (pixels) that form the image. The algorithm selects those pixel values from the exposure histogram that are likely to contain clinically relevant information. For this step, the computer uses a search algorithm that is seeking the region of the remaining data that looks like chest radiograph data; one can think of this as a search for the shape within the exposure histogram that matches the shape of a chest radiograph histogram. The data for different parts of the body are different. The algorithm has been set to look for the data patterns seen in different body parts and the different common variations that are seen for each body part. Once the algorithm identifies the appropriate shape, it then uses this to define the upper and lower boundaries of exposure data to be included in the formation of the image. This subset of the original data is then used to direct the next steps in image processing.

Poorly processed digital chest images usually result from problems occurring at these stages of the process. The most common causes are a failure to instruct the digital system as to the type of image to be processed or excessive scatter outside the edge of the collimated field. The digital system has to be told that the data set it is looking for is a chest radiograph. If it is told that a different part of the body is being imaged, it will look for data that looks like that body part and process the image data incorrectly. If there is a lot of scatter in the area outside the collimated field, it may not correctly define the edge of that field and may incorporate the scattered exposure into its defined exposure boundary. This is one of the reasons why it is important to avoid overexposure. On an overexposed image, the algorithm is more likely to include data that is due to scatter and is therefore not in the clinically relevant region of exposure.

Adjusting the Data for Differences in Exposure: The Fuji "S" Number, the Initial Adjustment for Display Optical Density

The method used by the system to define the "clinically relevant data" does not depend on the exposure used to obtain the original data set. In order to display the "clinically relevant data" as an image with proper display optical density or luminance, the system must correct for exposure differences. It does this by comparing the pixel values for the "clinically relevant data" to a stored expected range of pixel values. It then adjusts the "clinically relevant data" to lie within the range for proper display. The degree of adjustment is related to a number called "S." If the extracted "clinically relevant data" is underexposed compared to the range of pixel values for display, the "clinically relevant data" will be adjusted so that it falls within the display range by amplifying each pixel value. If it is overexposed, then the computer program will decrease each pixel value. The Fuji system was designed so that an "S" value of 200 corresponds to the correct level for display of the image. The "S" value is not the speed of the system. The "speed" of an analog system is defined as the exposure level required for a specific degree of film optical density. In the digital systems, the optical density of the display is not determined by the exposure of the digital receptor. There is no way to equate the speed of a screen-film system to the proper exposure for a digital system. An "S" of 200 may have originally been based on the exposure required for a 200-speed screen-film system, but as the Fuji systems evolved, the imaging plates have become more sensitive to X-ray photons while the "S" number system has remained the same.

Final Adjustment for Image Mean Optical Density

The "S" number adjustment will usually place the image data set close to the range for proper display. There is, however, some variability in laser printers and in soft-copy display devices, so the system makes it possible to adjust the final optical density or luminance and then store this change so it can be used for subsequent radiographs. In the Fuji system, this factor is called the GS factor.

Adjustment for Display Contrast

In the process of selecting the "clinically relevant data," the computer program selected the highest and lowest pixel values of this data. This constitutes an initial estimate of the contrast range for the final image. It does not define the shape of the contrast curve or the steepness of its midportion. The final adjustment is made by use of a conversion method called a look-up table. In this method, there is either a stored table or a stored formula that says for a data pixel value of "x," use a value of "y" for the display. The companies recommend specific look-up tables for specific parts of the body. The radiologist can accept the companies recommendations or choose different

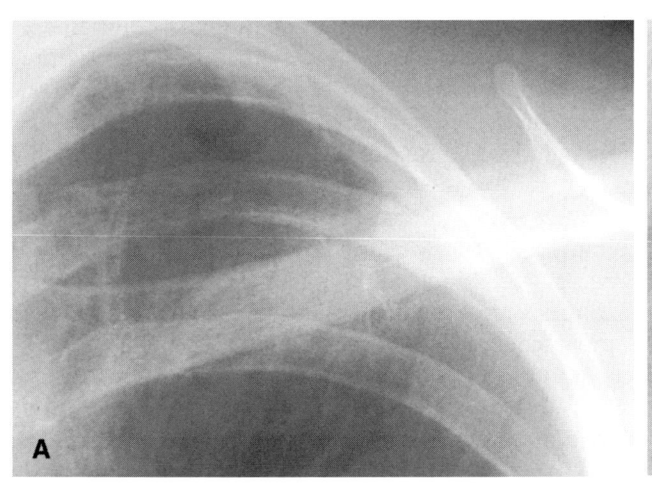

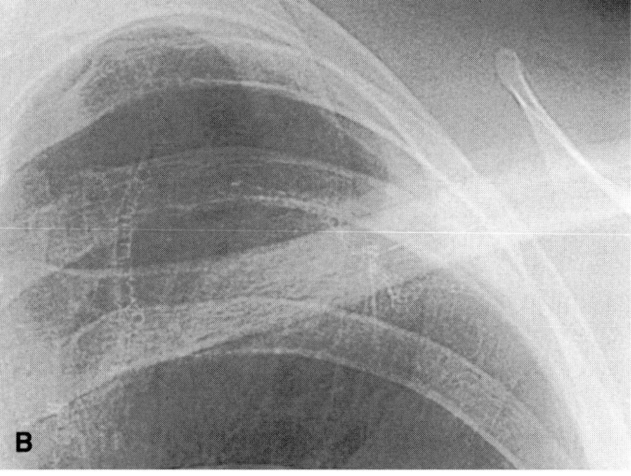

Figure 8 Improved visibility of pneumothorax using edge enhancement in a patient status postsurgery for recurrent spontaneous pneumothoraces. The surgical clips and the small residual pneumothorax are more conspicuous in (**B**) with mild edge enhancement than in (**A**) with no edge enhancement.

look-up tables. Once chosen, this selection can be stored in the computer memory so that the same look-up table can be consistently chosen. In the Fuji system, this factor is called the GT factor.

Once this overall look-up table has been selected, one can accept the companys default contrast setting or one can adjust the slope of the midportion of the characteristic curve. This factor is called the GA factor in the Fuji system. The higher the GA, the steeper the slope of the midportion of the characteristic curve is, and the less steep the bottom and top of the characteristic curve.

High-Spatial-Frequency Enhancement: Edge Enhancement

Mathematically, all images can be transformed (using the Fourier transform) into groups of sine and cosine waves. The waves are of different frequencies and it is therefore possible to describe images as having different spatial frequencies. All images are composed of parts with different spatial frequencies. High-spatial frequencies are seen where there are sharp edges; lower spatial frequencies are seen where there are blurred or unsharp edges. Filtering methods exist to enhance or diminish the intensity of specific groups of spatial frequencies in an image. By enhancing high-spatial frequencies in an image, sharp edges are enhanced and appear sharper, but since image noise is also of high-spatial frequency, it is also enhanced. If high-spatial frequencies are filtered from the image, then the edges of sharply defined objects and visible noise are decreased.

Edge enhancement is an important part of the image processing of digital chest radiographs. The edges of all objects in standard chest radiographs are somewhat blurred because of the penumbra caused by the X-ray tube focal spot size and often by slight patient motion and cardiac pulsation. Slight edge enhancement restores these edges toward the appearance they would have in a specimen radiograph with a very small focal spot X-ray tube. It enhances the conspicuity of blood vessels, interstitial markings, surgical staples, and pneumothoraces (Fig. 4. 8). This method also enhances the edges of catheters, making them easier to see. It is normally included as part of the recommendation for image-processing settings for film display. Some soft-copy display systems, however, do not provide the capabilities for edge enhancement and diagnostic accuracy in these systems may be less (27).

High-Spatial-Frequency Blurring: Noise Blurring

High-spatial-frequency blurring can be used to decrease the visibility of noise in digital images. Because noise from quantum mottle makes some digital images appear grainy, image-processing methods were provided so that the images would look smoother, more like screen-film images. If such processing were applied to the entire image, then fine interstitial lines would also blur and be more difficult to detect. For this reason, some programs apply the image blurring only to areas of relatively low pixel values (more transparent regions of the original image). These low pixel value areas are those with the least X-ray exposure and therefore the most noise. The use of these noise concealing programs unfortunately also blurs the edges of high-frequency structures, such as catheters in the mediastinum (Fig. 7D and F).

Optical Density Equalization: Methods to Bring the Entire Image to an Optical Density Where High-Contrast Display Is Possible

The range of optical densities on a chest radiograph is quite wide. This is the result of the differing proportions of water, calcium, and air in the path of the X-ray photons in different parts of the image. Because of this wide range of densities, all chest images represent a compromise: To have the lungs at a proper display density, the mediastinum is too light. If one wants to see tubes in the esophagus behind the heart, then one can increase the exposure, but the lungs become too dark. Optical density equalization image processing is used to partially correct for these density differences. Current methods are moderately good, but in the future, newer methods will probably be better.

The fundamental concept underlying methods for optical density equalization is that one can separate an image into components of different spatial frequencies. High-spatial frequencies show the edges of objects, medium-spatial frequencies demonstrate the shape of moderate-sized structures, and low-spatial frequencies tend to show broad effects across an image. It is the low-spatial-frequency information that is modified in optical density equalization. While different methods are used by different companies, in concept, if one takes the low-spatial-frequency image and changes areas that are black to white (and vice versa) and then partially adds it back into the original image, then larger areas of density differences will be decreased in their intensity and the whole image will show a lower range of optical densities. The resulting image will show a lower range of optical densities across the image allowing one to then enhance the contrast across the entire image. Image details become more conspicuous when contrast is enhanced. This method is very helpful for enhancing interpretation of bedside chest radiographs. It has the disadvantage that large areas of lung consolidation or large pleural effusions will also be affected by the processing, making them less intensely white. Sometimes faint but larger areas of airspace disease will be less conspicuous on these images. Also, the area over the liver sometimes looks more radiolucent and could appear similar to the radiolucency that can occur on supine films with free abdominal air.

Computer-Aided Detection and Diagnosis

Once the chest radiograph has been converted into a computer-readable form, the computer can be used to search for signs of specific diseases. There are two different types of approach: computer programs to help radiologists find abnormalities and computer programs to help radiologists arrive at the correct diagnosis of an abnormality. Experimentally, computer-aided detection methods for the chest radiograph have been used to identify lung nodules, interstitial disease, and cardiomegaly (28–36). Currently, there is one commercial system designed to help radiologists detect small pulmonary nodules (37). When using this system, radiologists showed an average increase in cancer detection of 11% for primary non–small cell lung cancers (NSCLCs) 9–27 mm in diameter. The radiologists did less well in detecting the smaller nodules without computer assistance. With the computer, radiologists showed a 21% improvement in the detection of NSCLCs 9–14.5 mm in diameter (37–40). (The author of this chapter receives sponsored program support from Riverain Medical Group, Miamisburg, Ohio, U.S.A. They manufacture the commercial computer-aided detection system for lung nodules on chest radiographs.)

Commercial computer systems that can help to detect other diseases and that help diagnosis radiographic findings are under development and should be available in the next few years (41).

Energy-Subtraction Imaging

Energy-subtraction imaging (also called dual-energy subtraction imaging) is based on the kilovolt dependence of absorption of calcium and water. At lower kilovolt levels, calcium absorbs or scatters moderately more X-ray photons than water. At higher kilovolt levels, the absorption levels are more similar. By obtaining a chest radiograph at two different energy spectra, one can process the images to create a bone-emphasis and a soft-tissue-emphasis image. This acquisition can be done either using one exposure where two imaging plates are exposed, but with a layer of copper or other absorber between them so that the energy spectra are different, or by taking two exposures one right after the other at different kilovolt peak settings. The images must then be closely matched so that the chest is exactly the same size and position. This is done by a process called warping, where one image is distorted (warped) to be the same size and shape as the other. Subsequently, the images are registered (matched in position) as closely as possible. They can then be processed through a complex series of steps that eventually yield the bone-emphasis and soft-tissue-emphasis images (Fig. 9 to Fig. 11). With the current commercial systems, slight image blurring occurs in this process, so that the finest interstitial lines may be less conspicuous. Several studies have shown that lung nodules become more difficult to detect when they are projected over bone structures (4,42,43). When radiologists review the soft tissue images obtained with energy subtraction, these small nodules become more conspicuous and more are detected (44–46).

AMBER System

The AMBER system is a special type of digital chest radiographic system that scans the chest adjusting the intensity of the X-ray beam according to how much radiation has penetrated the chest. It continually adjusts the amount of exposure so that more radiation

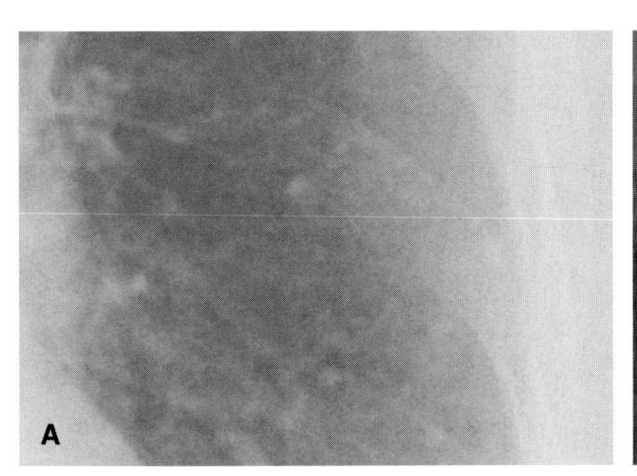

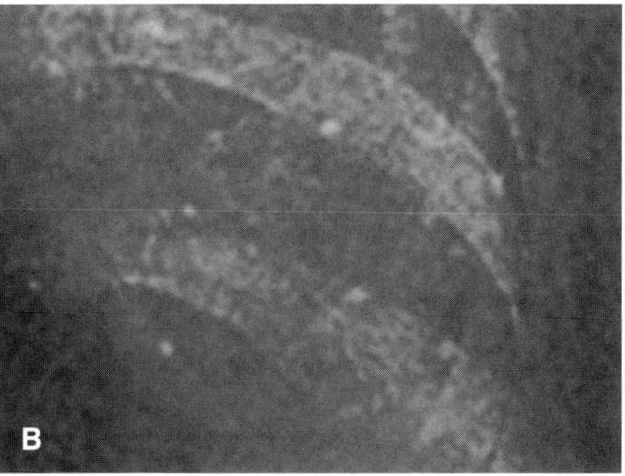

Figure 9 Energy subtraction used to confirm calcification in nodules. (**A**) Digital chest image with standard processing shows several small lung nodules. (**B**) The calcium emphasis image is shown and the small nodules (now appearing white) can be seen to contain calcium.

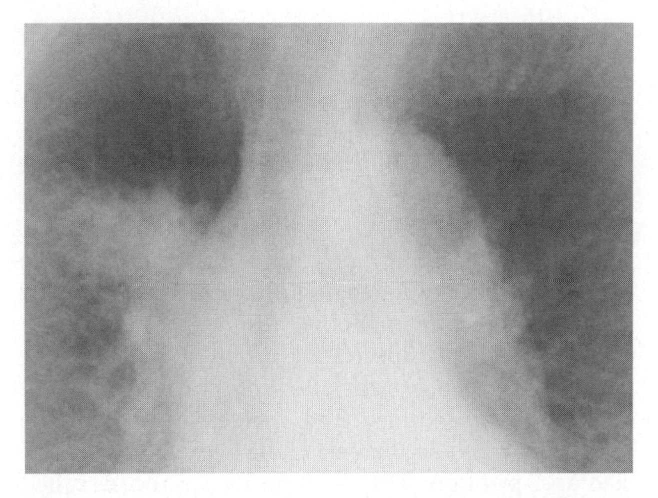

Figure 10 Energy subtraction used to enhance visibility of a central mass. A squamous-cell lung cancer involving the right upper hilum is seen. The energy subtraction processing has greatly decreased the visibility of the ribs and enhanced the conspicuity of the mass.

is applied where there is more absorption (as in the mediastinum) and less over the lungs. It produces very high-quality images.

IMAGE PROCESSING: FUTURE METHODS

Future developments in the image processing of digital chest radiographs are likely. While the following section cannot be complete, it describes several approaches that appear promising.

Image Segmentation for Anatomic Definition of Processing Parameters

Segmentation of an image is the process whereby an image is divided into separate regions, either by hand or computer, based on some identified difference between them. In the chest, work is underway to segment the mediastinum, rib boundary of the lungs, and the lungs themselves (47–49). Once these areas are segmented, different image-processing techniques could be applied to these different regions (Fig. 12). The segmented areas could be adjusted to have different black/white scales, different degrees of edge enhancement, and/or different contrast scales.

Sequential Subtraction: Change Detection

Computer programs are under development to enhance the detection of changes from one film to the next as a method to aid radiologists in their detection of disease (50–54). The processes involved include warping, registration, and subtraction. Because most nonobvious disease occupies only a small portion of the chest, the algorithms, which function on the whole chest, can warp one image to match the other in spatial dimensions, register them, and subtract them, enhancing only the area that showed local change (Fig. 13). A commercial system has been introduced into Japan, but not yet in the United States.

Disease-Specific Algorithms

A disease-specific algorithm is a preselected method for image processing that is optimized to identify a specific disease. An example would be that if one knows that a patient is at risk for a pneumothorax, one could have the computer enhance the image so that any pneumothorax would become more conspicuous. While disease-specific image-processing settings do not yet exist, situation-specific image-processing algorithms are commonly used. The clearest example is the use of histogram equalization to enhance the visibility of tubes and lines within the mediastinum and upper

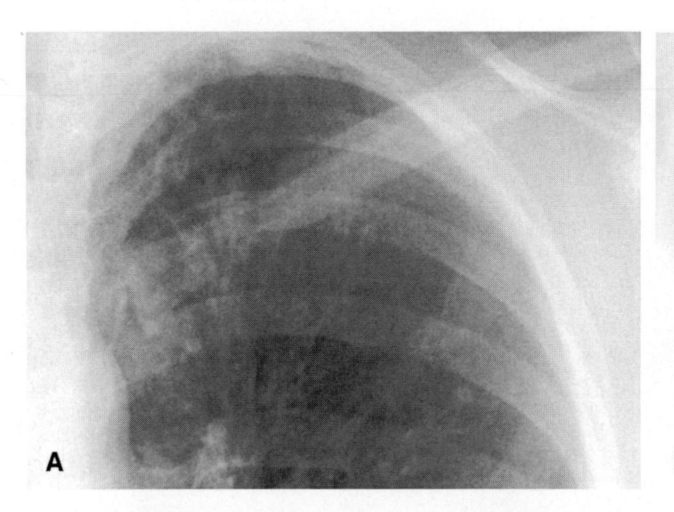

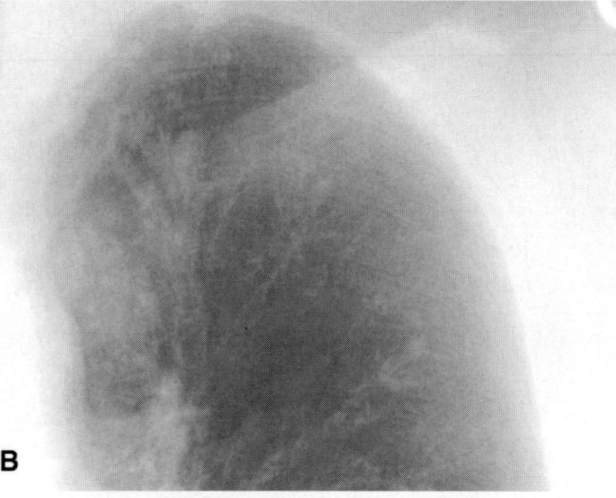

Figure 11 Energy subtraction used to enhance visibility of airways disease. Digital chest radiographs with (**A**) standard and (**B**) soft-tissue-emphasis energy-subtraction processing in a patient with mucus plugs and bronchiectasis from cystic fibrosis. The soft-tissue-emphasis image largely eliminates the conspicuity of the ribs. The lung disease is more conspicuous.

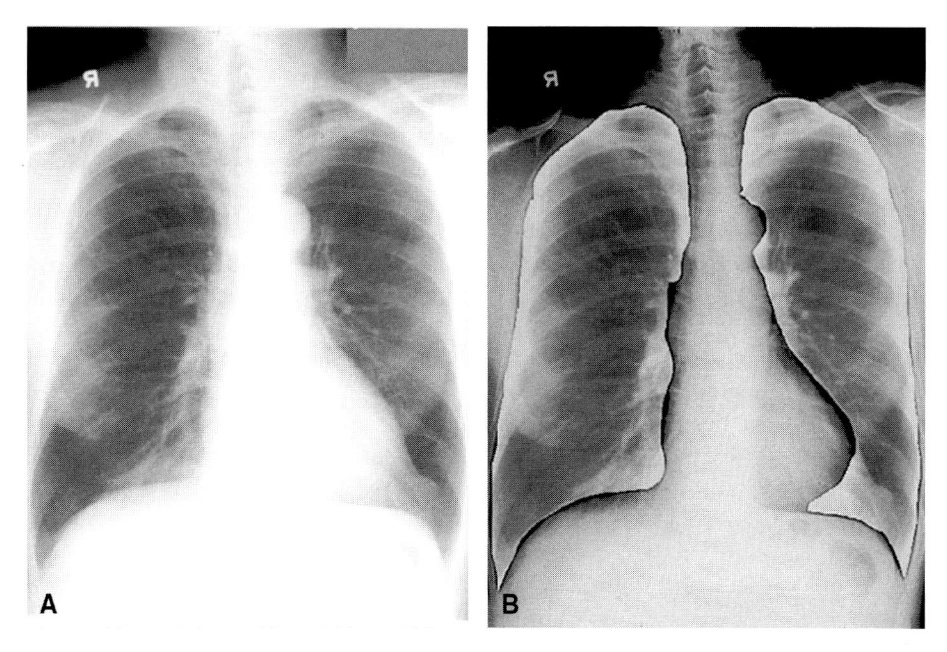

Figure 12 Segmentation for anatomy-based image processing. In this study, a normal screen-film chest radiograph has been digitized (**A**). It has then been processed so that the lungs are segmented from the image for organ-specific image processing (**B**). By doing this, the processing for the mediastinum and the lungs can be different. In this case, the mediastinum and upper abdomen were processed to have a greater optical density and more edge enhancement than the lungs. The retrocardiac region (particularly the vessels), chest wall, and abdomen have been enhanced. *Source*: Courtesy of Lo SCB and Zhao H, Georgetown University Medical Center.

abdomen. The settings used to enhance this visibility, but with some probable loss of information for subtle disease in the lungs. In the past, optimization methods have emphasized the desire to find image-processing settings that maximize the value of the chest radiograph for all diseases based on both how common the diseases are and their importance to the patient. In the future, it will be possible to have a system in which each chest radiograph goes through several different image-processing methods, each optimized for detection of a specific group of diseases. It has been proposed that one would use the input of clinical information to decide which image-processing method should be applied to each film. There is an inherent risk in this method in that if one only looks for what is expected, then one may fail to detect an unsuspected disease until it is more severe. Thus, I think that more than one image-processing method should be used on all images rather than a single method tailored to look for a specific diagnosis. In the future, computer-detected disease patterns are likely to be used to adjust the image processing or display parameters so that the detected disease is emphasized. The research goal is to have the computer adjust the image so that the radiologist is unlikely to miss the disease rather than have the computer place an arrow on the image directing the radiologists attention to a specific location.

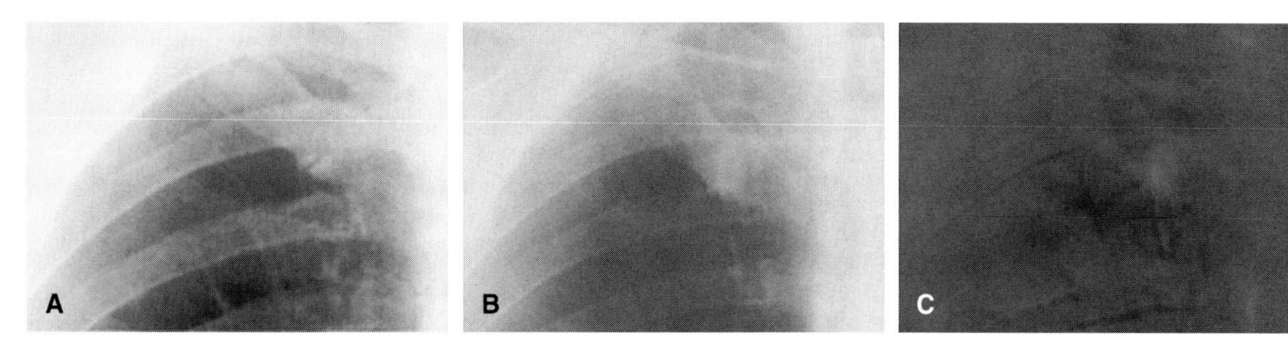

Figure 13 Sequential subtraction used to aid detection of lung nodule. (**A**) The lung apex 1 year before (**B**) was taken. (**B**) The lung apex on current image. (**C**) The subtraction image obtained after the images have been warped and registered. This subtraction image shows (as a white region) a change between the two films, which represented a small non–small cell lung cancer projected over the first-rib calcified cartilage. *Source*: Courtesy of Lo SCB and Zhao H, Georgetown University Medical Center.

Tomosynthesis

Tomosynthesis is a highly promising method in which multiple images are obtained of the chest at slightly differing angles of the X-ray tube. Using digital methods, tomosynthesis produces images similar to the type of conventional tomography used many years ago. Both methods produce a series of image layers through the chest that largely eliminate the shadows from adjacent layers. The advantage of digital tomosynthesis is that these multiple image layers are produced rapidly (in a few seconds) and at a radiation dose substantially less than used for conventional tomography (55,56). This method requires special equipment, but appears capable of aiding in the detection of lung disease.

DISPLAY METHODS

Printed On Film Vs. Soft-Copy Display

Digital chest radiographs can be viewed either by printing them on film or by viewing them on a computer screen. With current technology, there is no firm evidence that one method of viewing provides greater accuracy than the other. Display on film is a more mature technology and only limited technical improvements that would affect diagnostic quality are foreseen. Computer screen (or monitor) display is a moderately mature technology, but one where technical innovation is more likely. If the changes in computer screen display are favorable to the display of chest radiographs, then this method of display may eventually surpass that of the display on film. Some of the advantages that could make soft-copy display the diagnostically superior method are the ability to rapidly switch between image-processing settings, the incorporation of computer-aided detection and diagnosis, temporal subtraction of sequential images, and the ability to label an image that will be incorporated into the report to the patients treating physician. The optimum report in the future is likely to consist of annotations on an image with a final impression rather than the word-based descriptions currently used.

Image Size and Viewing Distance

Digital chest radiographs can be printed life-size or at a decreased size. Studies have shown that diagnostic accuracy on two-thirds size images is equivalent to screen-film chest images (5,9,57). One study showed no problems at 56% of life-size with a selenium detector system (58). On the other hand, half-size images have been reported to limit disease detection (59,60). When smaller images are used, the radiologist viewing them should be closer to see the fine detail. If one normally views a standard chest radiograph at 3 ft., the two-thirds-sized image should be viewed at 1.5–2 ft, for example.

SUMMARY

Digital chest radiography is a rapidly evolving method for imaging the chest. In its current form, it has been shown to be diagnostically equivalent to conventional chest radiography. Since analog screen-film chest radiography is technologically mature and digital chest radiography is still in a process of moderate innovation, it is likely that the diagnostic quality of digital chest radiography will, in the future, be superior to that of conventional chest radiography, replacing it for many uses. Digital chest radiographs can be produced by three competing methods: film digitization, systems that store the energy of the encoded X-ray photons for later extraction, and near-real-time systems for extracting the encoded X-ray information. For each of these methods, there are trade-offs in labor versus machine costs. To date, there is no evidence that any one method is diagnostically superior to the other, although digitized film requires that the original film be of high quality to achieve a high-quality digitized image. The two other types of digital acquisition are more robust to exposure differences. Once in digital form, image processing provides important advantages in correcting and improving disease conspicuity. Digital images are the input data for computer-aided detection systems. They allow digital storage, transmission, retrieval, and soft-copy display. Newer methods of image acquisition and image processing are quite promising. Dual-energy imaging, temporal subtraction imaging, and tomosynthesis each provide methods for removing the shadows of the ribs that can obscure lung disease. Further improvements in digital chest radiography are to be expected.

REFERENCES

1 Schaefer CM, Greene RE, Oestmann JW, et al. Improved control of image optical density with low-dose digital and conventional radiography in bedside imaging. Radiology 1989; 173:713–6.
2 Freedman M, Lo SCB, Nelson MC, Pe E, Mun SK. Comparative test of two storage phosphor plate imaging systems: the Agfa ADC and the Fuji AC-1+. In: Brody W, Johnston G, eds. Computer Applications to Assist Radiology. Carlsbad, CA: SCAR 92, Symposia Foundation, 1992.
3 International Labor Organization. Guidelines for the Use of the International Classification of Radiographs of Pneumoconiosis. Geneva: International Labor Organization, 1992.
4 Austin JHM, Romney BM, Goldsmith LS. Missed bronchogenic carcinoma: radiographic findings in 27 patients with a potentially respectable lesion evident in retrospect. Radiology 1992; 182:115–22.
5 MacMahon H, Sanada S, Doi K, et al. Direct comparison of conventional and computed radiography

with a dual-image recording technique. Radiographics 1991; 11:259–68.
6 Marglin SI, Rowberg AH, Godwin JD. Preliminary experience with portable digital imaging for intensive care radiography. J Thorac Imag 1990; 5:49–54.
7 Kehler M, Albrechtsson U, Andresdottier A, Larusdotti H, Lundin A. Accuracy of digital radiography using stimulable phosphor for diagnosis of pneumothorax. Acta Radiol 1990; 31:47–52.
8 Schaefer CM, Green RE, Oestmann JW, et al. Digital storage phosphor imaging versus conventional film radiography in CT-documented chest disease. Radiology 1990; 174:207–10.
9 Kehler M, Albrechtsson U, Andersson B, Larusdotti H, Lundin A, Pettersson H. Assessment of digital chest radiography using stimulable phosphor. Acta Radiol 1989; 30:581–6.
10 Schaefer CM, GreeneRE, Llewellyn HJ, et al. Interstitial lung disease: impact of postprocessing in digital storage phosphor imaging. Radiology 1991; 178:733–8.
11 Schaefer CM, GreeneRE, Hall DA, et al. Mediastinal abnormalities: detection with storage phosphor digital radiography. Radiology 1991; 178:169–73.
12 Woodard PK, SloneRM, Sagel SS, et al. Detection of CT-proved pulmonary nodules: comparison of selenium-based digital and conventional screen-film chest radiographs. Radiology 1998; 209:705–9.
13 van Heesewijk HP, van der Graaf Y, de Valois JC, et al. Chest imaging with a selenium detector versus conventional film radiography: a CT-controlled study. Radiology 1996; 200:687–90.
14 Muller RD, Von Koschitzki T, Hirche H, et al. Frequency-filtered image post-processing of digital luminescence radiographs in pulmonary nodule imaging. Clin Radiol 1996; 51:577–86.
15 Woodard PK, SloneRM, Sagel SS, et al. Detection of CT-proved pulmonary nodules: comparison of selenium-based digital and conventional screen-film chest radiographs. Radiology 1998; 209:705–9.
16 Krupinski EA, EvanoffM, Ovitt T, Standen JR, Chu TX, Johnson J. Influence of image processing on chest radiograph interpretation and decision changes. Acad Radiol 1998; 5:79–85.
17 Yang ZG, SoneS, Li F, et al. Detection of small peripheral lung cancer by digital chest radiography. Performance of unprocessed versus unsharp mask-processed images. Acta Radiol 1999; 40:505–9.
18 Awai K, KomiM, Hori S. Selenium-based digital radiography versus high-resolution storage phosphor radiography in the detection of solitary pulmonary nodules without calcification: receiver operating characteristic curve analysis. AJR Am J Roentgenol 2001; 177:1141–4.
19 Kim JH, ImJG, Han MC, Min BG, Lee CW. Improved visualization of simulated nodules by adaptive enhancement of digital chest radiography. Acad Radiol 1994; 1:93–9.
20 Garmer M, HennigsSP, Jager HJ, et al. Digital radiography versus conventional radiography in chest imaging: diagnostic performance of a large-area silicon flat-panel detector in a clinical CT-controlled study. Am J Roentgenol 2000; 174:75–80.
21 Muller RD, WahlingS, Hirche H, et al. ROC analysis of detection performance by analogue and digital plain film systems in chest radiography. Acta Radiol 1996; 37:847–54.
22 American College of Radiology. Standards 1999–2000. Reston VA: American College of Radiology, 2000.
23 Freedman MT, PeEV, Mun SK, Lo SCB, Nelson MC. Potential for unnecessary patient exposure from the use of storage phosphor imaging systems. SPIE Med Imag 1993; 1897:472–9.
24 Freedman MT, MunSK, Pe EV, Lo SCB, Nelson MC. Image optimization procedures for the Fuji AC-1. SPIE Med Imag 1993; 1897:480–502.
25 Freedman M, Artz DS. Image processing in digital radiography. Semin Roentgenol 1997; 32:25–37.
26 Freedman M, Artz DS. Digital radiography of the chest. Semin Roentgenol 1997; 32:38–44.
27 Kosuda S, KajiT, Kobayashi H, Watanabe M, Iwasaki Y, Kusano S. Hard-copy versus soft-copy with and without simple image manipulation for detection of pulmonary nodules and masses. Acta Radiol 2000; 41:420–4.
28 Xu XW, DoiK, Kobayashi T, et al. Development of an improved CAD scheme for automated detection of lung nodules in digital chest images. Med Phys 1997; 24:1395–403.
29 MacMahon H, EngelmannR, Behlen FM, et al. Computer-aided diagnosis of pulmonary nodules: results of a large-scale observer test. Radiology 1999; 213:723–6.
30 Lo SCB, FreedmanMT, Lin JS, Mun SK. Automatic lung nodule detection using profile matching and back-propagation neural network techniques. J Digit Imag 1993; 6:48–54.
31 Lo SCB, ChanHP, Lin JS, Li H, Freedman M, Mun SK. Artificial convolutional neural network for lung nodule detection. IEEE Trans Med Imag 1995; 14:711–8.
32 Lin JS, LoSCB, Hasegawa A, Freedman M, Mun SK. Reduction of false positives in lung nodule detection using a two-level neural classification. IEEE Trans Med Imag 1996; 15:206–17.
33 Lin JS, HasegawaA, Freedman M, Mun SK. Differentiation between nodules and end-on vessels using a convolutional neural network architecture. J Digit Imag 1995; 8:132–41.
34 Katsuragawa S, DoiK, MacMahon H. Image feature analysis and computer-aided diagnosis in digital radiography: classification of normal and abnormal lungs with interstitial disease in chest images. Med Phys 1989; 16:38–44.
35 Doi K, GigerML, MacMahon H, et al. Computer-aided diagnosis: development of automated schemes for quantitative analysis of radiographic images. Semin Ultrasound CT MR 1992; 13:140–52.
36 Kobayashi T, XuXW, MacMahon H, Metz CE, Doi K. Effect of a computer-aided diagnosis scheme on radiologists performance in detection of lung nodules on radiographs. Radiology 1996; 199:843–8.
37 Freedman M, LoSCB, Lure F, et al. Computer aided detection of lung cancer on chest radiographs:

algorithm performance vs radiologists performance by size of cancer. SPIE Med Imag: Visual, Display, Image-Guided Proc 2001; 4319:150–9.

38 Freedman M, LoSCB, Osicka T, et al. Computer aided detection of lung cancer on chest radiographs: effect of machine CAD false positive locations on radiologists behavior. Proc SPIE: Image Process 2002; 4684:698–703.

39 Freedman M, OsickaT, Lo SCB, et al. Methods for identifying changes in radiologists behavioral operating point of sensitivity-specificity trade-offs within an ROC study of the use of computer aided detection of lung cancer. Proc SPIE: Image Process Perform 2001; 4324:184–94.

40 Freedman MT. Digital chest radiography. In: Boiselle P, White C, eds. New Techniques in Thoracic Imaging. New York: Marcel Dekker, 2002:315–48.

41 Freedman MT, Osicka T. Computer aided diagnosis for decision support in thoracic imaging. In: Siegel E, Reiner B, Erickson B, eds. CAD in Thoracic Imaging: Decision Support in the Digital Medical Environment. SCAR (Society for Computer Applications in Radiology), Primer 2005; 6:53–68.

42 Stitik F, Tockman M. Radiographic screening in the early detection of lung cancer. Radiol Clin North Am 1978; 16:347–66.

43 Stitik F, TockmanM, Khouri N. Chest radiology. In: Miller AB, ed. Screening for Cancer. New York: Academic Press, 1985:163–91.

44 Ishigaki T, SakumaS, Ikeda M. One-shot dual-energy subtraction chest imaging with computed radiography: clinical evaluation of film images. Radiology 1988; 168:67–72.

45 Kelcz F, ZinkFE, Peppler WW, Kruger DG, Ergun DL, Mistretta CA. Conventional chest radiography vs dual-energy computed radiography in the detection and characterization of pulmonary nodules. AJR Am J Roentgenol 1994; 162:271–8.

46 Kido S, IkezoeJ, Naito H, et al. Clinical evaluation of pulmonary nodules with single-exposure dual-energy subtraction chest radiography with an iterative noise-reduction algorithm. Radiology 1995; 194: 407–12.

47 Hasegawa A, LoSCB, Lin JS, Freedman MT, Mun SK. A shift-invariant neural network for the lung field segmentation in chest radiography. J VLSI Sign Proc Sys 1998; 18:241–50.

48 Tsujii O, FreedmanMT, Mun SK. Anatomic region-based dynamic range compression for chest radiographs using warping transformation of correlated distribution. IEEE Trans Med Imag 1998; 17:407–18.

49 Tsujii O, FreedmanMT, Mun SK. Lung contour detection in chest radiographs using 1-D convolutional neural networks. J Electron Imag 1999; 8:46–53.

50 Difazio MC, MacMahonH, Xu XW, et al. Digital chest radiography: effect of temporal subtraction images on detection accuracy. Radiology 1997; 202:447–52.

51 Katsuragawa S, TagashiraH, Li Q, MacMahon H, Doi K. Comparison of the quality of temporal subtraction images obtained with manual and automatic methods of digital chest radiography. J Digit Imag 1999; 12: 166–72.

52 Kakeda S, NakamuraK, Kamada K, et al. Improved detection of lung nodules by using a temporal subtraction technique. Radiology 2002; 224:145–51.

53 Tsubamoto M, JohkohT, Kozuka T, et al. Temporal subtraction for the detection of hazy pulmonary opacities on chest radiography. AJR Am J Roentgenol 2002; 179:467–71.

54 Johkoh T, KozukaT, Tomiyama N, et al. Temporal subtraction for detection of solitary pulmonary nodules on chest radiographs: evaluation of a commercially available computer-aided diagnosis system. Radiology 2002; 223:806–11.

55 Dobbins JT III, Godfrey DJ. Digital x-ray tomosynthesis: current state of the art and clinical potential, Phys Med Biol 2003; 48:R65–106.

56 Godfrey DJ, McAdamsHP, Dobbins JT III. Optimization of the matrix inversion tomosynthesis (MITS) impulse response and modulation transfer function characteristics for chest imaging. Med Phys 2006; 33:655–67.

57 Kehler M, AlbrechtssonU, Arnadottier E, et al. Digital luminescence radiography in interstitial lung disease. Acta Radiol 1991; 32:18–23.

58 van Heesewijk HP, vad der Graff Y, de Valois JC, Vos JA, Feldberg MA. Digital chest imaging using a selenium detector: the impact of hard copy size on observer performance: a computed tomography-controlled study. Invest Radiol 1997; 32:363–7.

59 Schaefer CM, ProkopM, Oestmann JW, et al. Impact of hard-copy size on observer performance in digital chest radiography. Radiology 1992; 184:77–81.

60 Fisher PD, Brauer GW. Impact of image size on effectiveness of digital imaging systems. J Digit Imag 1989; 2:39–41.

5

Radiofrequency Ablation of Lung Tumors

Amita Sharma and Jo-Anne O. Shepard
Department of Radiology, Massachusetts General Hospital, Boston, Massachusetts, U.S.A.

INTRODUCTION

Radiofrequency ablation (RFA) has recently been introduced as a minimally invasive therapy for patients with lung cancer and lung metastases. It has been established in the treatment of hepatic and renal tumors (1). The successful ablation of 97.5% to 100% has been reported in patients with renal cell carcinoma, especially in small or exophytic lesions (2–5). In patients with liver tumors who are not surgical candidates RFA has a less successful but definite role in therapy (6).

The first lung RFA was performed in 1995 on rabbits (7), which documented the safety and feasibility of this technique in the lungs. Dupuy published the first report on three human subjects in 2000 (8). Implementation of this technique for treatment of primary and metastatic lung tumors and for palliation of pain from chest wall invasion has resulted in numerous clinical studies worldwide.

Surgical resection by lobectomy remains the gold standard for treatment of lung cancer (9). When compared with lobectomy limited pulmonary resections are associated with an increased mortality and higher local recurrence (9,10). Unfortunately, the majority of resectable patients have limited pulmonary reserve or severe comorbid states that preclude surgery.

Alternative treatments to surgery include chemotherapy and radiotherapy but success is limited. Local failure following radiotherapy has been reported in 42–57% of patients treated for lung cancer and this is the most common cause of death in these patients (11–13). Better response rates are seen in those patients receiving radiotherapy for smaller tumors and in those receiving higher doses (14). Chemotherapy is not generally used as a single agent in patients with localized lung cancer but is usually an adjunct to radiotherapy or surgery (15). Complications to radiotherapy and chemotherapy include radiation pneumonitis, esophagitis, and pulmonary fibrosis.

In addition to primary lung cancer, metastatic disease commonly spreads to the lungs. In approximately 20% of patients, metastatic disease is limited to the lungs and these patients are candidates for surgical resection (16). Over time, patients with metastatic disease are likely to develop multiple lesions. Repeated wedge resections in these patients can lead to significant loss of pulmonary tissue and function and are therefore less than ideal. Patients with peripheral lung tumors invading the chest wall and causing pain that is unresponsive to analgesia are considered candidates for RFA for palliation of symptoms. The lower morbidity and mortality of RFA compared with other forms of treatment, the lower procedure costs and ability to perform the ablation in an outpatient setting have resulted in great interest from patients and clinicians. The exact role of lung RFA in the treatment algorithm is yet to be determined, but experience is increasing and prospective multicenter trials are underway.

PRINCIPLE OF RADIOFREQUENCY ABLATION

The principle of RFA is to convert radiofrequency waves into heat within a tumor. This is achieved by placement of an electrode in a tumor, usually via image guidance. The electrode is a 14- to 17-gauge needle, which has an insulated metal shaft and an exposed tip measuring 1–3 cm in length. The RF generator is connected to the electrode and also to 2–4 large conductive pads placed on the thighs or the back of the chest, which dissipate the heat and complete the circuit. Low frequency RF voltage (less than 1 MHz) results in an alternating current at the exposed tip of the electrode, which causes the ions in adjacent tissues to rapidly oscillate, resulting in frictional heating. Heat extends through the tissues further from the electrode via conduction. Conduction is limited by air in the lungs, and this allows heat to become concentrated within the tumor itself (7). Heat is dissipated by moving fluids, such as blood in vessels, known as the "heat sink" effect (17), and to a lesser extent by moving air in the adjacent airways (18,19).

The results of tissue heating are determined by the temperature rise and the duration of heating (20,21). Cell function is maintained at temperatures up to 40°C. Between 40°C and 45°C, cells remain viable but are more susceptible to damage by other agents such as radiotherapy or chemotherapy. Temperatures of 46°C maintained for 60 min will result in irreversible cell death. At temperatures of 50–52°C, cell death occurs within 4–6 min. Between 60°C and 100°C, there is instantaneous cell death secondary to coagulation of protein complexes and intracellular enzymes. The coagulative necrosis can continue for several days after heating has ceased, and, therefore, biopsy immediately after RFA may underestimate the degree of necrosis that will ultimately occur. Temperatures greater than 100°C result in tissue vaporization and charring. Tissue charring adjacent to the electrode increases impedance and decreases radiofrequency output. The formation of carbon dioxide bubbles hinder tissue conductivity and also reduce the effectiveness of ablation. The optimum temperature range following RFA is 60–100°C, and the optimum time is determined by the type of generator used.

RADIOFREQUENCY ABLATION EQUIPMENT

The ideal electrode permits a maximal diameter of coagulation necrosis in a reproducible and safe manner. Early studies have evaluated the optimum needle gauge and exposed tip length in order to maximize ablation diameters and maintain reproducibility and safety (20).

Current clinical applications use three types of systems. The first system utilizes a 14-guage, multitined, expandable electrode, which consists of a trocar-style cannula from which multiple active tines can be deployed incrementally once placed within the center of the tumor (Fig. 1). The system is available from two vendors (RITA Medical Systems, Mountain View, California, U.S.A. and Boston Scientific, Natick, Massachusetts, U.S.A.). The alternating current is applied by the generator to several of the tines to increase the extent of the treatment zone. Treatment times vary between 15 and 40 min, and a diameter of 5 cm is achievable. The tip of the trocar and the inactive tines have temperature thermocouples that are used to monitor and control ablation. At the end of ablation, the tines are retracted back into the trocar needle prior to needle removal.

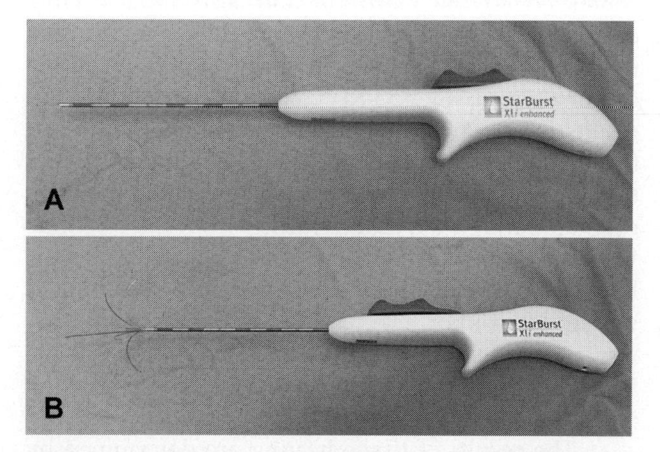

Figure 1 StarBurstTM expandable multitined electrode (RITA Medical, Freemont California, U.S.A.) (**A**). A 14-gauge needle electrode has nine retractable tines that can be deployed once the tip is within the tumor (**B**). Several tines act as an active electrode, thereby increasing the diameter of ablation.

The second system uses a straight, internally cooled electrode in which sealed tubes are positioned alongside the active electrode within a closed system (Valleylab, Boulder, Colorado, U.S.A.). A continuous perfusate of iced water or saline passes through the tubes and cools the electrode tip during ablation. This reduces tissue charring from heat deposition adjacent to the needle tip (22). The electrode is available as a single 17-gauge electrode or a cluster electrode consisting of three 17-gauge electrodes spaced 5 mm apart, working simultaneously. A radiofrequency generator, internal perfusion pump, electrode, and grounding pads form the system (Fig. 2) . Impedance feedback and pulsing of the alternating current results in ablation up to 5 cm in diameter (23). Temperature is measured at the tip of the electrode and should be greater than 60°C. When the perfusion pump is activated, temperatures less than 15°C should be recorded. Multiple single electrodes can also be inserted in different positions and connected to a switch box generator, which allows sequential ablation through the electrodes, thereby decreasing the total time for multiple treatments.

The third system (Berchtold, Tuttlingen, Germany) uses a perfusion electrode that contains multiple holes at the tip that allow dissipation of a conductive perfusate around the tumor tissue in order to improve electrical and thermal conductivity. Injection of 36% NaCl solution into a tumor immediately prior to RFA increased coagulation diameter from 3.1 to 5.2 cm in a canine tumor model (24).

A direct comparison between the different electrodes has been reported in porcine lungs (25). The RFA was performed with a single internally cold electrode (Valleylab), a saline perfusion electrode (Berchtold), and a multitined electrode (RITA Medical Systems). The area of coagulative necrosis was correlated with postablation CT scans. The perfusion electrode produced significantly larger ablation zones than either internally cooled electrode or the multitined electrode. However, it also produced an irregular ablation zone that was determined largely by the unpredictable distribution of hypertonic saline. In addition, normal lung rather than

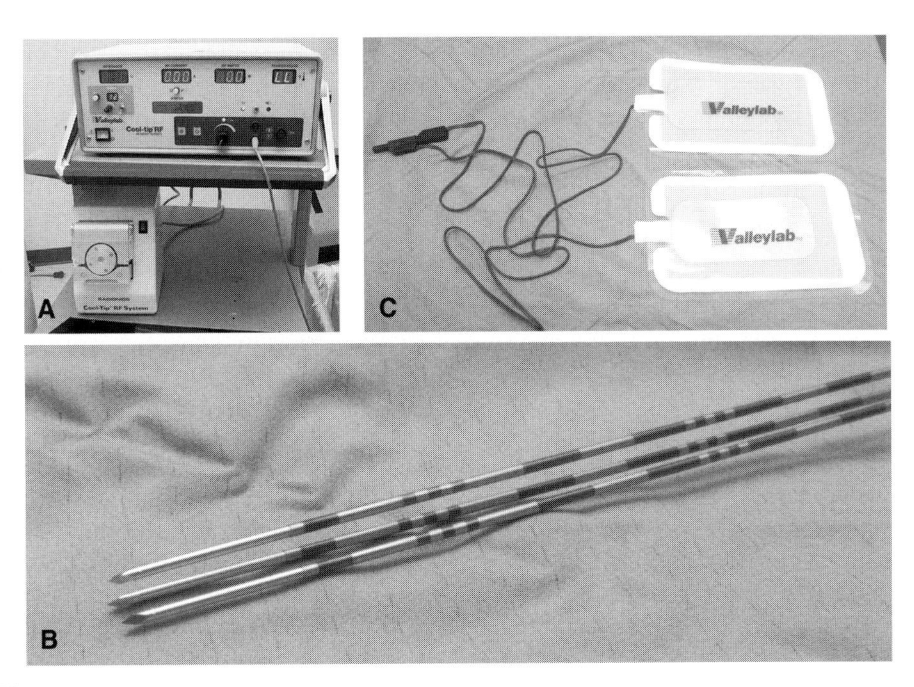

Figure 2 Cool-tip™ radiofrequency generator, pump (**A**), cluster electrode (**B**), and grounding pads (**C**) (ValleyLab, Boulder, Colorado, U.S.A.). The pump perfuses ice-cold water or saline through inflow and outflow tubes that run within the shaft of the electrode and cool the tip during ablation. The electrodes are available in 17 gauge single or cluster electrode, where three electrodes set 5 mm apart result in a larger ablation diameter.

tumors were ablated, making direct extrapolation of the findings to tumor ablation difficult.

The RFA of the lung produces larger ablation diameters than RFA of the liver or kidney, presumably due to the insulating effect of air (26). Increase in the diameter of ablation has been described in porcine liver by altering hepatic blood flow (17). In addition, manipulation of the lung environment has been recently studied in the animal model in an attempt to increase the diameter of ablation. Ablation diameters increase when the local blood flow and ventilation are reduced (18,19). Occlusion of the pulmonary artery results in a significantly larger ablation zone than occlusion of the segmental bronchi. Injection of hypertonic saline into lung has also resulted in larger ablation diameters, due to increased ionicity and conductivity of the environment (24,27,28)

HISTOLOGICAL CHANGES FOLLOWING RADIOFREQUENCY ABLATION OF LUNG

Histological Studies in Animals

The histological changes resulting from RFA of normal lung have been studied in rabbit and pig models (7,29,30) (31–35). Earlier studies using hemotoxylin and eosin stains underestimated the extent of coagulative necrosis because this stain does not identify "Ghost" cells that have undergone necrosis so rapidly that cell structure is maintained (36). Histological interpretation requires methods such as NADH stains that assess cell viability to reflect the extent of irreversible cell damage more accurately than conventional methodology (35).

The histological changes consist of three spherical zones of varying cell damage that encircle the electrode (35). The innermost layer consists of coagulative necrosis. Beyond the central layer is an intermediate layer where mitochondrial enzyme staining shows loss of cellular integrity. Surrounding the intermediate layer is an outer layer that consists of alveolar congestion and hemorrhage. Mixed viable and nonviable cells are present within this outer zone. During the following 10 days, the intermediate layer exhibits continuing necrosis while the outer layer heals with granulation and fibrous tissue.

Goldberg first correlated the histopathological changes of ablation with CT in rabbit lungs (7). Homogeneous opacification on CT immediately following ablation corresponded to all three layers of coagulative necrosis and peripheral inflammation. The changes in the lungs evolved for 3 days, when consolidation on CT was maximal. At 10 days, central low attenuation on chest CT corresponded to fibrosis in the lung.

The ablated area of lung contracts in size between 2 and 4 weeks as the zone of necrosis decreases. The lesion is more solid and may become wedge shaped on CT. It may also be associated with thickening in the adjacent pleura (34). Over time, the inner area of necrosis accounts for a smaller proportion of the total diameter, and, by 8 weeks, any remaining tissue is due to granulation tissue only, the necrotic tissue having been resorbed.

Angiographic studies have confirmed that the ablated lung becomes devascularized (37). Within the ablated zone, thrombi develop in vessels at around 7 days and the bronchial epithelium degenerates. This allows communication of the airways with the necrotic tissue at approximately 3 weeks, resulting in a sterile cavity surrounded by granulation tissue (31). Cavities are reported in 20–58% of ablated lesions (38,39).

After 4 weeks, CT may overestimate the degree of necrosis as the lesion seen on CT consists of ablated lung and possibly a peripheral pneumonitis, which is secondary to obstruction of the ablated bronchi (35).

The MRI appearances of normal lung following RFA have been studied in the porcine model (30,32,33). The central layer of coagulative necrosis is of low signal on T1W, isointense or high signal on T2W, with lack of enhancement following intravenous contrast. The outer layer of alveolar congestion is of isointense or increased signal intensity on T1W, increased signal intensity on T2W, and fast spin echo (FSE). Peripheral enhancement occurs following intravenous contrast injection. During follow up, decrease in lesion diameter occurs due to resorption of the inner layer of necrosis. MRI was reported to be more accurate than CT in reflecting the histological size of the ablated lesion (30).

Tumor models in rabbits (29,37,40) and dogs (41) confirm that the MRI, CT, and histological changes are comparable. Interestingly, the zone of coagulative necrosis is reported to be larger in a lung tumor than in ablated normal lung (29). The solid nature of the tumor results in lower impedance and improved ablation than aerated lung. Surrounding air will also insulate the tumor and concentrate the heat that is generated. High impedance in the lung decreases the ablated margin around the tumor and, therefore, increases the risk of residual disease. Viable tumor cells in the periphery following RFA were reported in up to 40% of cases (29,40). This may be due to improper positioning of the electrode or due to tumor abutting a large vessel (40).

Histological Studies in Humans

There have been very few studies of radiological–pathological correlation in humans as ablated tumors are rarely surgically excised. A prospective ablate and resect study was performed on 8 patients with stage I or II lung cancer (42). The RFA at thoracotomy was followed by lobectomy, and histological analysis performed, which included cell viability staining. Complete ablation was seen in 3 patients with tumors smaller than 2 cm. Incomplete ablation was seen in the remaining 5 patients but this may have been related to the use of palpation, rather than imaging, to place the electrode. In addition only a single treatment of short duration was utilized for lesions greater than 2 cm, which may not have been adequate. Also, immediate cell sampling did not allow the full extent of ablation to occur. An Italian study reported complete ablation in 6 of 9 patients treated with RFA by thoracotomy or percutaneous image guidance. The residual tumor group mean size was 3.1 cm, in contrast to the completely ablated group in which mean size was 2.3 cm (43).

Histological correlation has also been reported on 2 patients who underwent lobectomy or autopsy 3–4 months following RFA (44). Each patient had the expected postablation findings on follow-up CT, MRI, and PET, but residual viable cells were found adjacent to bronchovascular areas in both cases.

RADIOFREQUENCY ABLATION TECHNIQUE

There are a number of clinical studies describing the techniques, imaging findings, and outcomes for lung RFA for the treatment of lung cancers and metastatic disease (38,39,45–47). The patients form a heterogeneous group with varying tumor size, tumor types, and ablation techniques. Follow-up imaging varies from institution to institution, and determination of successful ablation, or diagnosis of recurrent disease, has not been standardized. However, these studies provide a rich source of information regarding current techniques and evolving knowledge.

Patient Selection

The RFA for the treatment of lung cancer is mainly for stage I or II disease, although stages III and IV disease has been included (47,49,56). Nodules range from 5 to 161 mm in diameter pretreatment. Most studies make a distinction between tumors less than 3 cm and those greater than 3 cm as this appears to be the size threshold for achieving complete necrosis using current technology. Suitable candidates for RFA of the lung include patients who are unresectable because of severe comorbidities such as emphysema or severe cardiac disease and those who have had prior surgical resections or radiation but are not eligible for further resection or radiation. Additionally, patients who refuse conventional therapies are potential candidates for RFA of the lung. In those patients with significant underlying pulmonary disease, such as emphysema and pulmonary fibrosis, clinical evaluation with pulmonary function tests is recommended prior to approval for RFA to assess if the patient can withstand a significant pulmonary hemorrhage or a tension pneumothorax. Patients who have had a pneumonectomy and those with FEV1 <1.0 L are considered relative contraindications to RFA. When patients are oxygen dependent, it is advisable to provide general anesthesia for sedation in order to safely achieve the necessary pain relief. Additionally, pulmonary arterial hypertension poses a risk for significant pulmonary hemorrhage particularly in patients with centrally located tumors. However, some patients with peripherally located tumors near the pleura may be considered as potential RFA candidates. Centrally located lesions adjacent to the hilum may be considered for treatment; however, there is a risk of developing a bronchopleural fistula when the lesion is adjacent to a lobar or main bronchus. Lesions adjacent to large central pulmonary arteries or veins may be incompletely treated due to the heat sink effect. Treatment of lesions adjacent to the pericardium may cause the development of a cardiac arrhythmia.

Patients are also evaluated for any coagulation disorders and any medications that affect coagulation should be discontinued. Abnormal prothrombin time (PT), partial thromboplastin time (PTT), and platelet count results preclude treatment with RFA until the clotting abnormality is corrected. Fatalities have been reported in the literature from platelet dysfunction and clopidrogel (58,59). Patients who have pacemakers or intracardiac defibrillators require evaluation prior to the procedure by cardiology or the electrophysiology laboratory. In certain instances, placement of a magnet on the chest wall over the pacemaker during the RFA procedure will be sufficient to prevent malfunction of the pacemaker. However, patients with pacemakers and implantable cardioverter-defibrilators (ICDs) should be reevaluated immediately following the RFA to assess whether there is interruption in the function of the pacemaker or defibrillator (60).

In patients being considered for RFA of the lung at our institution, confirmation of the tumor is performed by percutaneous needle biopsy. Patients are assessed by a multidisciplinary team. A thoracic surgeon and a thoracic oncologist first evaluate the patient for consideration of conventional therapies including surgery, radiation, and chemotherapy. The patient also consults with the thoracic radiologist and the interventional nurse to obtain informed consent and to discuss the RFA procedure, possible complications, and follow-up. All patients are staged with FDG–PET-CT to exclude metastatic disease within the mediastinum and extrathoracic sites.

Sedation

It is necessary to sedate all patients for RFA of the lung. Sedation is performed in order to allow the patient to be completely immobile for the procedure, which may last as long as 2 hours, and to prevent discomfort from the intense heat and pain during the ablation. The majority of patients can be adequately sedated with intravenous conscious sedation. Conscious sedation requires adherence to hospital sedation guidelines, advanced cardiovascular life support (ACLS) certification, dedicated nursing, and cardiopulmonary monitoring during the procedure. However, conscious sedation is contraindicated in patients with severe cardiac and pulmonary comorbidities, who are oxygen dependent, or who have very low ejection fractions. In addition, patients who have airway abnormalities may not be candidates for safe conscious sedation. In these patients or in patients in whom severe chest wall pain may be anticipated, general anesthesia should be considered. Patients should be evaluated by anesthesia prior to the procedure when these conditions exist. Additionally, general anesthesia with a double lumen tube is recommended in patients who may be at risk for pulmonary hemorrhage so that there can be occlusion of the main bronchus on the side of the procedure to contain pulmonary hemorrhage into the treated lung and thereby prevent spillage of blood into the contralateral lung. The double lumen tube can also reduce excursion of a single lung, therefore improving lung isolation (61). This is especially helpful in patients who have very small nodules near the diaphragm. Novel techniques have been described, such as protection of the trachea during ablation of a peritracheal tumor using an endotracheal tube cuff filled with cool distilled water, which was repeatedly exchanged to prevent mucosal injury (53). Sedation techniques at other centers vary between no sedation (54), conscious sedation (1,38,39,45,47–49,51,52,55,57), and general anesthesia (50,53,62). In addition, epidural anesthesia (45) and local nerve blocks (53) have been used.

Procedure

Choice of electrodes for this procedure depends largely on operator experience and nodule size and position. Both multitined electrodes (RITA Medical Systems and Boston Scientific) (39,48,51–54,57) and internally cooled single or cluster electrodes are used (Valleylab) (38,45,47–51,55,62). In lesions very close to a large vessel, central bronchus, or the heart and pericardium, the cool-tip electrode permits more precise placement of the tip than an expandable multitined electrode. The length of the electrode is selected to permit a long enough needle to reach the nodule if it should shift position during the procedure and to allow easy manipulation of the needle. In general, at least 5 cm of extra length should be selected.

The RFA is usually performed with CT guidance. The route of the electrode placement is selected to avoid fissures, central bronchi, large central vessels, bullae, or chest wall structures such as the brachial plexus and subclavian vessels. The appropriate access route is selected, and the patient is placed on the CT scanner in a prone or supine position. The decubitus position is less stable and reserved only for when it is the only feasible approach. The pneumothorax rate tends to be higher from the lateral approach (63).

Once the patient is placed on the CT table, the grounding pads are applied to the thighs. Normally, the pads become warm during the procedure. Proper application of the pads is necessary to avoid burning of the skin during the RFA treatment. Techniques to limit the risk of burns include placing the long edge of the pad closest to site of ablation and ensuring proper contact by shaving and cleaning of the skin (64).

Preliminary CT scans are performed once the patient has received initial sedation, allowing respirations to become reproducible, regular, and shallow. Once the proper plane of imaging has been determined, the skin is marked. In some patients, it is necessary to angle the gantry either cephalad or caudad to avoid intervening structures such as ribs, fissures, or large vessels or bronchi. Additionally, the patient may be rotated into a slight oblique position with placement of a wedge for similar reasons.

After having marked the patient's skin, the skin is prepped widely and draped in a sterile manner with surgical towels and sheets. When conscious sedation is employed, subcutaneous lidocaine is used to provide local anesthesia. A nick is made in the skin at the entry point for the single or cluster electrode to allow ease of placement of the electrode(s) through the skin into the chest wall. The electrode is then advanced incrementally with confirmatory CT scans to assess placement of the electrode. Once the electrode is aligned perfectly toward the nodule and has been placed just superficial to the pleural surface, the electrode is then passed deliberately through the pleura in a swift manner and beyond the pleura into the lung. Repeat imaging is useful to confirm adequate alignment as the electrode is advanced through the nodule. For proper treatment, the tip of the electrode is placed just distal to the far end of the nodule. Difficulty in puncturing the nodule can lead to increase in pneumothorax rate (65). The nodule can also move away from the electrode and toward vital structures (Fig. 3) (52). It may be necessary to place towels on the chest wall adjacent to the electrode in order to prop it into the desired position.

Once the electrode is properly placed, treatment can be initiated and the perfusion pump is started to cool the tip. An initial 12-min treatment is used. It may be necessary to administer additional narcotic sedation just prior to commencement of the treatment and during the actual ablation. It is advisable to place an oxygen mask on the patient at this time and to have suction available should there be pulmonary hemorrhage. A percutaneous chest tube kit should be immediately available for use should a pneumothorax develop.

Once ablation is instituted, the patient is closely monitored for adequate pain control, respiration, and oxygenation. The patient should never be unattended during this period because pain from the procedure

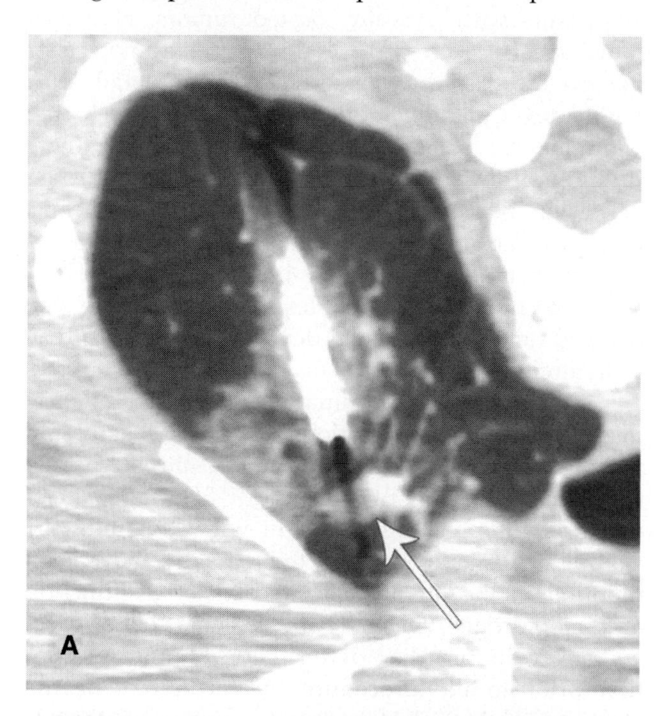

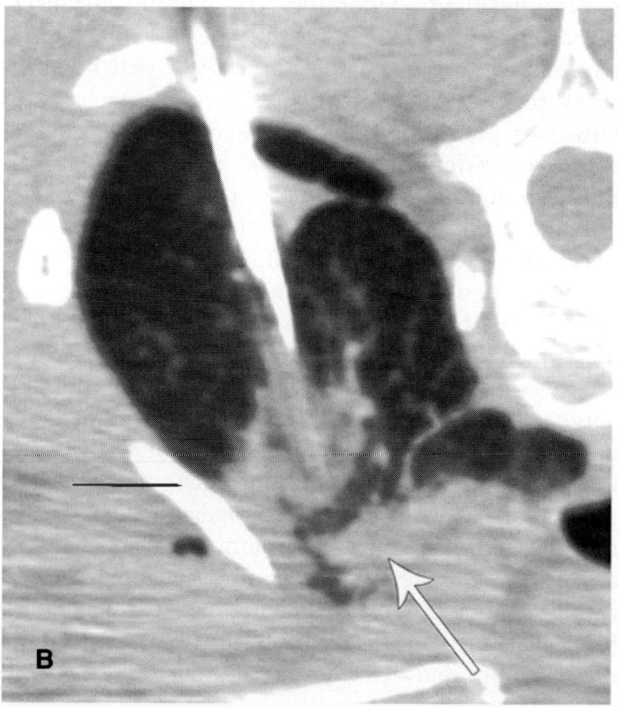

Figure 3 Prone axial CT scans in a 47-year-old woman with right upper-lobe adenocarcinoma (**A**) (*arrow*). The radiofrequency ablation (RFA) was complicated by difficulty in puncturing the nodule, which repeatedly moved away from the electrode toward the anterior chest wall (**B**) (*arrow*). Following RFA, the patient complained of right arm parasthesia, which resolved slowly over 6 months. This was attributed to heat conduction into the adjacent brachial plexus.

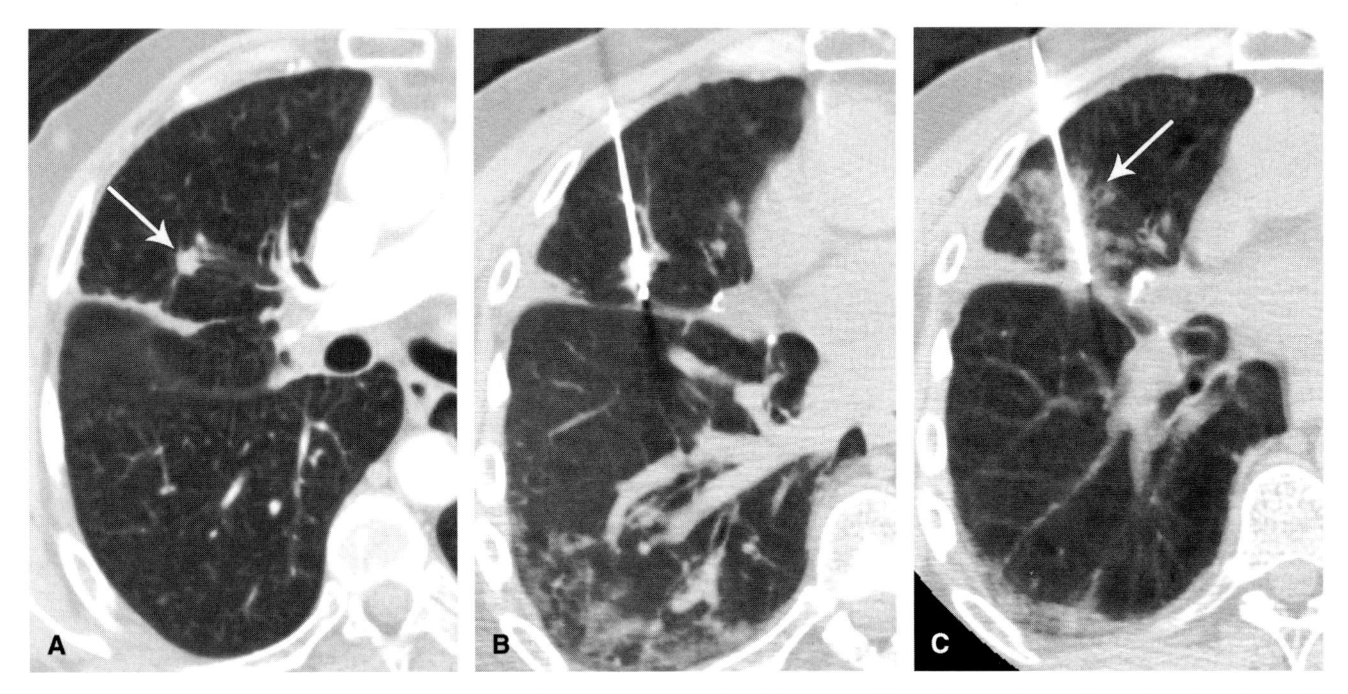

Figure 4 Axial CT scans in a 55-year-old man with a 9 mm, metastatic, right upper-lobe adenocarcinoma (*arrow*) undergoing radio frequency ablation (RFA) (**A**). A single electrode is seen within the nodule (**B**). Following RFA, a 4 cm ground-glass zone of ablation change is seen (*arrow*) (**C**).

may cause the patient to move or cough, resulting in movement of the electrode. Such movements may exacerbate pulmonary hemorrhage or pneumothorax. Many patients experience diaphoresis during RFA due to elevation of the internal body temperature that requires intravenous fluid replacement during and following the procedure.

Following termination of a 12-min ablation, the pump is turned off and the temperature within the lesion is measured. If the temperature exceeds 60°C, the lesion is considered adequately treated, otherwise a repeat of 6- to 12-min ablation will be necessary. The patient is scanned with the electrode in place to assess for the development of treatment response on the scan. Treatment response is seen as a zone of ground glass surrounding the nodule that generally appears immediately following the treatment and progresses within minutes to hours following the procedure (Fig. 4). Additionally, scanning is performed to detect any immediate complications such as pneumothorax, hemothorax, or pulmonary hemorrhage. If the treatment is insufficient, the electrode is repositioned appropriately and a second or third subsequent treatment is performed until adequate coverage is obtained. The electrode is left in until the procedure is completed and the patient is ready to move onto the stretcher.

Once the patient is ready to be transferred from the table to the stretcher, the drapes are removed and the skin is cleaned. The electrode is removed quickly, a bandage is applied to the skin, and the patient is rolled into a dependent position such that they are lying on the puncture site. A dependent position is a procedure routinely performed in order to minimize the complication of pneumothorax by allowing the dependent lung to become atelectatatic, decreasing respiration in the dependent lung, and therefore minimizing the chance for an air leak to develop. Patients are kept in the dependent position in a supine or prone position for 3 h following the procedure. They are given low flow nasal oxygen at 2 L/min and are required to lie still and not talk, move, or cough. If necessary, additional sedation is administered to improve patient compliance.

Ablation of the tract during electrode removal is performed at a few centers (39,48). Charring around the needle during ablation can inhibit the retractions of the tines. This can then cause injury to the lung and pleura when the needle is removed (66).

Postprocedure Care

Follow-up imaging is obtained with a portable chest radiograph at 1 and 3 h after the procedure. The radiographs are obtained in the supine or prone position with the patient remaining in the dependent position. If a substantial pneumothorax or hemothorax develop, the air or blood is drained appropriately. Patients are then admitted overnight for observation. Following overnight observation, patients receive an upright posteroanterior (PA) and lateral chest radiograph and are discharged from the hospital if they are asymptomatic. Patients are prescribed oral analgesic narcotics for treatment of potential pleuritic pain that may develop over the ensuing 2 weeks. Prophylactic antibiotic coverage is used in several centers but there is no consensus regarding its routine use (49,50,53–55,62). At our institution, antibiotics are administered prophylactically in patients who may have prosthetic cardiac valves, mitral valve prolapse, or joint prostheses. Patients are not treated routinely for the prevention of pneumonia. However, patients are instructed to carefully monitor for fever or sputum production that may signal a developing pneumonia and are treated as needed should these symptoms develop.

COMPLICATIONS OF RFA

Complications are similar in most institutions. The most common procedural complication reported is pneumothorax (11.9–60%) (38,39,45–57). The frequency of pneumothorax is similar to that reported with lung biopsy and is more common in patients with emphysema (67). Chest tube insertion is required in up to 58% following pneumothorax. Pleural effusions are generally small and self-limiting but are described in up to half of the cases. Low-grade fever (less than 39°C) is reported in 20–100% (65). Pneumonia occurs in 10% of patients and is more common with emphysema and obstructive lung disease. Abscess formation has occurred within large lesions (45,55). Hemoptysis occurs in 11%, although pulmonary hemorrhage is less common (Fig. 5) (39,65). Death due to massive hemoptysis occurred following RFA of a central lesion (57). Air leak and pneumomediastinum are unusual (45,47,68). Delayed pneumomediastinum and subcutaneous emphysema have been described 11 days after ablation of a peripheral tumor as a result of lesion cavitation. Both the cavity and tract were treated with fibrin sealant (68). Burns have occurred at the grounding pads (64) and at the needle insertion site due to a 22-gauge needle left in the patient during the ablation, allowing upward extension of heat into the skin, resulting in a 1 cm third degree burn (53). Temporary hoarseness from recurrent laryngeal nerve injury (53), pulmonary embolus, acute respiratory distress syndrome (ARDS) (49), hemothorax (45), renal failure (57), atrial fibrillation, and air embolus (53,69) have all been reported.

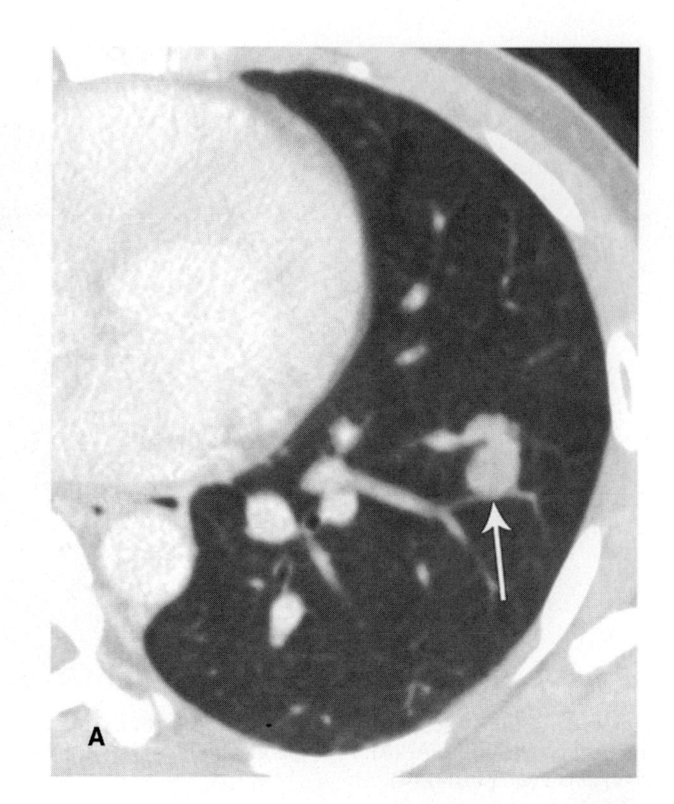

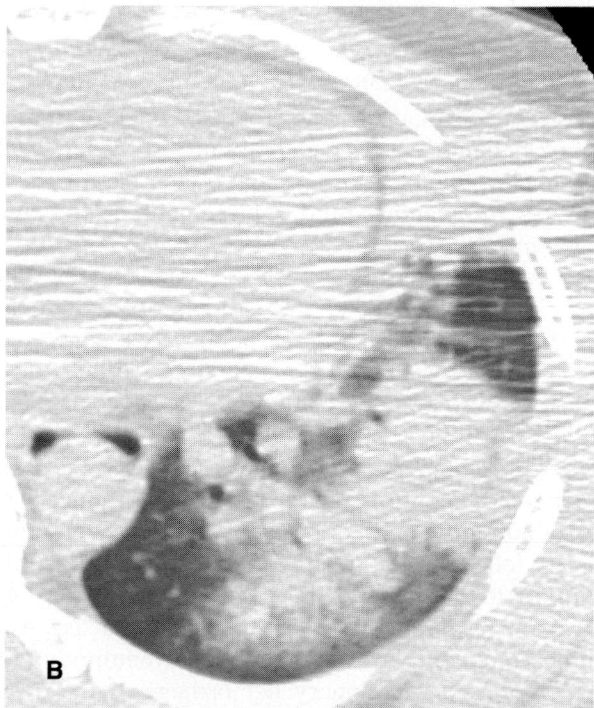

Figure 5 Axial CT scans in a 43-year-old man with metastatic tonsillar-adenocarcinoma (*arrow*) in the left lower lobe treated with radiofrequency ablation (**A**). Pulmonary hemorrhage occurred immediately following ablation, but the patient was asymptomatic (**B**).

IMAGING FINDINGS AT FOLLOW UP

Post-RFA follow-up protocols most often employ contrast-enhanced CT scans at regular, usually 3–6 month intervals. The aim is to detect complications from RFA, confirm the expected radiological findings over time, and identify recurrent or distal disease. MRI is used less frequently, but is documented to accurately demonstrate evolution of ablation changes (50,53). PET scanning has been used in selective cases (52,53,55–57).

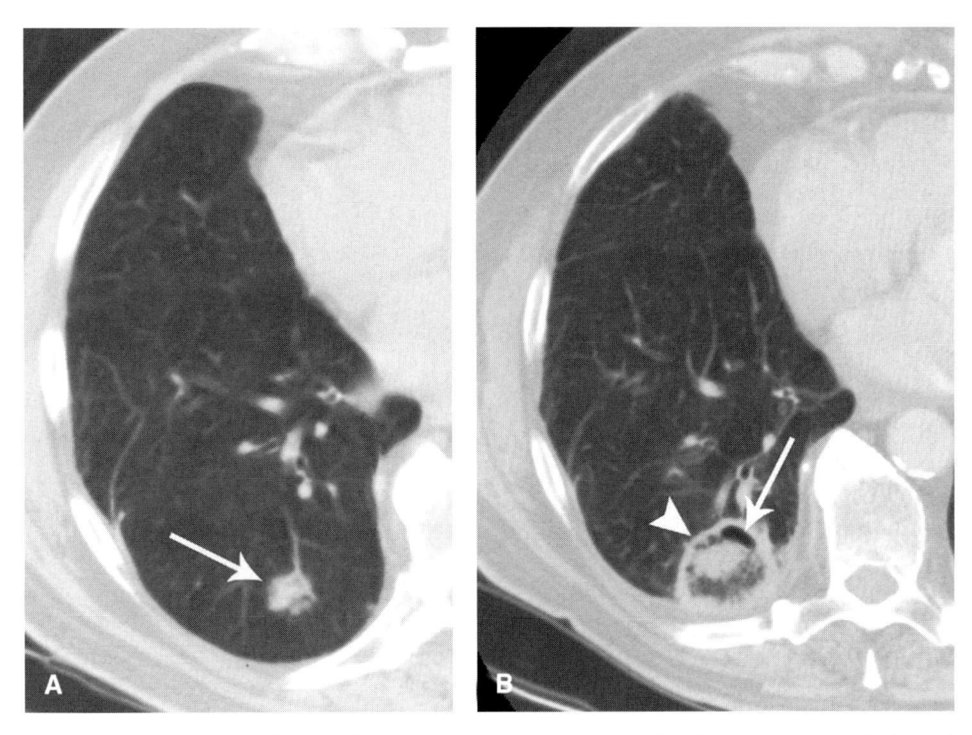

Figure 6 Axial CT Scans in an 81-year-old man with metastatic colon cancer to the right lower lobe (**A**) (*arrow*). One month post-radiofrequency ablation, ground glass opacity surrounds the nodule (*arrow*). The peripheral lung is seen as a peripheral rim of increased density (*arrowhead*). There is cavitation within the ablated lung parenchyma (**B**).

CT Imaging Following RFA

Immediate appearances on CT have been correlated with histological findings and are similar to the animal models described above (38,39,45,47–50,54). It is recommended that a safety margin of 5–10 mm of ground glass opacity is demonstrated around the lesion to confirm complete enclosure of the tumor within the central and intermediate layers of coagulative necrosis (Fig. 5) (39,45,47,49,54). The ablated lesion may continue to increase in size due to ongoing coagulation necrosis in the first few days following ablation (29,39,45). Ground glass opacity then becomes more solid or develops an initial peripheral ring of dense opacity (Fig. 6).

Cavitation was initially thought to represent a complication of RFA but was not associated with clinical infection and was concluded to be a normal expected finding (Fig. 5)(70). Cavitation is reported within the lesion in 20–58% of cases in the first month (38,39,45,49,53). It has been reported to be more common in central lesions than peripheral lesions, with the use of the cluster electrode rather than the single cool-tip electrode (38) and in patients with greater than 200% increase in size of the ablated lesion compared with baseline (39,65). In the absence of true cavitation, bubble-like lucencies may also been seen (38).

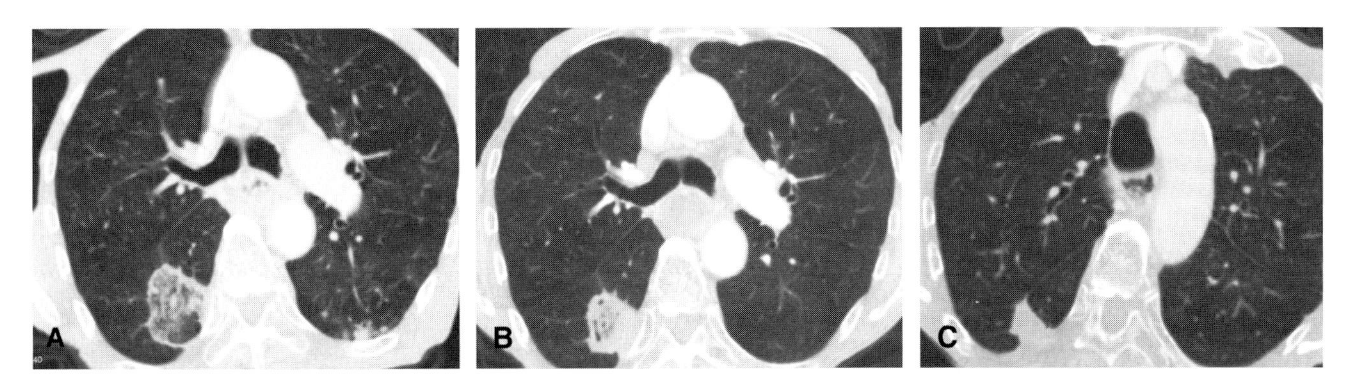

Figure 7 Axial CT scans in a 73-year-old man with bronchioalveolar cell carcinoma treated by radiofrequency ablation. Immediate ground glass opacity becomes more solid at 1-month follow up (**A**). Contraction of the ablation zone at 3 months is associated with pleural thickening (**B**) (*arrow*). At 6 months there is further contraction of the postablation lesion and adjacent pleural thickening consistent with expected posttreatment findings (**C**).

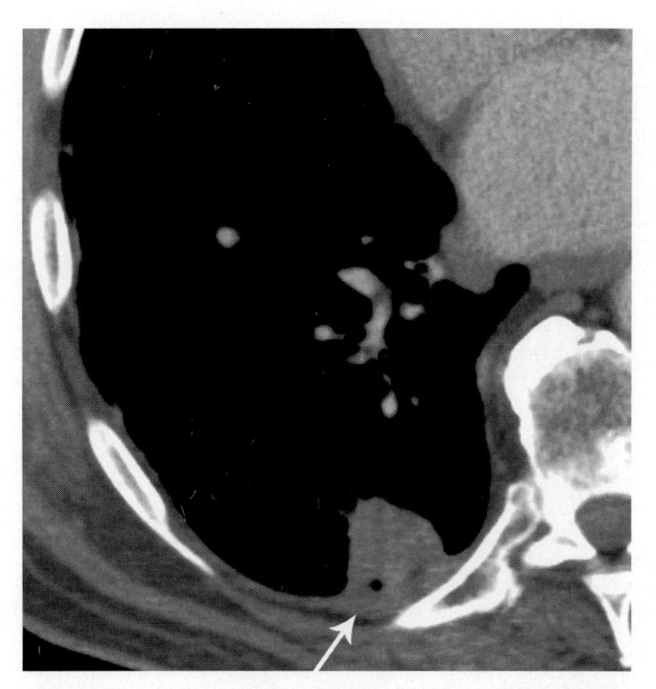

Figure 8 Axial CT scan in an 81-year-old man with metastatic colon cancer to the right lower lobe. Six months following radiofrequency ablation there has been contraction of the ablation zone and there is associated pleural thickening (*arrow*).

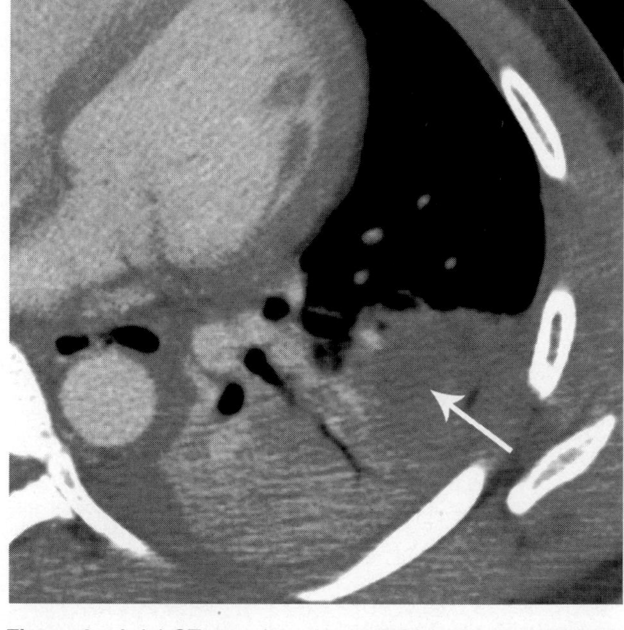

Figure 9 Axial CT scan in a 43-year-old man with metastatic tonsillar adenocarcinoma 24 h post-radiofrequency ablation of a left lower lobe nodule. The ablated lung nodule does not show enhancement (*arrow*). There is surrounding consolidation and a left pleural effusion that resolved spontaneously.

The postablation lesion has an expected appearance over time (Fig. 7). By 3 months, most studies report that the size of the lesion has reached a plateau but remains significantly larger than baseline (38,39,47,49,52). Between 3 and 6 months, the lesion decreases in size and at this stage any increase in diameter should be regarded as highly suspicious for tumor recurrence. The shape of the lesion also changes from spherical to a wedge-shaped mass. This can be explained by central necrotic tissue having been resorbed and peripheral lung granulation and fibrous tissue forming the residual lesion. This continues to contract down to form a solid triangular linear or wedge-shaped density consistent with a scar. In the treatment of small tumors, the residual scar may be larger than the original lesion. As the ablated lesion contracts there is associated volume loss. The lesion moves to the periphery and is often associated with pleural thickening (Fig. 8) (38).

Nodules from lung cancer and metastatic disease have been shown to enhance with intravenous contrast, which is thought to be due to neovascularization of the tumor cells and this is best demonstrated by nodule densitometry (71,72). Nodule densitometry is performed using limited thin section slices (1–3 mm prior to intravenous contrast and then dynamically following intravenous contrast at 45, 90, 180, and 300 s after intravenous contrast injection). The most solid portion of the lesion is used to calculate the nodule attenuation and the maximum post-contrast attenuation is subtracted from the precontrast to obtain nodule enhancement measurements. Swensen demonstrated 98% sensitivity in the detection of malignancy using a threshold of 15 HU enhancement of baseline (71). Loss of nodule enhancement has been used as a sign of successful ablation (Fig. 9) (47,48,54,55,72). Enhancement of the postablation lesion at 3 months should remain below baseline but may be greater than that seen at one month, presumably due to a recovering circulation in the surrounding ablated lung (48,52). Peripheral enhancement in surrounding lung has been documented to occur in successfully ablated lesions, presumably due to the reactive hyperemia that occurs in the surrounding ablated lung (39,49).

Focal or eccentric enhancement is interpreted as recurrent disease although biopsies are not performed for confirmation in most studies (Fig. 10) (49,52,54,55). In some cases, biopsy has been performed in patients with no evidence of enhancement and apparently successful ablation but viable cells have been detected. This suggests that residual disease is inadequately demonstrated by current imaging techniques (42,44,45).

MRI Imaging Following RFA

Limited human studies are available on the MRI appearances following radiofrequency ablation. One study comments on the necrosis following ablation

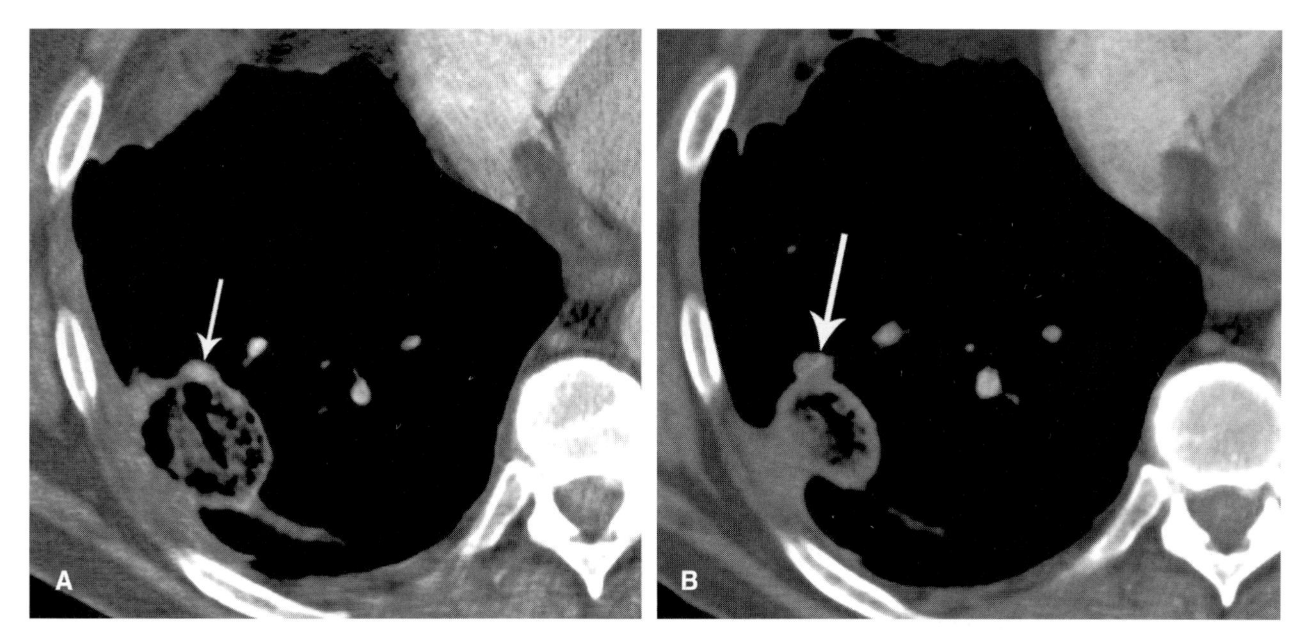

Figure 10 Axial CT scans of the right lower lobe in a 64-year-old man with right lower-lobe adenocarcinoma. One month following radiofrequency ablation a contrast-enhanced CT demonstrated eccentric enhancement at the periphery of the ablation zone (**A**) (*arrow*). The nodule increases in size at 3 months consistent with residual disease (**B**) (*arrow*).

being diagnosed by reduced or absent enhancement on dynamic MRI imaging (53).

PET Imaging Following RFA

The use of FDG-PET in the evaluation of lung RFA has been investigated in an animal model (73), in case reports and small studies (8,55,74).

The RFA of normal lungs was shown to result in a ring of increased activity on PET scans as early as 1 day following ablation. Activity decreased after 4 weeks. Histologically, this ring of activity corresponded to vascular congestion, pulmonary hemorrhage, and alveolar infiltration with neutrophils. Central low activity corresponded to the zone of coagulative necrosis (73).

As with contrast-enhanced CT, PET within hours of RFA may be the most accurate measure of residual disease, before inflammation in adjacent lung clouds interpretation.

In our experience, reactive changes in ablated lung last much longer in human subjects. One to three months post-RFA, a peripheral rim of activity is commonly seen on an FDG-PET scan (Fig. 11). Comparison with baseline PET scans or fusion of PET and CT images can confirm that this increase in activity surrounds the photopenic tumor necrosis and represents activity in ablated lung. Six months post-RFA, the central photopenic area often demonstrates a relative increase in activity. This may be due to the presence of reactive lung occupying the site of central necrotic tumor that has been resorbed. Eccentric areas of PET activity may suggest recurrent disease when associated with abnormal enhancement on CT or a focal increase in size. Further research into the most useful time to use PET post-RFA is clearly indicated (75).

Signs of Recurrent Disease

The confirmation of complete ablation is a challenge, as the lesion is not removed following RFA and actually increases in size due to the ablation of the tumor and adjacent lung parenchyma. Detection of residual tumor therefore relies on several factors.

Follow-up imaging demonstrates decrease in lesion size from 1 to 3 months. Residual disease should be suspected if there is increase in size of the ablated lesion or there is a focal bulge in the shape of the lesion beyond 3 months (Fig. 10) (38,39,52). In addition nodule enhancement has been shown to be associated with malignancy (71). Immediately following RFA enhancement should be absent or reduced to below baseline. Focal areas of enhancement are therefore suspicious of residual tumor (47–50,52,54,55,72).

FDG-PET imaging can demonstrate increased activity as a normal reaction to ablation of surrounding lung. Eccentric or focal areas of activity have been reported to represent residual or recurrent disease (55). In our experience, the PET findings need to be interpreted together with the CT findings. Coregistration can be useful in identifying areas of increased activity (Fig. 11).

Patients who have had successful RFA on all forms of imaging assessment have still been documented to show residual tumor cells by biopsy and long-term follow- up of all patients is needed (44,45).

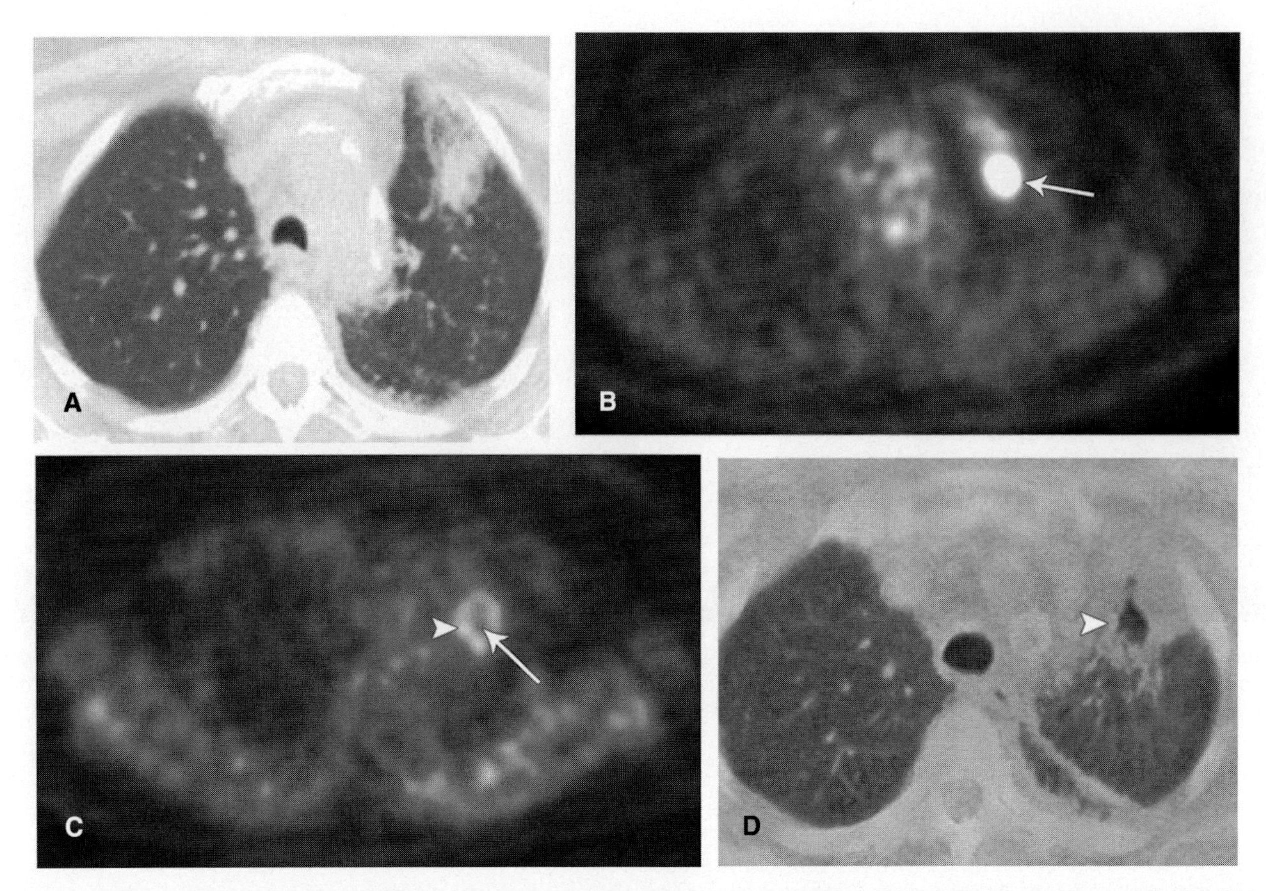

Figure 11 Axial CT scan (**A**), staging PET scan (**B**), 6 month post-radio frequency ablation (RFA)-PET (**C**), and fusion PET-CT (**D**) in a 76-year-old woman with recurrent, large-cell, left-upper lung cancer (*arrow*) (**B**). Prior to RFA, the nodule (*arrow*) demonstrates increased activity on FDG-PET. (**C**) Six months post-RFA, the tumor becomes photopenic (*arrow*) and the surrounding lung demonstrates increased PET activity consistent with inflammatory change within the ablated lung (*arrowhead*). (**D**) This corresponds to the lung surrounding a cavity on the PET-CT fusion study with registration (*arrowhead*).

RISK FACTORS FOR LOCAL PROGRESSION AFTER RFA

At this time, the most useful indicators of successful RFA include tumor size less than 3 cm (39,49–52,54, 55,76–78), a temperature rise of greater than 60°C within the tumor during RFA (38,39,45, 47,49,54,58) and development of ground glass opacities immediately post-RFA which, encompass a treated tumor with a safety margin of 5–10 mm (38,45,47,49,54,65). Histological type has not been found to be a risk factor for progression.

Success of 69–100% in ablating lesions less than 3 cm has been reported with average survival of 17.3–19.7 months (49,52,55). In lesions greater than 3 cm, only 23–39% achieved complete necrosis and mean survival was 8.7 months (49,55). Studies on survival post-RFA for metastases report slightly better results. The average survival for colorectal metastases was reported to be 33 months in one study, with acturial 1-, 2-, and 3-year survival of 85%, 64%, and 46%, respectively. Size greater than 3 cm was independently associated with reduced survival (76).

COMBINED TREATMENT

RFA is known to be less effective in tumors that are greater than 3 cm in diameter. This is due to the limitations in diameter of coagulative necrosis that can be achieved by the currently available systems. Overlapping ablations have been used for larger lesions but these may fail to entirely encompass the tumor especially if the lesion is an irregular shape. Viable tumors cells have been reported in the peripheral layer of ablated tumors where adequately high temperatures may not be achieved due to poor conduction or adjacent vessels or airways (78).

Combined treatment of RFA with radiotherapy or brachytherapy has been evaluated (79–81). Radiotherapy and RFA are postulated to have a synergistic effect; RFA works best on the center of a lesion, where relative hypoxia makes radiotherapy least effective. Peripheral hyperemia as a result of RFA would be expected to increase local oxygen pressure and thereby decrease the ratio of hypoxic cells, which are resistant to radiotherapy. The authors of one study did not find a difference in survival between patients with small and large tumors when RFA was combined with radiotherapy. This suggests that radiotherapy improves the effectiveness of RFA in larger lesions (79).

RFA during minithoracotomy has also been described in combination with video-assisted thoracoscopic surgery (82). RFA was performed in an attempt to prevent local recurrence that is a problem in patients with wedge resections rather than lobectomy for the treatment of lung cancer (9,10)

OTHER ABLATION MODALITIES

Microwave Ablation

Microwave ablation utilizes a 14.5-gauge single- or trio-microwave antenna that is placed in a tumor. Electromagnetic waves pass from a generator (60 W power at 915 MHz) (Vivawave System, Vicant Medical, Mountain View, California, U.S.A.) to the antenna's noninsulated tip. The electromagnetic waves agitate surrounding water molecules causing frictional heating and coagulation necrosis. No grounding pads are necessary and the system does not suffer from the heat sink affect that reduces the efficacy of RFA near large vessels.

Microwave is reported to produce higher intratumoral temperatures with larger ablation volumes and faster ablation times than RFA (83). A prospective study of patients with lung cancer receiving microwave ablation followed by lobectomy demonstrated complete tumor coagulation and absence of viable cells (83). A study of peripheral lung cancers treated with microwave ablation under ultrasound guidance confirmed that this is a feasible and safe method in the lung (84).

Cryoablation

Cryoablation has been investigated in a handful of centers for the treatment of lung tumors (85,86). A 2–3 mm sheath is passed into a tumor under imaging guidance into which is inserted a cryoprobe. High-pressure argon and helium gas are used to freeze and thaw the lesion, respectively.(87). Freezing initially results in a very small ice ball as air is a poor conductor and contains little water to propagate freezing. On thawing intense intraalveolar hemorrhage occurs, which increases the local water content and magnifies the size of the subsequent ice ball. Two to three cycles of freezing and thawing are performed that result in ice balls 2.5–3 cm in diameter. The percutaneous tract measure 3 mm in diameter and fibrin glue is employed to plug the tract following ablation thereby reducing the risk of pneumothorax and bleeding.

The advantages of cryoablation over RFA are its low-pain complication, excellent visualization of the ice ball during treatment and the lack of damage to adjacent vessels and bronchi. A report of 20 patients treated with tumors measuring less than 3 cm indicated a successful ablation rate of 30% during a follow-up period of 21 months.

Complications were low, and included pneumothorax, small pleural effusion, hemoptysis, and temporary phrenic nerve palsy. Hemoptysis was more common than with RFA, reported in 41% of patients with cryoablation. This is thought to be due to the rupture of the capillary wall and hemorrhage on thawing, as demonstrated on animal studies (88).

Laser Ablation

Laser ablation has been described as an alternative method of percutaneous ablation (89). Single or multiple laser fibers are introduced through a small caliber applicator, such as 5.5 French Teflon tube. Cooling fluid is perfused along the applicator in order to prevent charring of the laser fibers during treatment. The fluid may include tumoricidal agents, such as chemotherapy or radioisotopes. Technical success is related to lesion size with recurrence rates of 15% reported in lesions less than 4 cm and 42% in lesions greater than 4 cm (89).

Complications are similar to other percutaneous techniques with pneumothorax being the most common. Pulmonary hemorrhage and hemoptysis are relatively common, reported in 12% and 10.5% of cases, respectively, which may be related to the laser technique or the deposition of fluid in the lung parenchyma.

CONCLUSION

Radiofrequency ablation and other methods of tumor ablation are new rapidly developing therapies for patients with lung tumors. Tumor ablation will undoubtedly form an important part in the management of patients with malignancy but as with any new technique, rigorous study is imperative in ensuring a safe and efficacious practice. Standardization of the terminology used will enhance communication between investigators and clinicians and allow greater comparison between the many clinical studies that are underway (90).

REFERENCES

1 Curley SA, Izzo F, Delrio P, et al. Radiofrequency ablation of unresectable primary and metastatic hepatic malignancies: results in 123 patients. Ann Surg 1999; 230(1):1–8.
2 Matsumoto ED, Johnson DB, Ogan K, et al. Short-term efficacy of temperature-based radiofrequency ablation of small renal tumors. Urology 2005; 65(5):877–81.

3 Hegarty NJ, Gill IS, Desai MM, Remer EM, O'Malley CM, Kaouk JH. Probe-ablative nephron-sparing surgery: cryoablation versus radiofrequency ablation. Urology 2006; 68(1 Suppl):7–13.
4 Gervais DA, McGovern FJ, Arellano RS, McDougal WS, Mueller PR. Radiofrequency ablation of renal cell carcinoma: part 1, Indications, results, and role in patient management over a 6-year period and ablation of 100 tumors. AJR 2005; 185(1):64–71.
5 McDougal WS, Gervais DA, McGovern FJ, Mueller PR. Long-term followup of patients with renal cell carcinoma treated with radio frequency ablation with curative intent. J Urol 2005; 174(1):61–3.
6 Sutherland LM, Williams JA, Padbury RT, Gotley DC, Stokes B, Maddern GJ. Radiofrequency ablation of liver tumors: a systematic review. Arch Surg 2006; 141(2): 181–90.
7 Goldberg SN, Gazelle GS, Compton CC, McLoud TC. Radiofrequency tissue ablation in the rabbit lung: efficacy and complications. Acad Radiol 1995; 2 (9):776–84.
8 Dupuy DE, Zagoria RJ, Akerley W, Mayo-Smith WW, Kavanagh PV, Safran H. Percutaneous radiofrequency ablation of malignancies in the lung. AJR 2000; 174 (1):57–9.
9 Ginsberg RJ, Rubinstein LV. Randomized trial of lobectomy versus limited resection for T1 N0 non-small cell lung cancer. Lung Cancer Study Group. Ann Thorac Surg 1995; 60(3):615–22; discussion 22–3.
10 Martini N, Bains MS, Burt ME, et al. Incidence of local recurrence and second primary tumors in resected stage I lung cancer. J Thorac Cardiovas Surg 1995; 109 (1):120–9.
11 Morita K, Fuwa N, Suzuki Y, et al. Radical radiotherapy for medically inoperable non–small cell lung cancer in clinical stage I: a retrospective analysis of 149 patients. Radiother Oncol 1997; 42(1):31–6.
12 Sibley GS, Jamieson TA, Marks LB, Anscher MS, Prosnitz LR. Radiotherapy alone for medically inoperable stage I non–small-cell lung cancer: the Duke experience. Int J Radiat Onc Biol Phys 1998; 40(1): 149–54.
13 Zierhut D, Bettscheider C, Schubert K, van Kampen M, Wannenmacher M. Radiation therapy of stage I and II non–small cell lung cancer (NSCLC). Lung Cancer 2001; 34 Suppl 3:S39–43.
14 Rowell NP, Williams CJ. Radical radiotherapy for stage I/II non–small cell lung cancer in patients not sufficiently fit for or declining surgery (medically inoperable): a systematic review. Thorax 2001; 56(8):628–38.
15 Alam N, Darling G, Shepherd FA, Mackay JA, Evans WK. Postoperative chemotherapy in nonsmall cell lung cancer: a systematic review. Ann Thorac Surg 2006; 81 (5):1926–36.
16 U P. Long-term results of lung metastasectomy: prognostic analyses based on 5206 cases. The International Registry of Lung Metastases. J Thorac Cardiovas Surg 1997; 113(1):37–49.
17 Goldberg SN, Hahn PF, Halpern EF, Fogle RM, Gazelle GS. Radio-frequency tissue ablation: effect of pharmacologic modulation of blood flow on coagulation diameter. Radiology 1998; 209(3):761–7.
18 Anai H, Uchida BT, Pavcnik D, et al. Effects of blood flow and/or ventilation restriction on radiofrequency coagulation size in the lung: an experimental study in swine. Cardiovasc Intervent Radiol 2006; 29(5):838–45.
19 Oshima F, Yamakado K, Akeboshi M, et al. Lung radiofrequency ablation with and without bronchial occlusion: experimental study in porcine lungs. J Vasc Interv Radiol 2004; 15(12):1451–6.
20 Goldberg SN, Gazelle GS, Dawson SL, Rittman WJ, Mueller PR, Rosenthal DI. Tissue ablation with radiofrequency: effect of probe size, gauge, duration, and temperature on lesion volume. Acad Radiol 1995; 2 (5):399–404.
21 Goldberg SN, Gazelle GS, Halpern EF, Rittman WJ, Mueller PR, Rosenthal DI. Radiofrequency tissue ablation: importance of local temperature along the electrode tip exposure in determining lesion shape and size. Acad Radiol 1996; 3(3):212–8.
22 Goldberg SN, Gazelle GS, Solbiati L, Rittman WJ, Mueller PR. Radiofrequency tissue ablation: increased lesion diameter with a perfusion electrode. Acad Radiol 1996; 3(8):636–44.
23 Goldberg SN, Gazelle GS, Dawson SL, Rittman WJ, Mueller PR, Rosenthal DI. Tissue ablation with radiofrequency using multiprobe arrays. Acad Radiol 1995; 2 (8):670–4.
24 Ahmed M, Lobo SM, Weinstein J, et al. Improved coagulation with saline solution pretreatment during radiofrequency tumor ablation in a canine model. J Vasc Interv Radiol 2002; 13(7):717–24.
25 Lee JM, Han JK, Chang JM, et al. Radiofrequency ablation in pig lungs: in vivo comparison of internally cooled, perfusion and multitined expandable electrodes. Br J Radiol 2006; 79(943):562–71.
26 Ahmed M, Liu Z, Afzal KS, et al. Radiofrequency ablation: effect of surrounding tissue composition on coagulation necrosis in a canine tumor model. Radiology 2004; 230(3):761–7.
27 Lee JM, Youk JH, Kim YK, et al. Radio-frequency thermal ablation with hypertonic saline solution injection of the lung: ex vivo and in vivo feasibility studies. Eur Radiol 2003; 13(11):2540–7.
28 Lee JM, Kim SW, Li CA, et al. Saline-enhanced radiofrequency thermal ablation of the lung: a feasibility study in rabbits. Korean J Radiol 2002; 3(4):245–53.
29 Goldberg SN, Gazelle GS, Compton CC, Mueller PR, McLoud TC. Radio-frequency tissue ablation of VX2 tumor nodules in the rabbit lung. Acad Radiol 1996; 3 (11):929–35.
30 Wacker FK, Nour SG, Eisenberg R, Duerk JL, Lewin JS. MRI-guided radiofrequency thermal ablation of normal lung tissue: in vivo study in a rabbit model. AJR 2004; 183(3):599–603.
31 Nomori H, Imazu Y, Watanabe K, et al. Radiofrequency ablation of pulmonary tumors and normal lung tissue in swine and rabbits. Chest 2005; 127(3):973–7.
32 Morrison PR, vanSonnenberg E, Shankar S, et al. Radiofrequency ablation of thoracic lesions: part 1,

experiments in the normal porcine thorax. AJR 2005; 184(2):375–80.

33 Oyama Y, Nakamura K, Matsuoka T, et al. Radiofrequency ablated lesion in the normal porcine lung: long-term follow-up with MRI and pathology. Cardiovasc Intervent Radiol 2005; 28(3):346–53.

34 Tominaga J, Miyachi H, Takase K, et al. Time-related changes in computed tomographic appearance and pathologic findings after radiofrequency ablation of the rabbit lung: preliminary experimental study. J Vasc Interv Radiol 2005; 16(12):1719–26.

35 Yamamoto A, Nakamura K, Matsuoka T, et al. Radiofrequency ablation in a porcine lung model: correlation between CT and histopathologic findings. AJR 2005; 185(5):1299–306.

36 Zervas NT, Kuwayama A. Pathological characteristics of experimental thermal lesions. Comparison of induction heating and radiofrequency electrocoagulation. J Neurosurg 1972; 37(4):418–22.

37 Miao Y, Ni Y, Bosmans H, et al. Radiofrequency ablation for eradication of pulmonary tumor in rabbits. The Journal of surgical research 2001; 99(2):265–71.

38 Bojarski JD, Dupuy DE, Mayo-Smith WW. CT imaging findings of pulmonary neoplasms after treatment with radiofrequency ablation: results in 32 tumors. AJR 2005; 185(2):466 71.

39 Steinke K, King J, Glenn D, Morris DL. Radiologic appearance and complications of percutaneous computed tomography-guided radiofrequency-ablated pulmonary metastases from colorectal carcinoma. J Comput Assist Tomogr 2003; 27(5):750–7.

40 Lee JM, Jin GY, Li CA, et al. Percutaneous radiofrequency thermal ablation of lung VX2 tumors in a rabbit model using a cooled tip-electrode: feasibility, safety, and effectiveness. Invest Radiol 2003; 38(2): 129–39.

41 Ahrar K, Price RE, Wallace MJ, et al. Percutaneous radiofrequency ablation of lung tumors in a large animal model. J Vasc Interv Radiol 2003; 14(8):1037–43.

42 Nguyen CL, Scott WJ, Young NA, Rader T, Giles LR, Goldberg M. Radiofrequency ablation of primary lung cancer: results from an ablate and resect pilot study. Chest 2005; 128(5):3507–11.

43 Ambrogi MC, Fontanini G, Cioni R, Faviana P, Fanucchi O, Mussi A. Biologic effects of radiofrequency thermal ablation on non–small cell lung cancer: results of a pilot study. J Thorac Cardiovas Surg 2006; 131(5): 1002–6.

44 Hataji O, Yamakado K, Nakatsuka A, et al. Radiological and pathological correlation of lung malignant tumors treated with percutaneous radiofrequency ablation. Intern Med (Tokyo, Japan) 2005; 44(8):865–9.

45 Yasui K, Kanazawa S, Sano Y, et al. Thoracic tumors treated with CT-guided radiofrequency ablation: initial experience. Radiology 2004; 231(3):850–7.

46 Hiraki T, Tajiri N, Mimura H, et al. Pneumothorax, pleural effusion, and chest tube placement after radiofrequency ablation of lung tumors: incidence and risk factors. Radiology 2006; 241(1):275–83.

47 Jin GY, Lee JM, Lee YC, Han YM, Lim YS. Primary and secondary lung malignancies treated with percutaneous radiofrequency ablation: evaluation with follow-up helical CT. AJR 2004; 183(4):1013–20.

48 Suh RD, Wallace AB, Sheehan RE, Heinze SB, Goldin JG. Unresectable pulmonary malignancies: CT-guided percutaneous radiofrequency ablation—preliminary results. Radiology 2003; 229(3):821–9.

49 Lee JM, Jin GY, Goldberg SN, et al. Percutaneous radiofrequency ablation for inoperable non–small cell lung cancer and metastases: preliminary report. Radiology 2004; 230(1):125–34.

50 Gadaleta C, Catino A, Ranieri G, et al. Radiofrequency thermal ablation of 69 lung neoplasms. J Chemother 2004; 16 Suppl 5:86–9.

51 Belfiore G, Moggio G, Tedeschi E, et al. CT-guided radiofrequency ablation: a potential complementary therapy for patients with unresectable primary lung cancer—a preliminary report of 33 patients. AJR 2004; 183(4):1003–11.

52 Ambrogi MC, Lucchi M, Dini P, et al. Percutaneous radiofrequency ablation of lung tumours: results in the mid-term. Eur J Cardiothorac Surg 2006; 30(1):177–83.

53 VanSonnenberg E, Shankar S, Morrison PR, et al. Radiofrequency ablation of thoracic lesions: part 2, initial clinical experience—technical and multidisciplinary considerations in 30 patients. AJR 2005; 184(2):381–90.

54 Rossi S, Dore R, Cascina A, et al. Percutaneous computed tomography-guided radiofrequency thermal ablation of small unresectable lung tumours. Eur Respir J 2006; 27(3):556–63.

55 Akeboshi M, Yamakado K, Nakatsuka A, et al. Percutaneous radiofrequency ablation of lung neoplasms: initial therapeutic response. J Vasc Interv Radiol 2004; 15(5):463–70.

56 Fernando HC, De Hoyos A, Landreneau RJ, et al. Radiofrequency ablation for the treatment of non–small cell lung cancer in marginal surgical candidates. J Thorac Cardiovas Surg 2005; 129(3):639–44.

57 Herrera LJ, Fernando HC, Perry Y, et al. Radiofrequency ablation of pulmonary malignant tumors in nonsurgical candidates. J Thorac Cardiovas Surg 2003; 125(4):929–37.

58 Dupuy DE, Mayo-Smith WW, Abbott GF, DiPetrillo T. Clinical applications of radio-frequency tumor ablation in the thorax. Radiographics 2002; 22 Spec No:S259–69.

59 Vaughn C, Mychaskiw G, 2nd, Sewell P. Massive hemorrhage during radiofrequency ablation of a pulmonary neoplasm. Anesth Analg 2002; 94(5):1149–51; table of contents.

60 Hayes DL, Charboneau JW, Lewis BD, Asirvatham SJ, Dupuy DE, Lexvold NY. Radiofrequency treatment of hepatic neoplasms in patients with permanent pacemakers. Mayo Clin Proc 2001; 76(9):950–2.

61 Elliott BA, Curry TB, Atwell TD, Brown MJ, Rose SH. Lung isolation, one-lung ventilation, and continuous positive airway pressure with air for radiofrequency ablation of neoplastic pulmonary lesions. Anesth Analg 2006; 103(2):463–4, table of contents.

62 Gadaleta C, Mattioli V, Colucci G, et al. Radiofrequency ablation of 40 lung neoplasms: preliminary results. AJR 2004; 183(2):361–8.

63 Ko JP, Shepard JO, Drucker EA, et al. Factors influencing pneumothorax rate at lung biopsy: are dwell time and angle of pleural puncture contributing factors? Radiology 2001; 218(2):491–6.
64 Steinke K, Gananadha S, King J, Zhao J, Morris DL. Dispersive pad site burns with modern radiofrequency ablation equipment. Surg Laparosc Endosc Percutan Tech 2003; 13(6):366–71.
65 Steinke K, King J, Glenn DW, Morris DL. Percutaneous radiofrequency ablation of lung tumors with expandable needle electrodes: tips from preliminary experience. AJR 2004; 183(3):605–11.
66 Steinke K, King J, Glenn D, Morris DL. Percutaneous radiofrequency ablation of lung tumors: difficulty withdrawing the hooks resulting in a split needle. Cardiovasc Intervent Radiol 2003; 26(6):583–5.
67 Yamagami T, Kato T, Hirota T, Yoshimatsu R, Matsumoto T, Nishimura T. Pneumothorax as a complication of percutaneous radiofrequency ablation for lung neoplasms. J Vasc Interv Radiol 2006; 17 (10):1625–9.
68 Radvany MG, Allan PF, Frey WC, Banks KP, Malave D. Pulmonary radiofrequency ablation complicated by subcutaneous emphysema and pneumomediastinum treated with fibrin sealant injection. AJR 2005; 185 (4):894–8.
69 Ghaye B, Bruyere PJ, Dondelinger RF. Nonfatal systemic air embolism during percutaneous radiofrequency ablation of a pulmonary metastasis. AJR 2006; 187(3):W327–8.
70 Marchand B, Perol M, De La Roche E, et al. Percutaneous radiofrequency ablation of a lung metastasis: delayed cavitation with no infection. J Comput Assist Tomogr 2002; 26(6):1032–4.
71 Swensen SJ, Viggiano RW, Midthun DE, et al. Lung nodule enhancement at CT: multicenter study. Radiology 2000; 214(1):73–80.
72 Berber E, Foroutani A, Garland AM, et al. Use of CT Hounsfield unit density to identify ablated tumor after laparoscopic radiofrequency ablation of hepatic tumors. Surg Endosc 2000; 14(9):799–804.
73 Okuma T, Matsuoka T, Okamura T, et al. 18F-FDG small-animal PET for monitoring the therapeutic effect of CT-guided radiofrequency ablation on implanted VX2 lung tumors in rabbits. J Nucl Med 2006; 47 (8):1351–8.
74 Okuma T, Okamura T, Matsuoka T, et al. Fluorine-18-fluorodeoxyglucose positron emission tomography for assessment of patients with unresectable recurrent or metastatic lung cancers after CT-guided radiofrequency ablation: preliminary results. Ann Nucl Med 2006; 20 (2):115–21.
75 Avril N. 18F-FDG PET after radiofrequency ablation: Is timing everything? J Nucl Med 2006; 47(8):1235–7.
76 Yan TD, King J, Sjarif A, Glenn D, Steinke K, Morris DL. Percutaneous radiofrequency ablation of pulmonary metastases from colorectal carcinoma: prognostic determinants for survival. Ann Surg Oncol 2006; 13(11): 1529–37.
77 Steinke K, Glenn D, King J, Morris DL. Percutaneous pulmonary radiofrequency ablation: difficulty achieving complete ablations in big lung lesions. Br J Radiol 2003; 76(910):742–5.
78 Hiraki T, Sakurai J, Tsuda T, et al. Risk factors for local progression after percutaneous radiofrequency ablation of lung tumors: evaluation based on a preliminary review of 342 tumors. Cancer 2006; 107(12):2873–80.
79 Grieco CA, Simon CJ, Mayo-Smith WW, DiPetrillo TA, Ready NE, Dupuy DE. Percutaneous image-guided thermal ablation and radiation therapy: outcomes of combined treatment for 41 patients with inoperable stage I/II non–small-cell lung cancer. J Vasc Interv Radiol 2006; 17(7):1117–24.
80 Jain SK, Dupuy DE, Cardarelli GA, Zheng Z, DiPetrillo TA. Percutaneous radiofrequency ablation of pulmonary malignancies: combined treatment with brachytherapy. AJR 2003; 181(3):711–5.
81 Dupuy DE, DiPetrillo T, Gandhi S, et al. Radiofrequency ablation followed by conventional radiotherapy for medically inoperable stage I non–small cell lung cancer. Chest 2006; 129(3):738–45.
82 Fukuse T, Ogawa E, Chen F, Sakai H, Wada H. Limited surgery and radiofrequency ablation for recurrent lung cancer. Ann Thorac Surg 2006; 82(4):1506–8.
83 Simon CJ, Dupuy DE, Mayo-Smith WW. Microwave ablation: principles and applications. Radiographics 2005; 25 Suppl 1:S69–83.
84 He W, Hu XD, Wu DF, et al. Ultrasonography-guided percutaneous microwave ablation of peripheral lung cancer. Clin Imag 2006; 30(4):234–41.
85 Ahmed A, Littrup P. Percutaneous cryotherapy of the thorax: safety considerations for complex cases. AJR 2006; 186(6):1703–6.
86 Wang H, Littrup PJ, Duan Y, Zhang Y, Feng H, Nie Z. Thoracic masses treated with percutaneous cryotherapy: initial experience with more than 200 procedures. Radiology 2005; 235(1):289–98.
87 Kawamura M, Izumi Y, Tsukada N, et al. Percutaneous cryoablation of small pulmonary malignant tumors under computed tomographic guidance with local anesthesia for nonsurgical candidates. J Thorac Cardiovas Surg 2006; 131(5):1007–13.
88 Izumi Y, Oyama T, Ikeda E, Kawamura M, Kobayashi K. The acute effects of transthoracic cryoablation on normal lung evaluated in a porcine model. Ann Thorac Surg 2005; 79(1):318–22; discussion 22.
89 Weigel C, Rosenberg C, Langner S, Frohlich CP, Hosten N. Laser ablation of lung metastases: results according to diameter and location. Eur Radiol 2006; 16 (8):1769–78.
90 Goldberg SN, Grassi CJ, Cardella JF, et al. Image-guided tumor ablation: standardization of terminology and reporting criteria. J Vasc Interv Radiol 2005; 16(6): 765–78.

6

Cardiac CT and MRI: State of the Art

Charles S. White
Department of Diagnostic Radiology, University of Maryland Medical Center, Baltimore, Maryland, U.S.A.

INTRODUCTION

The coronary arteries are difficult to image noninvasively because of the small size of even the larger vessels (2–4 mm), the tortuous course of the vessels along the epicardial surface, and physiologic movement related to cardiac and respiratory motion. Excellent temporal resolution is required for high-quality images of the coronary arteries and to assess indices of left ventricular function such as ejection fraction and wall motion. Whereas diagnostic invasive coronary angiography has reached a high state of development over the past three decades, noninvasive coronary imaging has progressed more slowly.

Most initial work with noninvasive coronary assessment was performed with electron beam tomography (EBT). Developed in the early 1980s, the EBT configuration has no moving parts and thus permits temporal resolution of approximately 100 ms (1). EBT has proved valuable in the evaluation of coronary calcium burden, but its inferior spatial resolution and moderate image noise have prevented its widespread adoption for detailed delineation of the coronary arteries.

Dual-slice helical CT first became available in 1992, but it was the development and widespread commercial dissemination of quad-slice multidetector CT (MDCT) with ECG-gating beginning in 1998 that signaled a focused effort to evaluate the coronary arteries noninvasively. The current generation of MDCT provides 64 slices per rotation, a spatial resolution of 0.625 mm or less in the *z*-axis, and a temporal resolution of 50–200 ms (2). These advances make possible routine visualization and characterization of the coronary tree using coronary CT angiography (CTA). This chapter focuses on issues of technique and patient preparation related to acquisition of cardiac CT, and the use of cardiac CT to perform calcium scoring, to assess the coronary arteries, and to evaluate non-coronary cardiac structures.

TECHNIQUE AND PATIENT PREPARATION

Protocols for cardiac CT acquisition differ from other MDCT protocols because of the requirement for ECG-gating (2,3). With ECG-gating, electrodes are attached to the patient and a waveform is generated. Specialized software detects the R wave of the ECG tracing, the most prominent rise in the tracing. As data are acquired, they can be sorted into their respective portions of the cardiac cycle based on elapsed time since the previous R wave, effectively freezing physiologic motion of the heart. The R–R interval refers to the duration between one R wave and the next, and intermediate times are designated as a percentage of the R–R interval (0–100%). The early part of the R wave from 0% to 40% corresponds roughly to systole and the later part corresponds to diastole. The precise distinction depends on multiple factors such as patient heart rate and physiologic status, and the lag between the electrical onset (R wave) and mechanical onset (left ventricular contraction) of systole.

Two types of ECG-gating or triggering are commonly used, prospective and retrospective. In prospective gating, imaging is performed at a single preselected interval after the R wave, usually in mid-diastole (approximately 60–75%). The major advantage of prospective ECG-gating is a reduction in radiation dose due to limitation of the acquisition to diastole. Substantial disadvantages include the inabi. lity to select other parts of the cardiac cycle if image quality of the coronary arteries is suboptimal, inability to assess left ventricular function because of the absence of other parts of the cardiac cycle, and susceptibility to ectopic beats such as premature ventricular contractions. In practice, prospective gating is applied mainly to calcium scoring of the coronary arteries because complete cessation of coronary artery motion is not as crucial for this indication as it is for assessment of coronary artery stenosis.

The second major type of ECG-triggering is retrospective gating. With this approach, imaging is performed throughout the cardiac cycle and image reconstruction can take place at any point in the cardiac cycle. Typically, images are reconstructed at each 10% increment of the cardiac cycle, generating 10 evenly spaced phases from 0% to 100% (3). Some centers use 10 phases beginning at 5%. Such complete coverage of the cardiac cycle permits selection of the optimal phase for analysis of the coronary arteries following coronary CTA, calculation of left ventricular ejection fraction based on end-diastolic and end-systolic images, and assessment of ventricular wall motion in a cine movie loop.

The major disadvantage of retrospective ECG-gating is the high radiation exposure to the patient, which may be fourfold or more than that of annual background radiation or approximately 15 mSv (4). Commercial vendors have introduced dose modulation as a method of reducing exposure. With dose modulation, the current is substantially reduced during the part of the cardiac cycle least important for coronary artery imaging, typically systole. Dose modulation may decrease radiation exposure by as much as 40% (5).

Coronary CTA is best performed in patients with a slow heart rate, ideally less than 65 beats per minute. As heart rate increases, the R–R interval decreases and diastole is disproportionately shortened. Optimal coronary images are typically obtained during diastole, when there is relatively little cardiac motion. Although diagnostic images are achievable at higher heart rates, particularly with improved temporal resolution of recent generation CT scanners, the shorter duration of diastole increases the likelihood of motion artifacts that degrade the image quality of the coronary arteries.

Pharmacologic intervention is often used to decrease the heart rate to acceptable levels. Most commonly, the beta-blocker metoprolol is administered. Metoprolol can be given by mouth or intravenously, and repeat doses can be used depending on heart rate response (3). In general, metoprolol is a safe drug; however, it should not be used in patients with clinically significant asthma or known or suspected heart block. Other beta-blockers and anxiolytics such as valium are sometimes used to reduce heart rate. Recently, many centers have begun to use sublingual nitroglycerin, a coronary vasodilator, immediately prior to scanning. The use of nitroglycerin is thought to improve image quality without affecting diagnostic accuracy.

Another important component of a successful cardiac CTA is the method of contrast injection. In general, a high osmolar contrast agent is preferred and a rapid infusion is recommended. Prior to injection, it is critical to assure that the central venous line is correctly positioned within the vein to prevent extravasation, as with any contrast injection. This is usually accomplished with a test injection of saline. Proper timing of the injection is achieved in one of two ways. In the first approach, a test injection using a small amount of intravenous contrast material is administered with a region of interest placed over the aorta and a time-contrast curve is plotted. The delay from injection to initiation of scanning is set manually based on the peak or upslope of this curve plus an additional delay of several seconds. In the second approach, a region of interest is placed over the ascending or descending aorta and the full contrast is tracked through the region in an automated fashion. Scanning is triggered when enhancement in the region of interest reaches a predetermined threshold, often set around 150 HU. With this latter technique it is critical that the region of interest be placed properly or the scan will not automatically initiate. The CT technologists should be trained to follow the time-contrast curve and should be prepared to initiate the scan manually if a problem arises.

There are multiple approaches to the particulars of contrast injection (3). In some cases this is dependent on the type of injector that is used. If a dual-head injector is available, contrast can be administered followed by saline, which is sometimes termed a biphasic injection. The purpose of saline use is to maximize contrast use by washing contrast in from the peripheral veins and to minimize opacification in the right heart. Too much right heart opacification may create streak artifacts that interfere with visualization of the right coronary system. It is possible to completely wash out contrast from the right heart. Some consider this to be undesirable because of the loss of right heart landmarks. Another option available on some injectors is to inject a combination of contrast and saline for a portion of the injection. This triple injection of pure contrast, followed by a mixture of contrast and saline, concluding with a saline flush is often termed a triphasic injection. The dual-head injection protocol used at University of Maryland is listed in Table 1. If only a single-head injector is available, a saline flush can be performed by layering the saline immediately atop the contrast in the injector.

A coronary CTA scan is typically obtained from a cranial to caudal direction. Since cessation of respiration is extremely important, we have adopted an approach where the technologists instruct the patient simply to stop breathing as the scanning starts. Presumably this leads to maintenance of breath-holding at the most comfortable part of the cardiac cycle, rather than doing preparatory breaths or using machine instructions that in our previous experience have caused confusion and breathing artifacts.

Table 1 Injection Protocol—Coronary CTA

Test injection—20 mL at 6 cc/s
Injection protocol
80 mL (100% contrast) at 6 cc/s
then
40 mL (50%/50%) at 5 cc/s
then
50 mL (saline) at 5 cc/s
Automated bolus tracking

Our protocol for coronary CTA is included in Table 2. The protocol should be modified for certain indications. For bypass graft assessment, the scan should extend to the take-off the internal mammary arteries if they are used as grafts. This may necessitate scanning in a caudal–cranial direction to ensure that the heart is imaged during suspension of breathing. A similar consideration applies to the global assessment or triple rule-out protocol (defined as the triple rule-out of coronary artery disease, pulmonary embolism, and aortic dissection in a single examination) used in the emergency department in which a wider field of view is also used. For some extracoronary cardiac indications, the use of thicker reconstruction sections is acceptable. Examples include CTA prior to radiofrequency ablation of the left atrium and assessment of valve morphology or left ventricular function.

IMAGE POST-PROCESSING

The reconstructed images of the axial dataset are typically post-processed using an independent workstation with dedicated software (3). Curved planar images in the plane of each of the coronary artery typically are generated (Fig. 1). These reformatted images are analyzed for calcified or non-calcified plaque as well as for areas of luminal stenosis. Luminal stenosis is measured using dedicated software on the workstation, freehand using digital calipers by the interpreting physician, or by visual estimation. Curved planar reconstructions can provide an accurate assessment of coronary artery status but are subject to error due to malposition of the centerline used to reconstruct the images. Thus, it is imperative that the interpreting physician view the dataset, including the reconstructed axial images, in an interactive manner. The interactive evaluation may also include cross-sectional or longitudinal views of the coronary arteries with thin maximum-intensity-projection images. Volumetric images may occasionally prove valuable to show the three-dimensional orientation and relationship of the coronary arteries to the remainder of the cardiac anatomy (Fig. 2).

Table 2 CTA Scanning Protocol

Parameter	Coronary CTA (64-slice)
KV	120
MA	>500
FOV (mm)	250
Collimation (mm)	0.625
Reconstruction (mm)	0.675
Direction	Cranial–caudal
Time (s)	8

Abbreviations: FOV, field of view; KV, kilovoltage; MA, milliamperage.

Setting Up a Service

A cardiac CT service can take several forms, involving radiologists, cardiologists, or a combination of these. Both the American College of Radiology and the American College of Cardiology have developed credentialing guidelines for individual practitioners (6,7). There are several types of single specialty and hybrid arrangements. It is important to recognize that Medicare will not reimburse more than one physician per study. Thus, shared reading arrangements between specialties should be reviewed carefully so as not to run afoul of relevant legal regulations (8).

Because of the time required for post-processing, many practices have employed an individual with specific training in the use of the more sophisticated tools required to perform post-processing. A background and familiarity with CT is a useful prerequisite. Therefore, many post-processing technologists are former or part-time CT technologists.

Marketing of the cardiac CT practice is essential. In addition to providing printed material, members of the cardiac CT team should present lectures to potential referrers. Such potential referrers include not only cardiologists, but also internists, family physicians, surgeons, and other practitioners.

Reimbursement by third-party insurance carriers of cardiac CT examinations currently is sporadic. Medicare has developed billing codes for various cardiac studies but these are considered investigational and are not yet uniformly reimbursed. Several societies recently published a joint consensus document outlining indications for cardiac CT (9). It remains to be seen which of these indications will receive payment by insurers.

CARDIAC CT APPLICATIONS

Calcium Scoring

Calcium scoring has been used for nearly two decades to provide a quantitative assessment of subclinical atherosclerotic coronary artery disease. Whereas traditional factors, such as age, hypertension, diabetes, smoking, and hypercholesterolemia, are valuable to assess risk in coronary artery disease, unlike

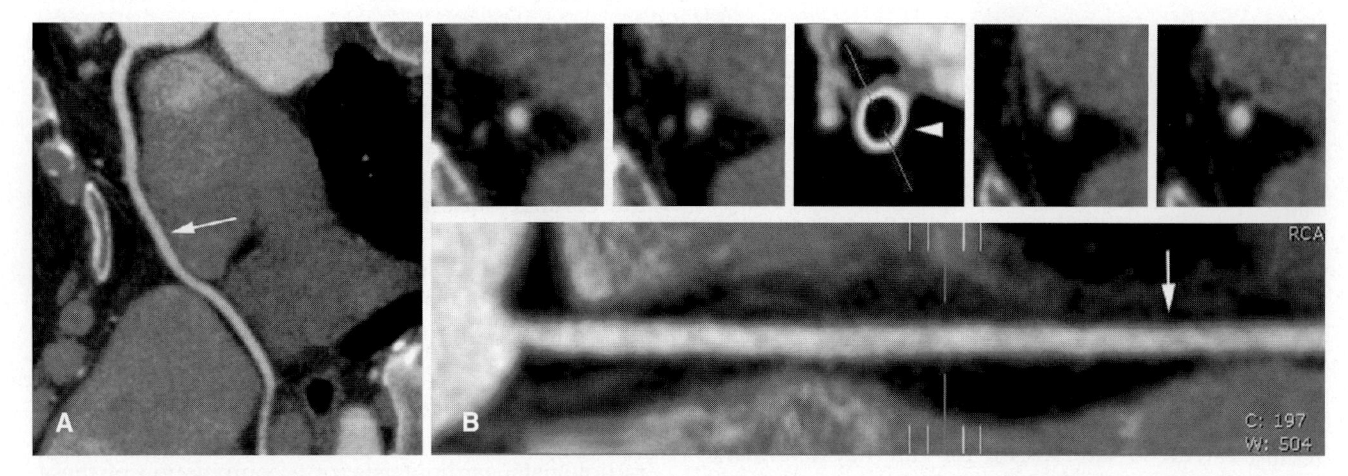

Figure 1 52-year-old woman with chest pain. (**A**) Curved planar reconstruction from a coronary CTA demonstrates no evidence of coronary artery disease. (**B**) Straightened coronary artery view allows measure of caliber along the length of the artery (*arrow*). Cross-sectional view (*arrowhead*) shows the arterial wall and lumen in a projection similar to intravascular ultrasound.

coronary calcification, they do not provide direct visualization of the status of the coronary arteries (10). Coronary calcified plaque is a marker of the total atherosclerotic plaque burden. There is a strong association between the amount of coronary calcification and likelihood of significant stenosis, but this relationship is not linear (11). From histological studies, it is estimated that calcified plaque accounts for only about 20% of total plaque burden (12). Thus, significant plaque and, uncommonly, stenosis can occur in the absence of visible calcification, and, conversely, stenoses may be absent in the presence of extensive calcification (13).

Much of the investigative work on calcium scoring has been reported with EBT. The most widely used quantitative method of assessing coronary calcium is the Agatston score. This score represents the product of the number of pixels with calcification and the density weighting of the calcification on a sliding scale (14). A threshold of 130 HU is used to designate calcification (Fig. 3). The Agatston score is calculated by means of standard software and results are normalized for age and gender with a percentile rank generated based on a large database. The Agatston score remains in wide use because of its incorporation in multiple large population-based studies (15).

With the nearly complete replacement of EBT by MDCT, considerable interest has focused on scoring methods that take into account the volumetric characteristics of the latter technique. Much interest has centered on whether MDCT provides as accurate and reproducible calcium score as EBT (16). A recent critical analysis of the literature suggests that MDCT correlates well with EBT, except possibly at low levels of coronary calcium. Two newer measurements, calcium volume and calcium mass, better account for volumetric characteristics and thus may provide more reproducible calcium scores among different scanners (17).

It is also important to review the non-cardiac portions of the images, including the mediastinum, lungs, and bony structures. Several studies have demonstrated a substantial rate of incidental findings (5–10%) in patients who undergo calcium scoring studies (18,19).

Coronary Artery Evaluation

Coronary artery assessment using CTA is often performed in the outpatient setting in patients with atypical chest pain who have risk factors for coronary artery disease. In addition, patients who have an equivocal stress testing also may be referred for evaluation.

Reliable coronary artery visualization is increasingly being achieved with the latest generation of CT scanners. In general, images reconstructed between 40% and 90% of the R–R interval are used for interpretation based on visual inspection. The optimal phase for right and left coronary arteries visualization frequently differ and there is no consistent phase at which the coronaries are best visualized. As described above, coronary artery images may be viewed using curved planar, thin slab maximum intensity projection or volumetric techniques (Fig. 4). Automated software permits extraction of the coronary arteries and assessment of the extent of coronary artery stenosis using a preselected reference point.

Multiple studies have assessed the diagnostic accuracy of coronary CTA in comparison to coronary angiography. Studies performed using a 4-slice CT scanner showed sensitivity and specificity values of 80–95% but had a high number of non-evaluable segments (up to 28%) (20–22). With 64-slice CT scanners, the number of nonevaluable segments has decreased, with continued high sensitivity. Nearly all of these studies were performed at a single site (23–25). Only one multicenter trial has been reported (26). This study used 16-slice CT scanners and included 187

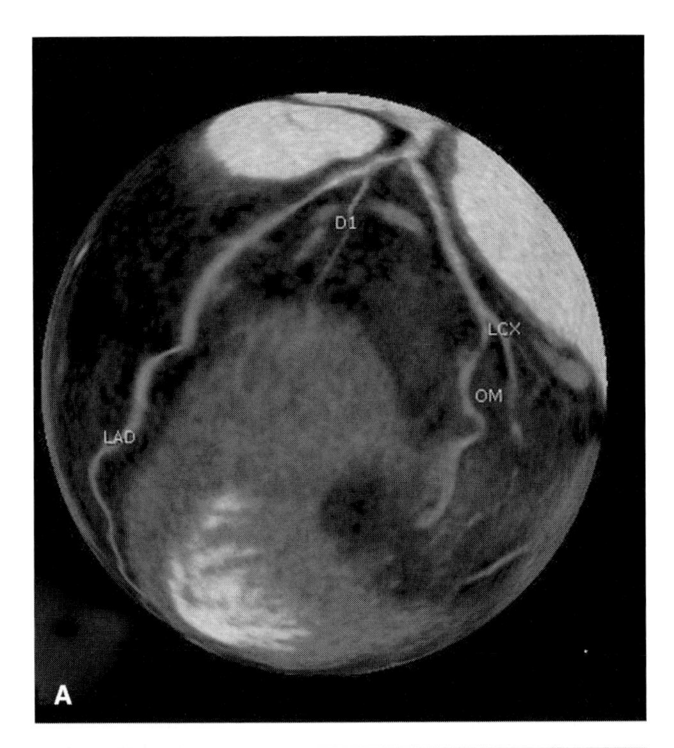

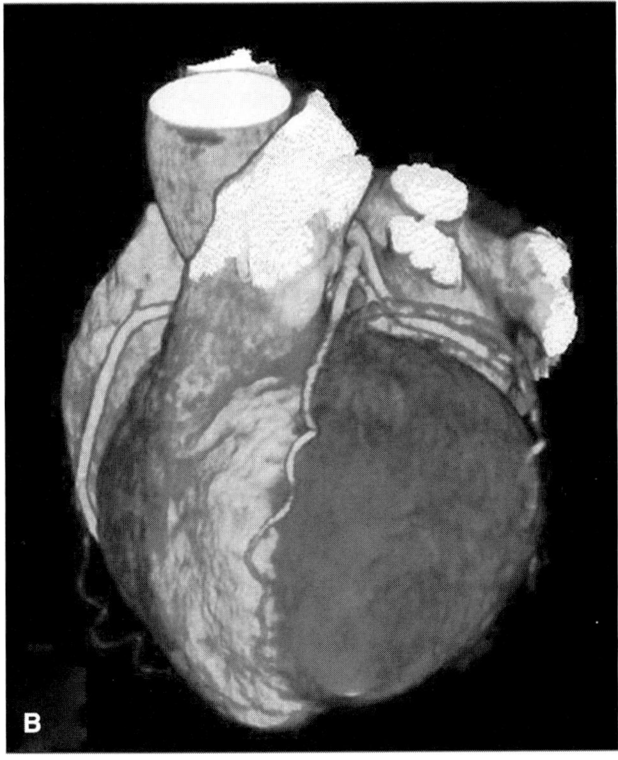

Figure 2 48-year-old man with atypical chest pain. (**A**) Globe rendering from a normal coronary artery study. (**B**) Volumetric rendering from a normal coronary artery study. (*See color insert for* **B**.)

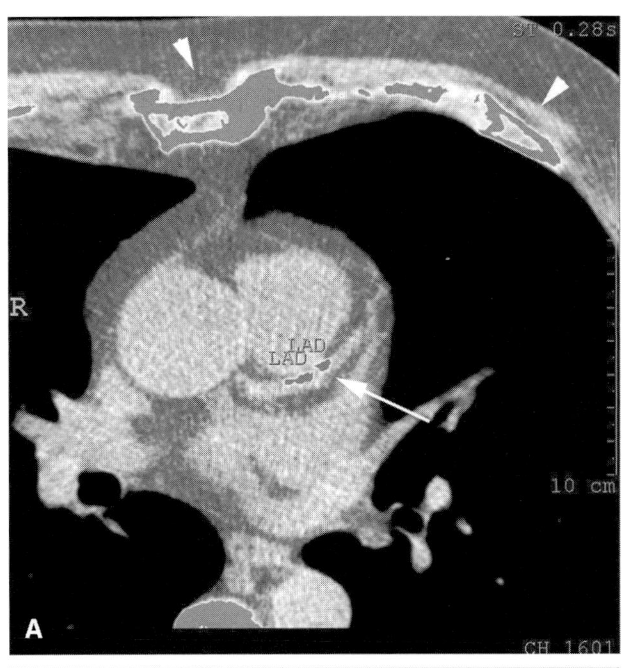

	ROI#	AreaSq.	Score	Score CDI	Mass*	Mass CDI
L.MAIN	0	0.0	0.0	0.0	0.0	0.0
LAD	2	31.5	104.8	52.4	19.4	9.7
CRX	0	0.0	0.0	0.0	0.0	0.0
RCA	0	0.0	0.0	0.0	0.0	0.0
PDA	0	0.0	0.0	0.0	0.0	0.0
Total	2	31.5	104.8	52.4	19.4	9.7

B

Figure 3 60-year-old man who underwent coronary calcium scoring as part of a clinical study. (**A**) The calcium scoring software in this unenhanced, prospectively ECG-gated, cardiac CT automatically highlights areas with Hounsfield Unit values greater than 130 with pink shading (*arrowheads*). The operator circles highlighted areas corresponding to the coronary artery, which are then re-shaded blue (*arrow*). (**B**) Agatston score, here listed under the column Score, as well as the column Mass*. (*See color insert for* **A**.)

patients from 11 sites with varying levels of experience in the performance of coronary CTA. The authors found a patient-based sensitivity of 98% and a specificity of 54%. Although the study used technology that is now outdated, the results suggest that there will be greater variability in outcomes as coronary CTA becomes more widely disseminated. An important additional consideration in assessing coronary CTA is that the use of invasive coronary angiography may not be an appropriate standard of reference. This may have adversely affected the results of these studies because catheter-based angiography assesses only the lumen and may under- or overestimate the true extent of coronary artery stenosis.

The ability of coronary CTA to detect both calcified and non-calcified plaque suggests that it may have a role in noninvasive detection of plaque

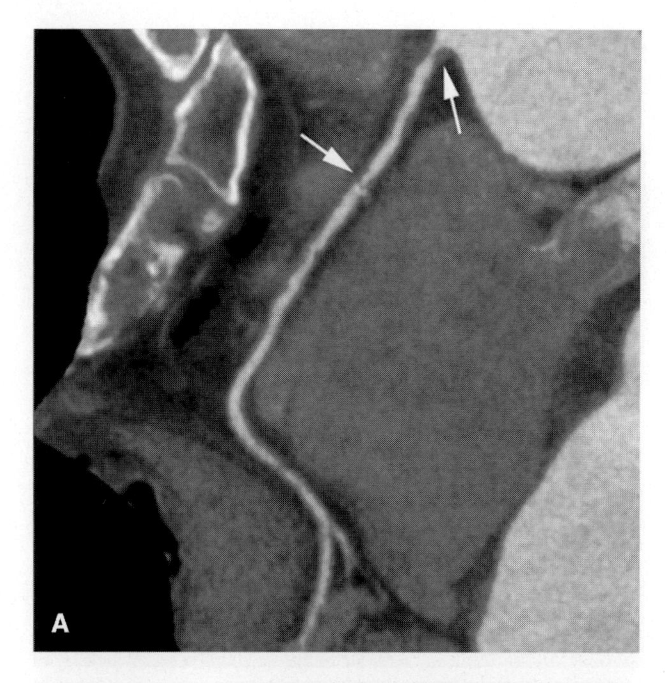

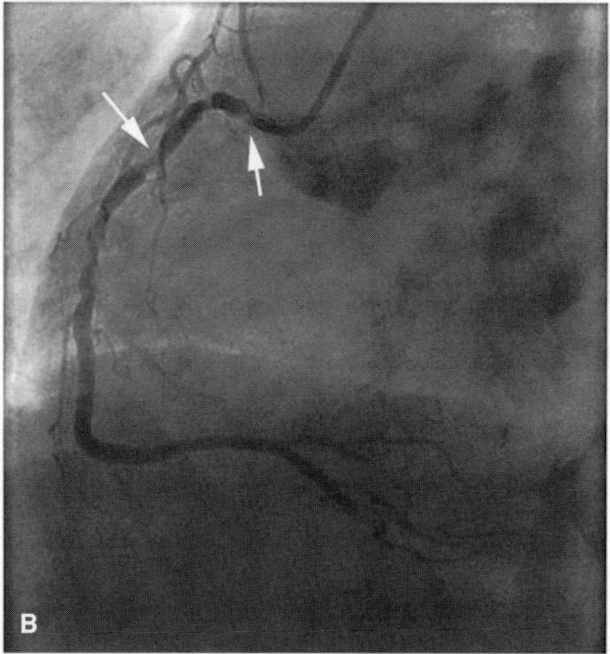

Figure 4 83-year-old man with chest pain. (**A**) Curved planar reconstructed image of the right coronary artery from a coronary CTA demonstrates multiple areas of proximal stenosis (*arrows*). (**B**) Coronary angiogram with injection of the right coronary artery shows similar areas of stenosis (*arrows*).

that is at risk for rupture, so-called vulnerable plaque. The concept of vulnerable plaque is not fully defined but is thought to consist of fatty components with a thin fibrous covering. Thrombosis formed from vulnerable plaque rupture may lead to occlusive coronary disease and myocardial infarction, even in patients with less than 50% coronary artery stenosis prior to plaque rupture. Although it is clear that CT can detect and to some extent characterize non-calcified plaque, it is less certain that it can distinguish vulnerable plaque from stable non-calcified plaque (27).

Another compelling indication for coronary CTA is the detection of coronary anomalies. Coronary artery anomalies occur in approximately 1% of patients and are the second leading cause of structural cardiac death in young athletes (28). Anomalies range from minor variations in coronary take-off to significant abnormalities of coronary course. The most dangerous adult anomaly is one in which a left or right anomalous coronary artery arises from the contralateral sinus of Valsalva and courses between the aorta and pulmonary artery to reach its standard distribution. This configuration may cause sudden death due to ischemia resulting from ostial stenosis due to a small, kinked, or angulated coronary orifice. Surgery is often recommended in these patients. In contrast, anomalous vessels that course anterior to the pulmonary artery or posterior to the aorta are nearly always benign (Fig. 5) (29).

Most anomalies are discovered using catheter-based angiography. The majority of coronary variants are readily dismissed as benign but anomalies of course may be problematic to assess due to difficulty in establishing their relationship with the unopacified great vessels. Coronary CTA provides precise and reliable delineation of the take-off of the affected coronary artery and its course in relation to the great vessels (30). Coronary CTA also provides excellent depiction of coronary artery aneurysms caused by atherosclerosis, Kawasakis disease, and other etiologies (Fig. 6) (31).

Cardiac CT is also useful to assess the patency of coronary artery bypass grafts. The most common types of grafts are internal mammary artery and saphenous vein grafts. Internal mammary grafts have a better long-term patency and are generally used to bypass the left anterior descending artery, which provides blood to the anterior-apical portion of the left ventricle. Saphenous vein grafts are typically used to bypass other branches of the coronary artery circulation, such as diagonal, obtuse marginal, and posterior descending arteries (32).

CT angiography readily depicts bypass grafts (33). In general, saphenous vein grafts are larger in caliber than internal mammary grafts. Occlusion of grafts is recognized as absence of flow in the affected graft. Stenosis can also be detected as luminal narrowing and plaque in the affected graft. The distal graft anastamosis is the most difficult portion of the graft to evaluate. Sensitivity and specificity of 95–100% for detection of occlusion has been reported using 16-slice CT, with somewhat lower rates for detection of stenosis (34,35).

Coronary CTA also may be used to assess stent patency with variable accuracy due to interference by

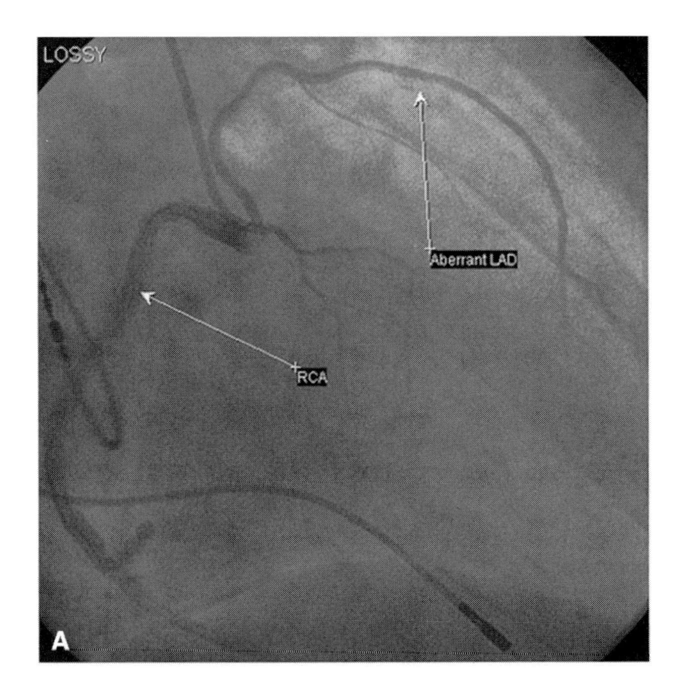

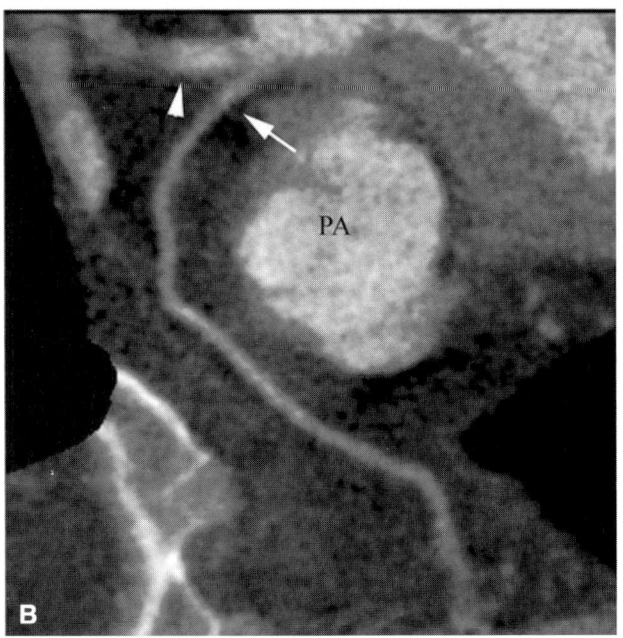

Figure 5 59-year-old woman with a coronary artery anomaly found on invasive angiography. (**A**) Coronary angiogram shows an anomalous left coronary artery (LAD) arising from or adjacent to the origin of the right coronary artery (RCA). (**B**) Curved planar reformatted image from coronary CTA shows common origin of the right coronary (*arrowhead*) and anomalous left anterior descending arteries (*arrow*) with passage of the anomalous vessel anterior to the pulmonary artery (PA), a nonmalignant configuration.

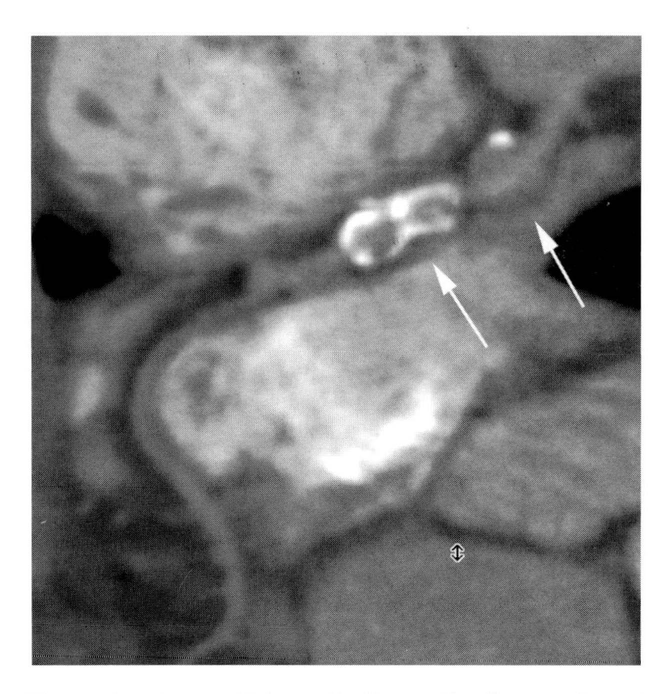

Figure 6 10-year-old boy with Kawasakis disease. Curved planar reformatted image from coronary CTA shows two proximal coronary aneurysms (*arrows*), with substantial calcification of the more distal aneurysm.

the metallic struts of the stent (36). The best results are achieved with large stents, particularly those 3.5 mm or greater in diameter (37). Use of a sharp reconstruction kernel and adjustment of window/level settings to decrease the intensity of strut artifacts are necessary for optimal interpretation (36). Thrombosis within the stent is often identified by lack of contrast within its lumen (Fig. 7). Absence of flow distal to the stent is an indication of stent occlusion, although the presence of distal flow, which may be due to collateral sources, suggests but does not ensure stent patency.

Chest Pain in the Emergency Department

Approximately 6 million patients present to the emergency department (ED) annually with chest pain. In many, the cause remains undetermined after initial evaluation with history and physical, electrocardiography, and cardiac enzymes. In this indeterminate group, further evaluation is often undertaken with radionuclide stress testing or echocardiography. While often permitting a diagnosis, these techniques are limited by a comparatively lengthy time needed to obtain the test. Thus, patients may remain in the ED for 12 or more hours awaiting disposition. Many who are admitted ultimately prove not to have a cardiac etiology of chest pain.

The improvements in MDCT technology and the increasing installation of scanners in or near the ED suite have led to suggestions that MDCT may have a role in evaluating the ED patient with chest pain. The two protocol approaches that have been recommended are dedicated coronary CTA and comprehensive or triple rule-out CTA. The latter approach may be used if the suspected cause of chest pain is not limited to the coronary arteries. The triple rule-out refers to the assessment of coronary artery disease, pulmonary embolism, and aortic dissection in a single examination. It consists of an ECG-gated protocol that

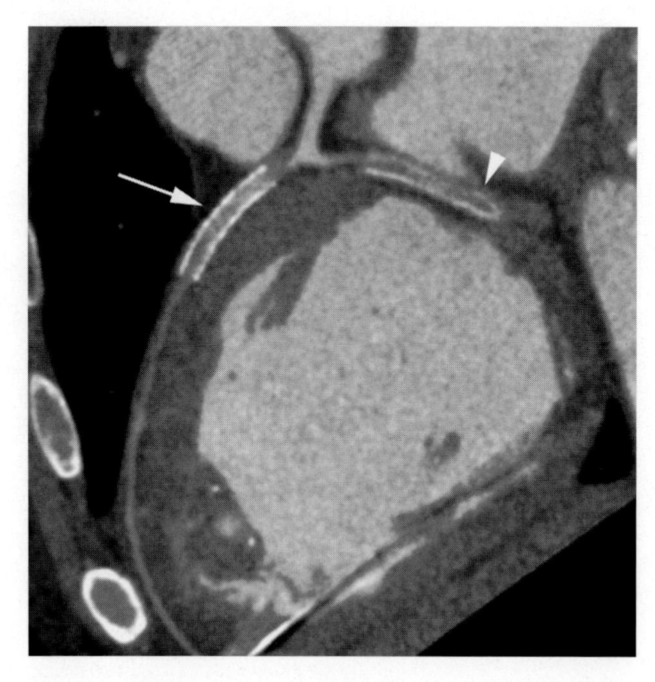

Figure 7 56-year-old man with chest pain and multiple stents. Curved planar reformatted image from coronary CTA demonstrates stents in the left anterior descending (*arrow*) and left circumflex arteries (*arrowhead*). The circumflex stent is occluded as shown by thrombus within its lumen and absence of distal flow. The contrast distal to the anterior descending stent suggests that this stent is patent.

represents a compromise between a dedicated coronary CTA and non-gated pulmonary embolism study. Because of the time required for the scan, the triple rule out is best performed using at least a 64-slice scanner.

Early results suggest a role for MDCT in evaluation of ED patients with chest pain who are considered to be at low to intermediate risk for serious coronary disease, potentially decreasing the number who require admission (38,39). However, considerable uncertainty remains, including the extent of increased CT volume and its economic impact, radiation concerns, and labor and technical issues that may affect turnaround time (38). Thus, widespread adoption awaits further investigation in this area (40).

Non-coronary Cardiac Assessment

Cardiac CT is used for many non-coronary applications such as assessment of the cardiac chambers and valves, tumor and thrombus, cardiac function and perfusion, and congenital heart disease.

Cardiac Chambers and Valves

Cardiac CTA provides an accurate assessment of cardiac chamber morphology including size and thickness. Left atrial evaluation before and after radiofrequency ablation is a specific application for which cardiac CTA is often used (Fig. 8). Radio-frequency ablation is used increasingly to treat refractory atrial fibrillation. The procedure involves ablation of various

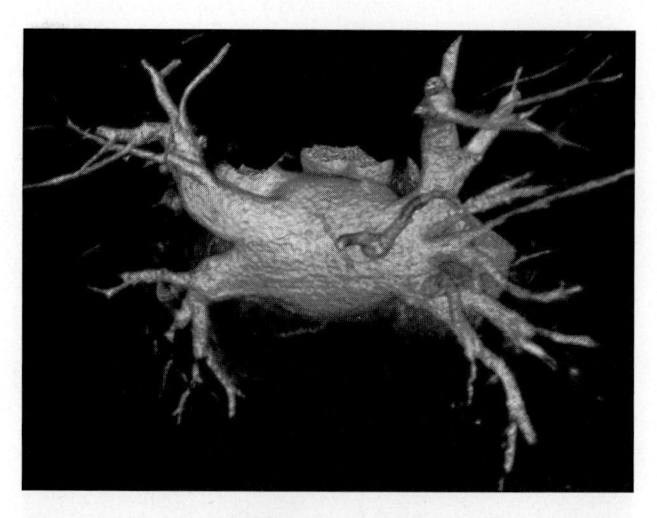

Figure 8 51-year-old woman with history of atrial fibrillation imaged prior to radiofrequency ablation. Volume rendered image shows the pulmonary venous drainage into the left atrium.

aberrant foci of electrical activity, many of which are located near the pulmonary veins, under fluoroscopic guidance. The classic pulmonary venous configuration consists of two right and two left pulmonary veins that enter the left atrium. However, there are numerous variations (41,42).

CT angiography is used to provide a roadmap of the pulmonary veins for the interventional cardiologist during the procedure (43). Several vendors have introduced a CTA electrophysiology package that permits rapid segmentation of the left atrium that facilitates determination of the pulmonary vein arrangement. Radiofrequency ablation has been associated with a reported 1–10% rate of pulmonary vein stenosis, a complication well-demonstrated on CTA (44).

Echocardiography is the principal technique for assessment of cardiac valves. Coronary CTA may be obtained in specific instances because it provides excellent delineation of valve thickness and extent of calcification. In this respect, it may be used to evaluate aortic stenosis prior to replacement surgery (Fig. 9). A movie loop containing the 10 cardiac phases permits dynamic measurement of the extent of stenosis (45). One important limitation of valvular assessment using cardiac CTA in comparison to other techniques is the inability to directly determine valvular gradients.

Cardiac Thrombus and Tumor

Thrombus is the most common cause of a filling defect. Thrombus in the apex of the left ventricle and the left atrial appendage is easily visualized on cardiac CTA and can readily be quantified (46). Left atrial thrombus is considered a contraindication to cardioversion and radiofrequency ablation.

Cardiac thrombus can be difficult to distinguish from cardiac tumors. The most common primary

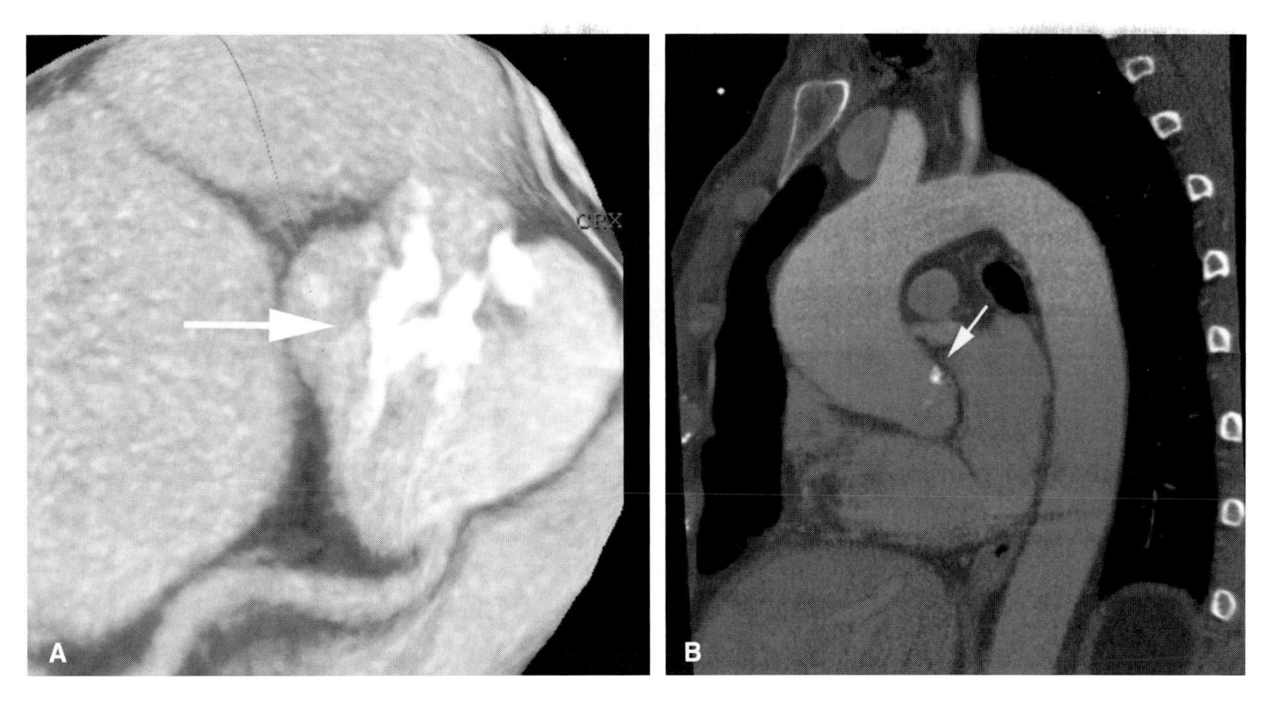

Figure 9 56-year-old man with aortic stenosis and a bicuspid aortic valve. (**A**) Multiplanar reconstruction from cardiac CTA through the aortic valve demonstrates extensive calcification of the valve leaflets (*arrow*). (**B**) Oblique sagittal image through the aorta shows aortic valve calcification (*arrow*) and poststenotic dilatation of the ascending aorta.

cardiac tumor is myxoma, which is most commonly located in the left atrium. On cardiac CTA, a left atrial myxoma is typically visualized as a pedunculated mass arising from the atrial septum in the region of the fossa ovalis. Large masses may prolapse into the left ventricle during ventricular diastole as seen on a cine-loop (47). Another characteristic benign abnormality frequently identified on CTA is lipomatous hypertrophy of the atrial septum, which manifests as an area of unencapsulated fat density that spares the region of the fossa ovalis. In addition, there are multiple other benign, malignant, and metastatic tumors that have fairly non-specific appearances (46). Cardiac CTA is also valuable for defining the extent of tumor encroachment into the heart from adjacent organs (Fig. 10).

Cardiac Function and Perfusion

Current MDCT scanners include software packages that permit assessment of multiple functional parameters, including ejection fraction, stroke volume, wall-motion, and wall thickening, and provide a detailed output display. An automated edge detection program provides an initial estimate of cardiac margins, but some operator input is usually necessary to define appropriate endo- and epicardial borders. A left ventricular ejection fraction similar to that of other methods may be obtained with cardiac CTA, but its lower temporal resolution may decrease its accuracy. Nevertheless, several investigators have shown a strong correlation between ejection fraction calculated with CT in comparison to MRI as well as echocardiography, ventriculography, and radionuclide imaging (48,49).

Cardiac ischemia or infarction may cause differential perfusion of the left ventricular myocardium on cardiac CTA. Decreased attenuation is observed in

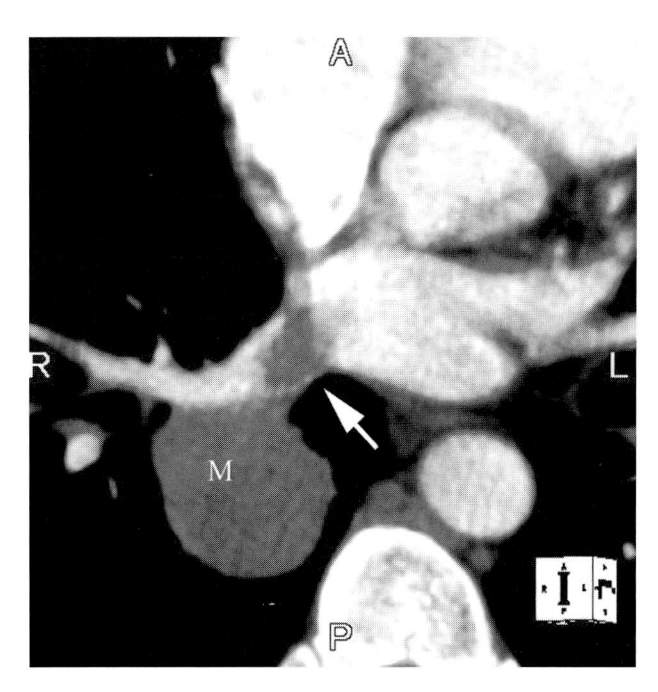

Figure 10 43-year-old man with a new lesion on chest radiography. Off-axial multiplanar reconstruction from cardiac CTA demonstrates a right lower lobe mass (M) invading the right inferior pulmonary vein (*arrow*).

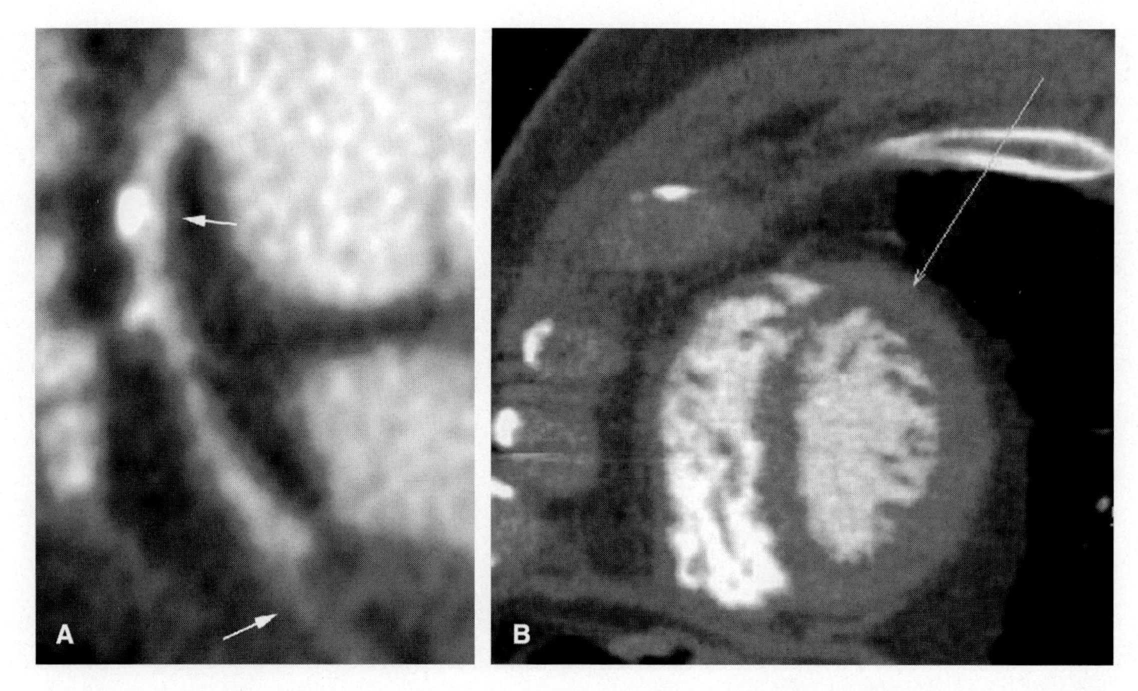

Figure 11 55-year-old man with previous myocardial infarction and chest pain. (**A**) Curved planar reconstructed image of the left anterior descending artery from a coronary CTA demonstrates multiple areas of calcified plaque and stenoses (*arrows*). (**B**) Thin maximum intensity projection through the short axis of the left ventricle shows an area of subendocardial low attenuation (*arrow*) indicating a perfusion defect. This finding is consistent with a prior myocardial infarction.

ischemic areas and may be subendocardial or transmural (Fig. 11). It is uncertain if acute ischemia is different in appearance than chronic ischemia or infarction. Preliminary investigation suggests that delayed enhancement after intravenous contrast administration may occur in patients with infarcted myocardium similar to that seen on viability studies on cardiac MRI (50).

Congenital Heart Disease

The high-spatial resolution and isotropic imaging provided by MDCT is optimal for anatomic evaluation of congenital heart disease (CHD) either preoperatively or after repair. Cardiac CTA is usually a second tier technique for this indication because of radiation dose, requirement for iodinated contrast material, and inability to provide flow and velocity information. Because of radiation concerns, it is used more comfortably in adults than children with congenital heart disease. Notwithstanding these limitations, cardiac CTA can provide exquisite two- and three-dimensional images of simple CHD, such as atrial and ventricular septal defects (Fig. 12), and more complex lesions, such as transposition of the great vessels and heterotaxy syndromes (51).

Cardiac CT in Comparison to other Noninvasive Cardiac Imaging Techniques

Over the past five years, the technological developments for cardiac CT have been much more rapid than for other cardiac imaging techniques. Currently, CT provides the best three-dimensional anatomic information of any competing technology. Cardiac CT suffers from relatively few artifacts. Disadvantages include the inability to obtain direct flow and velocity information, as well as the need to use of ionizing radiation and iodinated intravenous contrast.

Echocardiography remains a powerful tool for the assessment of myocardial and valvular function and does not require contrast or ionizing radiation. Limitations include operator dependence and a restricted field-of-view. Radionuclide imaging with single photon emission computed tomography (SPECT) and positron emission tomography (PET) can provide important information on myocardial perfusion and viability that is not easily obtained with the current generation of CT scans. However, spatial resolution of these techniques is substantially inferior to that of cardiac CT.

Cardiac MRI has superior temporal and contrast resolution as compared to CT, does not rely on iodinated contrast, has no ionizing radiation, and can measure velocities and assess valvular regurgitation. The use of MRI to assess myocardial viability is well-established, whereas the clinical utility of CT for this purpose is unproved. However, in comparison to CT, MRI is more expensive, has inferior spatial resolution, is prone to artifact-related image degradation, and generally cannot be performed in the presence of pacemakers and defibrillators. Table 3 provides a

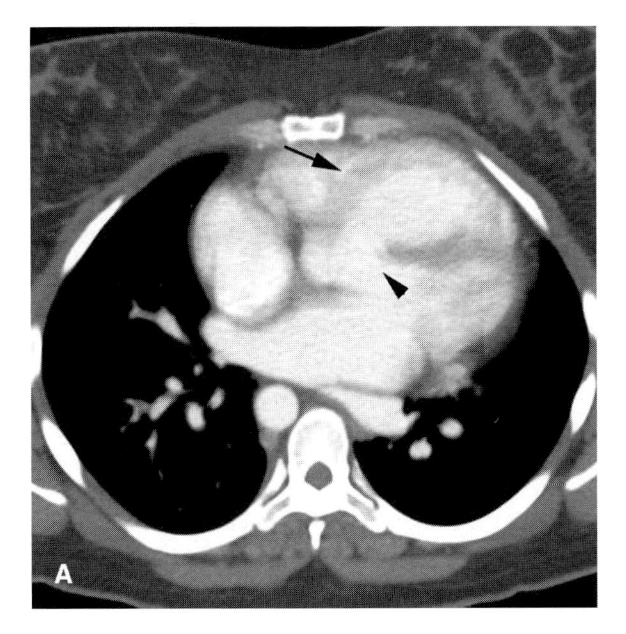

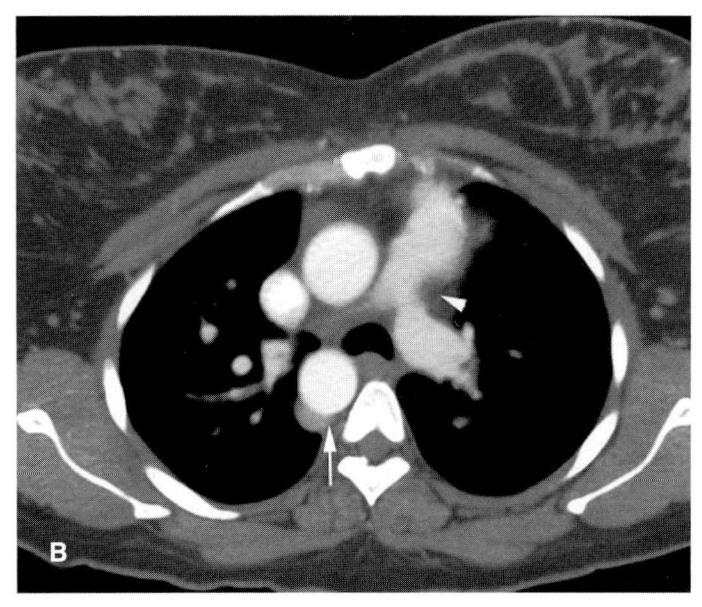

Figure 12 30-year-old woman with tetralogy of Fallot. (**A**) Axial image from a cardiac CTA shows a ventricular septal defect (*arrowhead*) with the aorta overriding the defect and right ventricular hypertrophy (*arrow*). (**B**) An image more cephalic than (**A**) shows pulmonic stenosis (*arrowhead*) the aorta descending on the right (*arrow*) in this patient with a right aortic arch.

summary of cardiac CT in comparison to other commonly used noninvasive cardiac imaging techniques.

Future Directions

The rapid advance in cardiac CTA technological development is likely to continue for the foreseeable future. Both hardware and software enhancements to cardiac CTA have been announced or are forthcoming. One vendor has introduced a dual-tube configuration in which the tubes are placed 90 from each other, permitting a temporal resolution of 83 ms (52). A second vendor has demonstrated images from a 256-slice scanner. Further improvements will likely occur in gantry rotation speed.

Workstation technology is also advancing rapidly. Better workflow patterns are in the offing. More rapid techniques are becoming available to extract coronary arteries from the data and calculate measures of cardiac function such as ejection fraction. Improvements in data transport increasingly permit remote viewing and interpretation of CT images.

Summary

Cardiac CTA has undergone rapid development in the last several years. There is now a wide range of coronary and extracoronary indications. As the body of literature in this area grows, third-party insurers are taking notice and assessing which of these myriad indications should be deemed reimbursable.

CARDIAC MRI

General Considerations

Cardiac MRI remains an important part of the imaging armamentarium because of its versatility and lack of ionizing radiation and iodinated contrast material (53). However, an adequate study requires

Table 3 Cardiac Imaging: Comparison of Different Noninvasive Techniques

	Coronary arteries	Valves	Function	Perfusion/ viability	Comments
CT scan	***	*	**	*	Ionizing radiation Iodinated contrast
Echocardiography	–	***	**	*	Limited field of view Operated dependence
Radionuclide perfusion	–	–	***	***	Ionizing radiation Inferior spatial resolution
MRI	**	**	***	***	Artifact prone Expensive

***, Excellent; **, good; *, fair; –limited or no usefulness.

that the patient remain in the magnet for some length of time. Acquisition of a diagnostic examination may be challenging in patients who are uncooperative or disoriented. However, if the patient is only mildly uncooperative, it is possible to obtain much useful information with fast imaging techniques, depending on the indication. Similar to MRI studies of other parts of the body, cardiac MRI is contraindicated in patients with a variety of foreign devices, including certain aneurysm clips, cochlear implants, and penile prostheses. MRI is also contraindicated in patients who have pacemakers or implantable cardioverter defibrillator (ICD) devices, although this limitation is being reconsidered. In general, MRI can be performed in patients who have prosthetic cardiac valves. Patients who have undergone recent cardiac surgery (coronary artery bypass graft or valve surgery) can probably be studied 1–2 weeks after the procedure, although this has not been documented conclusively.

Cardiac MRI Set Up

ECG-gating is mandatory in order to achieve a study of good quality (54). Gating is triggered to the R-wave, and thus image degradation occurs in patients who have irregular cardiac rhythms, such as atrial fibrillation, in which the R-R interval is highly variable. Because a high quality study depends on effective ECG triggering, it is advisable to ensure that the technologist obtains a good ECG-tracing, both outside and inside the machine, prior to beginning the examination. The tracing is often somewhat degraded due to the hydromagnetic effect in flowing blood once the patient is moved into the machine bore. To achieve a proper tracing it may be necessary to relocate the ECG leads on the patient. If no ECG-tracing can be obtained, a less desirable alternative is to gate from the pulse oximeter (peripheral gating).

Respiratory artifact may also substantially degrade the image. One technique employs respiratory compensation, which consists of reordering the sequence information to smooth out respiratory variations. A respiratory bellows is wrapped around the abdomen to perform these techniques. Another approach uses "navigator" pulses to track the diaphragm. Only imaging with the diaphragm in a predefined window is accepted.

For most situations, cardiac imaging is obtained by using a specialized phased-array cardiac coil. Parallel acquisition techniques (PAT) have substantially increased the speed of image acquisition. For infants, a head coil can be used.

Overview of Sequences Used in Cardiac MRI

Cardiac sequences can be divided generically into dark- or black-blood and bright-blood (gradient-echo) sequences. For dark-blood imaging, multislice T1-weighted spin-echo sequences have largely given way to double-inversion sequences that are faster and can be done in a breath hold. Fast T2-weighted images are used infrequently but may be appropriate in patients with cardiac masses or pericardial disease.

Bright-blood sequences (gradient-echo) are valuable to supplement dark-blood sequences. They can be used to perform fast imaging and obtain physiologic information. Bright-blood images can be placed in a cine format that allows visualization of cardiac motion at a single level in any plane throughout the cardiac cycle. With gradient techniques, the entire cardiac cycle is imaged in a single breathhold. Cardiac views are often obtained, including vertical-, horizontal-, and short-axis views. Gradient-echo techniques are sensitive to turbulence, which causes loss of signal. This characteristic can be employed to detect areas of turbulent flow due to stenosis or regurgitation. Gradient-echo techniques can be phase-encoded so that information regarding blood flow and velocity can be acquired. Steady-state, free-precession (True FISP, balanced FFE) sequences are now used widely to improve segmentation between myocardium and blood pool.

Three-Tesla (3T) magnets are increasingly available and have substantially greater signal-noise-ratio (nearly 1.5X) as compared to 1.5T. Early experience indicates that images of equal or superior quality can be acquired, but significant challenges remain, including artifacts from field inhomogeneity, and the necessity of coil technology and sequence programming to adapt to the newer technology.

Cardiac MRI—Specific Applications

Cardiac and Paracardiac Lesions

Thrombi are a frequent cause of cardiac lesions. They are particularly common in the left atrium in patients with atrial fibrillation, and are often located along the posterior wall or in the atrial appendage. Thrombi may be difficult to distinguish from cardiac tumors. Enhancement after gadolinium chelate administration is more typical of tumors than thrombi. Metastatic cardiac lesions are about ten- to forty-times more prevalent than primary cardiac tumors. Common origins of metastatic lesions include lung, breast, and skin. Lymphomatous involvement of the heart is also common. Spread of extracardiac tumors may occur through the systemic (renal cell carcinoma, hepatocellular carcinoma) or pulmonary (lung carcinoma) veins (Fig. 13).

The most common primary cardiac tumors are myxomas, which are almost always histologically benign (55). Seventy-five percent are located in the left atrium, where most are attached by a pedicle to the atrial septum near the fossa ovalis. These tumors

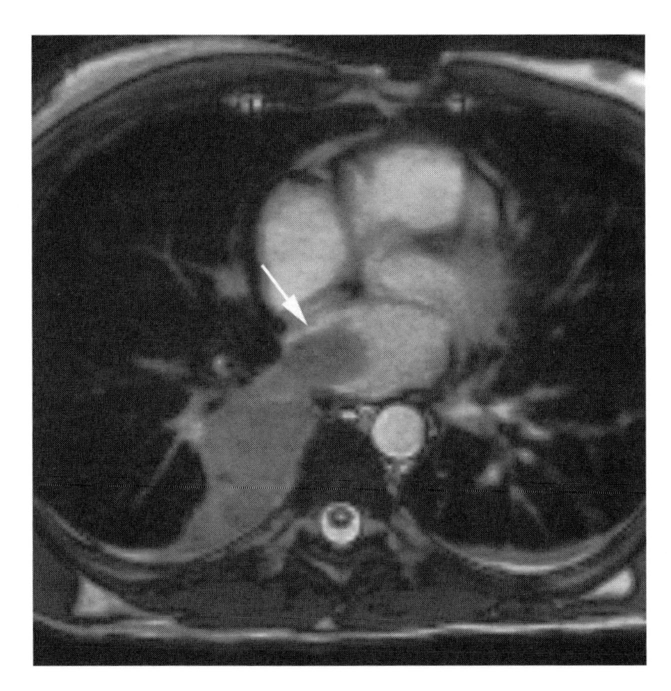

Figure 13 43-year-old man with lung cancer and cardiac invasion. Axial gradient echo MR image shows a left lower lobe mass extending into the left atrium (*arrow*) through the inferior pulmonary vein.

occur in the right atrium in about 20% of patients and are occasionally found in a ventricle (Fig. 14). Atrial myxomas are usually pedunculated and may prolapse through valves, causing regurgitation. Tumor fragments may embolize and cause systemic or pulmonary symptoms. Rhabdomyomas are less common tumors that typically manifest in infancy and have a strong association with tuberous sclerosis. Another tumor-like condition is lipomatous hypertrophy of the atrial septum, which consists of a large quantity of unencapsulated fat that is deposited in and widens the atrial septum, and may even project into the right atrium. On T1-weighted images, bright signal measuring at least 2 cm in transverse diameter is characteristic. Sparing of the region of the fossa ovalis is typical. Malignant primary tumors of the heart are rare, and consist of sarcomatous lesions, particularly angiosarcoma, other mesenchymal tumors, and lymphoma.

Pericardial Disease

The pericardium is well-visualized on dark-blood images as a low-signal intensity structure that is highlighted by the bright-signal intensity of the surrounding epicardial and mediastinal fat (56). The normal pericardium measures no more than 3 mm in width. A simple (transudative) pericardial effusion appears as widening of the pericardium with maintenance of the low signal intensity on T1-weighted images. It is particularly well-seen anterior to the heart and lateral to the left ventricle. Pericardial fluid usually appears bright on T2-weighted gradient-echo images (Fig. 15). Hemorrhagic or exudative fluid may show medium- or high-signal intensity on T1-weighted images.

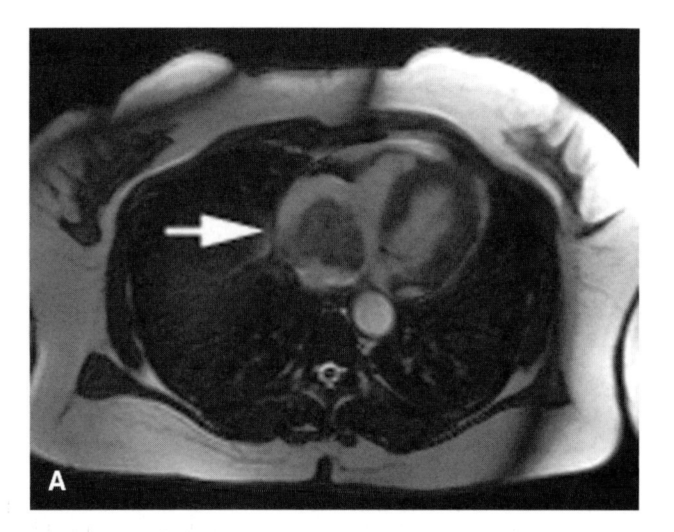

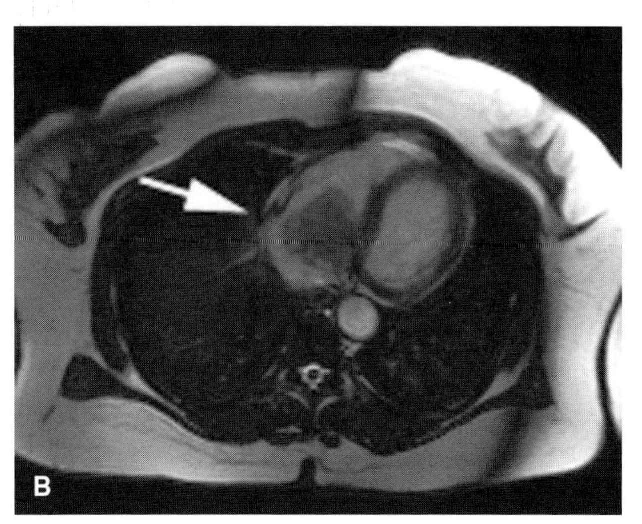

Figure 14 62-year-old woman with a right atrial myxoma. Axial bright-blood MR images in ventricular systole (**A**) and diastole (**B**) show the mass (*arrow*) in the right atrium prolapsing into the right ventricle.

Echocardiography is the primary technique used to detect pericardial effusions, but it is less optimal in defining pericardial thickening due to constriction. Pericardial constriction has a similar clinical and hemodynamic profile to restrictive cardiomyopathy. Moreover, treatment for restrictive cardiomyopathy is directed at the underlying cause, whereas surgical stripping is often performed for pericardial constriction. MRI is the technique of choice to make this distinction, although ECG-gated CT can also be used. The finding of a thickened pericardium confirms the diagnosis of pericardial constriction, along with ancillary signs of dilated venae cavae and sigmoid septum. Impairment of diastolic relaxation by the abnormal pericardium may also be evident on cine imaging.

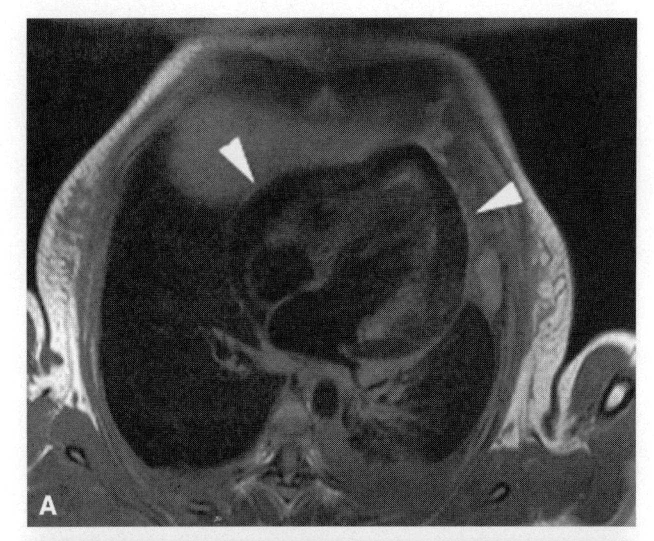

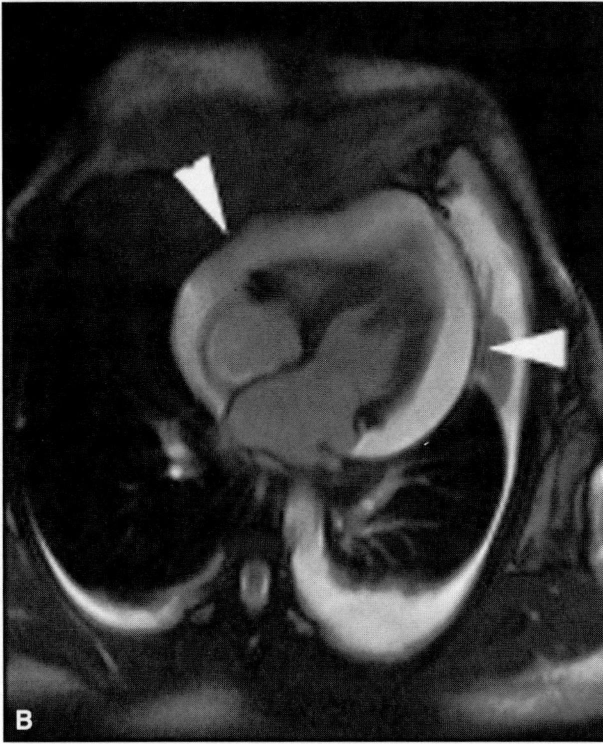

Figure 15 23-year-old woman with pericardial effusion. Axial dark-blood (**A**) and bright-blood (**B**) MR images show an area of low- and high-signal intensity (*arrowheads*), respectively, surrounding the heart. The signal characteristics are consistent with a transudate.

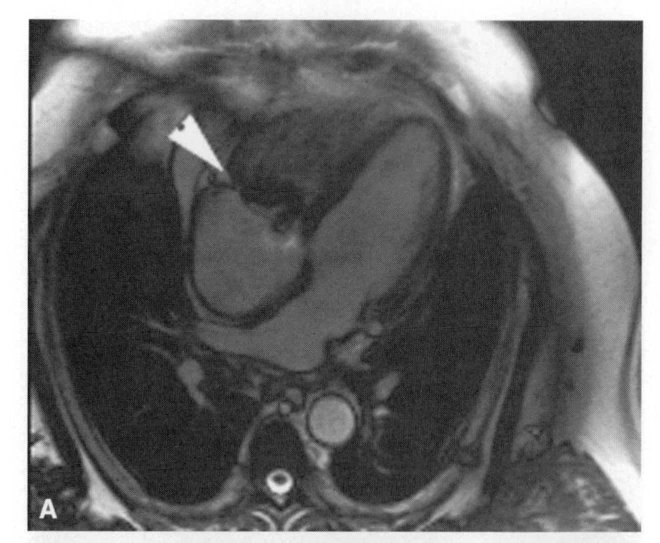

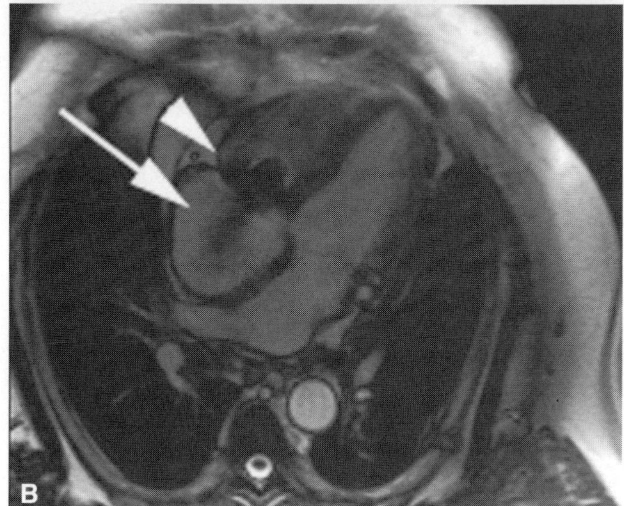

Figure 16 50-year-old man with tricuspid regurgitation from a prosthetic tricuspid valve. Diastolic (**A**) and systolic (**B**) axial gradient-echo MR images show the prosthetic valve as an area of signal absence (*arrowhead*). On the systolic image, an area of signal loss in the right atrium (*arrow*) corresponds to the regurgitant jet caused by tricuspid valve regurgitation.

Valvular Heart Disease

Echocardiography remains the principal technique to evaluate valvular disease. Both the valve diameter and estimate of the gradient across the valve can be measured with echocardiography. On MRI, it is possible to detect valvular stenosis or regurgitation on gated gradient-echo images (cine MRI). Stenosis or regurgitation is identified on this bright-blood sequence as a plume of low-signal intensity that emanates from the valve in the direction of blood flow during the appropriate part of the cardiac cycle (57). The low-signal intensity is caused by dephasing that occurs in the turbulent jet (Fig. 16). Some physiologic low-signal intensity may be observed in otherwise normal patients, but it is usually less extensive and of shorter duration. Valvular vegetations are difficult to identify on MRI, but perivalvular abscess or septic pseudoaneurysm is more readily shown.

Cardiomyopathies and Dysplasias

Three major types of cardiomyopathy are recognized: hypertrophic, dilated, and restrictive. Most patients with cardiomyopathy undergo echocardiography and/or angiocardiography, and MRI is used in a secondary role (58). The most common type of hypertrophic cardiomyopathy is characterized by asymmetric thickening of the septum in comparison with the lateral wall of the left ventricle. There is (paradoxical) systolic anterior motion (SAM) of the anterior leaflet of the mitral valve that may contribute to the outflow obstruction in the subaortic region. MRI shows striking thickening of the septum and, often, lateral wall of the left ventricle, with nearly complete obliteration of the ventricular cavity during systole. MRI can also demonstrate the turbulent flow in left ventricular outflow track and SAM of the mitral valve. Other forms of nonobstructive hypertrophic cardiomyopathy that can be visualized on MRI are apical, midventricular, and hypertensive hypertrophic cardiomyopathy.

Dilated cardiomyopathy is caused by ischemia and a variety of toxic and infectious agents that lead to severe compromise of the left ventricular ejection fraction. MRI typically shows a markedly dilated left ventricle that is hypokinetic. Restrictive cardiomyopathy is due to several infiltrative diseases (amyloidosis, sarcoidosis, hemochromatosis) that impair diastolic filling. On MRI, it appears as slight myocardial thickening with relatively preserved myocardial function. Myocardial edema may be evident (Fig. 17). Delayed enhancement imaging (see below) may, in some cases, demonstrate areas of fibrosis within the myocardium. An important role of MRI is to distinguish restrictive cardiomyopathy from pericardial constriction.

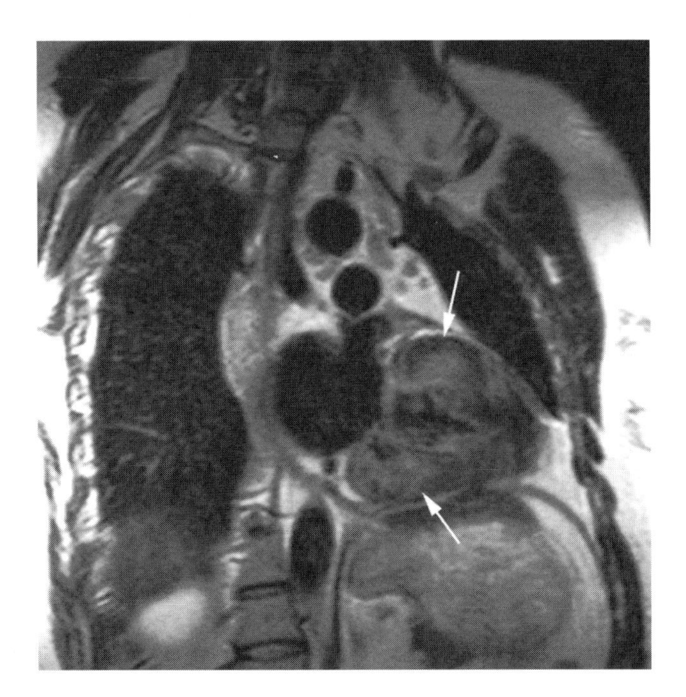

Figure 17 43-year-old woman with restrictive cardiomyopathy due to sarcoidosis. Vertical long axis T2-weighted spin-echo MR image shows high-signal intensity in the myocardium (*arrow*), consistent with myocardial edema due to infiltration with non-caseating granulomas.

A condition for which MRI has proved to be a primary technique is arrhythmogenic right ventricular dysplasia (ARVD). ARVD is an abnormality that occurs predominantly in adolescents and young adults and may cause ventricular tachycardia or sudden death. Pathologically, it is caused by replacement of the right ventricular free wall myocardium by fat or fibrosis. MRI findings in this condition include areas of fatty replacement, marked thinning of the free wall, and abnormalities on delayed enhancement sequences (59). Cine imaging may reveal abnormalities of wall motion.

Functional Cardiac Imaging

A further indication for cardiac MRI is to provide functional information about cardiac status (60). Left ventricular ejection fraction (end-diastolic volume-end-systolic volume/end-diastolic volume) can be calculated by acquiring multiphase images contiguously through the heart along its short axis. The end-diastolic and end-systolic volumes can be determined for each section, allowing determination of a global left ventricular ejection using a modification of Simpson's rule. Alternatively, the ejection fraction can be estimated from a single long-axis image. As noted above, valvular heart disease can be detected with gradient-echo imaging. The severity of the lesion correlates qualitatively with the extent of loss of signal that emanates from the valve. Another capability of MRI is to calculate the extent of shunting in patients with septal lesions (61). This measurement is obtained using a phase encoded gradient echo sequence to measure blood flow in the aorta and pulmonary artery. The proportion of flow in the two vessels indicates the amount of shunting (i.e. a left-to-right shunt demonstrates more flow in the pulmonary artery).

Myocardial Perfusion and Viability Imaging

One of the most important capabilities of MRI is its ability to provide important information about the status of the myocardium (62). In the setting of ischemia, the myocardium can respond in different ways. If acute ischemic thrombosis of a coronary artery is followed by rapid reperfusion, either spontaneously or after therapeutic reopening of the vessel, the affected myocardium may remain viable but demonstrate poor contractility. This is termed "stunned" myocardium. Another form of myocardial compromise occurs in the setting of chronic ischemia, in which there is a compensatory decrease in myocardial metabolism, a status referred to as myocardial hibernation. In the most severe situation, the myocardium is infarcted and non-viable. The distinction between a hibernating and infarcted myocardium, in particular, is critical because revascularization only improves a hibernating myocardium.

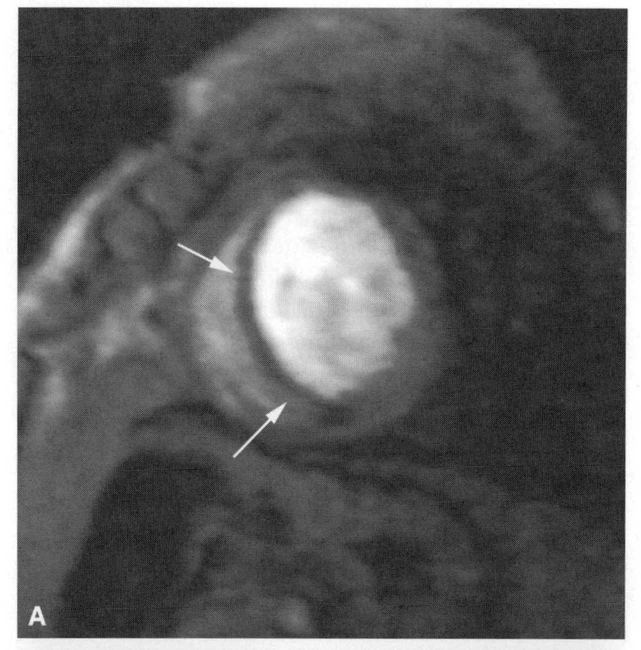

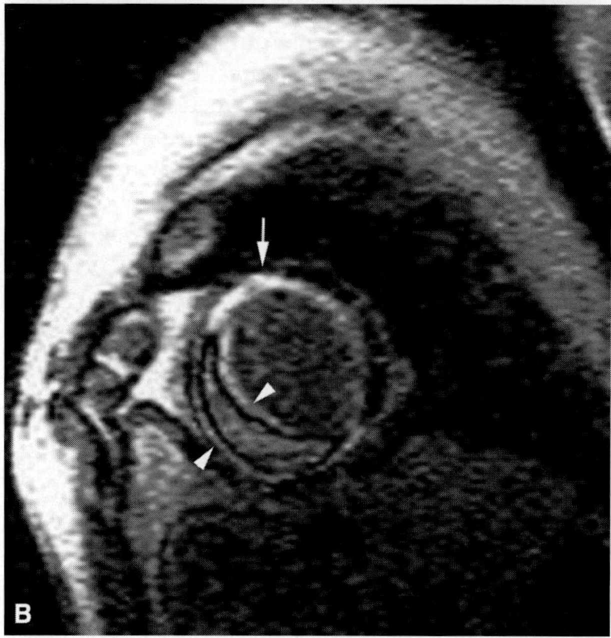

Figure 18 63-year-old with man a history of a large, anterior-wall, myocardial infarction who underwent a myocardial perfusion/viability study. (**A**) Short-axis gradient echo MR image from the myocardial perfusion study shows an area of low-signal intensity in the septum (*arrow*), indicating absence of perfusion. (**B**) Vertical, long-axis, MR image from a myocardial viability study ten minutes after injection of gadolinium chelate shows an area of high-signal intensity in the anterior myocardium (*arrow*), corresponding to myocardial infarction. Left ventricular thrombus is present (*arrowheads*).

PET is considered the standard reference technique to assess myocardial viability, but it is limited by expense and relatively inferior spatial resolution. MRI is well-suited for this purpose because its superior spatial resolution permits assessment of the transmural extent of myocardial damage. A typical acquisition consists of first pass perfusion imaging after administration of intravenous gadolinium chelate, wall motion evaluation, and myocardial viability assessment (Fig. 18). Myocardial viability imaging is usually obtained 10 to 15 minutes after contrast administration. An inversion-recovery, gradient-echo sequence is used, and the myocardium is nulled (i.e., a delay is introduced such that myocardial signal is absent). Non-viable myocardium is visualized as an area of high-signal intensity or hyperenhancement on these delayed images. The extent of transmural involvement of enhancement correlates with the likelihood of successful revascularization, with involvement limited to the subendocardial myocardium having the best prognosis. A stunned myocardium shows normal perfusion but abnormal wall motion. A hibernating myocardium shows abnormal perfusion and wall motion. Neither a stunned nor a hibernating myocardium shows enhancement on viability imaging.

It is well-recognized that myocardial delayed enhancement correlates pathologically with areas of fibrosis and scarring. The finding is not specific to ischemic myocardial infarction, but may be encountered with other conditions that cause fibrosis, such as myocarditis, hypertrophic cardiomyopathy, infiltrative cardiomyopathy, cardiac neoplasm, and arrhythmogenic, right-ventricular dysplasia (63). However, the distribution of infarct-related enhancement is typically segmental, whereas it is often more patchy in other conditions.

CONCLUSION

Both cardiac CT and MRI have important roles to play in the imaging assessment of cardiac disease. The most important contribution of cardiac CT is its ability to provide noninvasive assessment of the coronary arteries. For cardiac MRI, assessment of myocardial viability may offer its greatest impact. Continuing investigation will undoubtedly lead to improved capabilities for both of these noninvasive techniques.

REFERENCES

1 Thompson BH, Stanford W. Imaging of coronary calcium: a case for electron beam computed tomography. J Thorac Imag 2001; 16:8–15.
2 Wintersperger BJ, Nikolaou K. Basics of cardiac MDCT: techniques and contrast application. Eur Radiol 2005; 15(Suppl. 2):B2–9.
3 Lawler LP, Pannu HK, Fishman EK. MDCT evaluation of the coronary arteries, 2004: how we do it—data acquisition, postprocessing, display, and interpretation. AJR Am J Roentgenol 2005; 184:1402–12.

4 Hausleiter J, Meyer T, Hadamitzky M, et al. Radiation dose estimates from cardiac multislice computed tomography in daily practice: impact of different scanning protocols on effective dose estimates. Circulation 2006; 113:1305–10.
5 Poll LW, Cohnen M, Brachten S, Ewen K, Modder U. Dose reduction in multi-slice CT of the heart by use of ECG-controlled tube current modulation ("ECG pulsing"): phantom measurements. Rofo 2002; 174:1500–5.
6 ACR practice guideline for the performance and interpretation of cardiac computed tomography (CT). Available at: ACR website http://www.acr.org/s_acr/doc.asp?CID=2601&DID=24881.
7 Budoff MJ, Cohen MC, Garcia MJ, et al. American College of Cardiology Foundation; American Heart Association; American College of Physicians Task Force on Clinical Competence; American Society of Echocardiography; American Society of Nuclear Cardiology; Society of Atherosclerosis Imaging; Society for Cardiovascular Angiography & Interventions; Society of Cardiovascular Computed Tomography. ACCF/AHA clinical competence statement on cardiac imaging with computed tomography and magnetic resonance. Circulation 2005; 112:598–617.
8 Mulaik MW. Everybodys doing a brand new dance now...CT/CTA coronary. Radiol Manage 2006, 28: 12–5.
9 Hendel RC, Patel MR, Kramer CM, et al. ACCF/ACR/SCCT/SCMR/ASNC/NASCI/SCAI/SIR 2006 appropriateness criteria for cardiac computed tomography and cardiac magnetic resonance imaging: a report of the American College of Cardiology Foundation Quality Strategic Directions Committee Appropriateness Criteria Working Group, American College of Radiology, Society of Cardiovascular Computed Tomography, Society for Cardiovascular Magnetic Resonance, American Society of Nuclear Cardiology, North American Society for Cardiac Imaging, Society for Cardiovascular Angiography and Interventions, and Society of Interventional Radiology. J Am Coll Cardiol 2006; 48:1475–97.
10 Berman DS, Hachamovitch R, Shaw LJ, et al. Roles of nuclear cardiology, cardiac computed tomography, and cardiac magnetic resonance: noninvasive risk stratification and a conceptual framework for the selection of noninvasive imaging tests in patients with known or suspected coronary artery disease. J Nucl Med 2006; 47:1107–18.
11 Arad Y, Spadaro LA, Goodman K, et al. Predictive value of electron beam computed tomography of the coronary arteries. 19-month follow-up of 1173 asymptomatic subjects. Circulation 1996; 93:1951–3.
12 Rumberger JA, Simons DB, Fitzpatrick LA, et al. Coronary artery calcium area by electron-beam computed tomography and coronary atherosclerotic plaque area: a histopathologic correlative study. Circulation 1995; 92:2157–62.
13 Budoff MJ, Georgiou D, Brody A, et al. Ultrafast computed tomography as a diagnostic modality in the detection of coronary artery disease: a multicenter study. Circulation 1996; 93:898–904.
14 Agatston AS, Janowitz WR, Hildner FJ, Zusmer NR, Viamonte M Jr, Detrano R. Quantification of coronary artery calcium using ultrafast computed tomography. J Am Coll Cardiol 1990; 15:827–32.
15 Hoff JA, Chomka EV, Krainik AJ, Daviglus M, Rich S, Kondos GT, Age and gender distributions of coronary artery calcium detected by electron beam tomography in 35,246 adults. Am J Cardiol 2001; 87: 1335–9.
16 Rumberger JA. Clinical use of coronary calcium scanning with computed tomography. Cardiol Clin 2003; 21:535–47.
17 Becker CR, Kleffel T, Crispin A, et al. Coronary artery calcium measurement: agreement of multirow detector and electron beam CT. AJR Am J Roentgenol 2001; 176:1295–8.
18 Horton KM, Post WS, Blumenthal RS, Fishman EK. Prevalence of significant noncardiac findings on electron-beam computed tomogrpahy coronary artery calcium screening examinations. Circulation 2002; 106:532–7.
19 Schragin JG, Weissfeld JL, Edmundowicz D, Strollo D, Fuhrman CR. Non-cardiac findings on coronary electron beam computed tomography Scanning. J Thorac Imag 2004; 19:82–6.
20 Achenbach S, Giesler T, Ropers D, et al. Detection of coronary artery stenoses by contrast-enhanced, retrospectively electrocardiographically-gated, multislice spiral computed tomography. Circulation 2001; 103:2535–8.
21 Nieman K, Cademartiri F, Lemos PA, Raaijmakers R, Pattynama PM, de Feyter PJ. Reliable noninvasive coronary angiography with fast submillimeter multislice spiral computed tomography. Circulation2002; 106:2051–4.
22 Ropers D, Baum U, Pohle K, et al. Detection of coronary artery stenoses with thin-slice multi-detector row spiral computed tomography and multiplanar reconstruction. Circulation 2003; 107:664–6.
23 Leschka S, Alkadhi H, Plass A, et al. Accuracy of MSCT coronary angiography with 64-slice technology: first experience. Eur Heart J 2005; 26:1482–7.
24 Raff GL, Gallagher MJ, ONeill WW, Goldstein JA. Diagnostic accuracy of noninvasive coronary angiography using 64-slice spiral computed tomography. J Am Coll Cardiol 2005; 46:552–7.
25 Nikolaou K, Knez A, Rist C, et al. Accuracy of 64-MDCT in the diagnosis of ischemic heart disease. AJR Am J Roentgenol 2006; 187:111–7.
26 Garcia MJ, Lessick J, Hoffmann MH; CATSCAN Study Investigators. Accuracy of 16-row multidetector computed tomography for the assessment of coronary artery stenosis. JAMA 2006; 296:403–11.
27 Becker CR, Nikolaou K, Muders M, et al. Ex vivo coronary atherosclerotic plaque characterization with multi-detector-row CT. Eur Radiol 2003; 13:2094–8.
28 Maron BJ. Sudden death in young athletes. N Eng J Med 2003; 349:1064–75.
29 Greenberg MA, Fish BG, Spindola-Franco H. Congenital anomalies of the coronary arteries. Classification and significance. Radiol Clin North Am 1989 27:1127–46.

30 Datta J, White CS, Gilkeson RC, et al. Anomalous coronary arteries in adults: depiction at multi-detector row CT angiography. Radiology 2005; 235:812–8.
31 Murthy PA, Mohammed TL, Read K, Gilkeson RC, White CS. MDCT of coronary artery aneurysms. AJR Am J Roentgenol 2005; 184(Suppl. 3):19S–20.
32 Goldman S, Zadina K, Moritz T. Long-term patency of saphenous vein and left internal mammary artery grafts after coronary artery bypass surgery: results from a Department of Veterans Affairs Cooperative Study. J Am Coll Cardiol 2004; 44:2149–56.
33 Frazier AA, Qureshi F, Read KM, Gilkeson RC, Poston RS, White CS. Coronary artery bypass grafts: assessment with multidetector CT in the early and late postoperative settings. Radiographics 2005; 25:881–96.
34 Schlosser T, Konorza T, Hunold P, Kuhl H, Schmermund A, Barkhausen J. Noninvasive visualization of coronary artery bypass grafts using 16-detector row computed tomography. J Am Coll Cardiol 2004; 44:1224–9.
35 Stein PD, Beemath A, Skaf E, et al. Usefulness of 4-, 8-, and 16-slice computed tomography for detection of graft occlusion or patency after coronary artery bypass grafting. Am J Cardiol 2005; 96:1669–73.
36 Maintz D, Seifarth H, Raupach R, et al. 64-slice multidetector coronary CT angiography: in vitro evaluation of 68 different stents. Eur Radiol 2006; 16:818–26.
37 Rixe J, Achenbach S, Ropers D, et al. Assessment of coronary artery stent restenosis by 64-slice multi-detector computed tomography. Eur Heart J 2006; 27:2567–72.
38 White CS, Kuo D, Kelemen M, et al. Chest pain evaluation in the emergency room: can multi-slice CT provide a comprehensive evaluation? AJR 2005; 185:533–40.
39 Dorgelo J, Willems TP, Geluk CA, van Ooijen PM, Zijlstra F, Oudkerk M. Multidetector computed tomography-guided treatment strategy in patients with non-ST elevation acute coronary syndromes: a pilot study. Eur Radiol 2005; 15:708–13.
40 White C, Read K, Kuo D. Assessment of chest pain in the emergency room: what is the role of multidetector CT? Eur J Radiol 2006; 57:368–72.
41 Schwartzman D, Lacomis J, Wigginton WG. Characterization of left atrium and distal pulmonary vein morphology using multidimensional computed tomography. J Am Coll Cardiol 2003; 41:1349–57.
42 Marom EM, Herndon JE, Kim YH, McAdams HP. Variations in pulmonary venous drainage to the left atrium: implications for radiofrequency ablation. Radiology 2004; 230:824–9.
43 Cronin P, Sneider MB, Kazerooni EA, et al. MDCT of the left atrium and pulmonary veins in planning radiofrequency ablation for atrial fibrillation: a how-to guide. AJR Am J Roentgenol 2004; 183:767–78.
44 Packer DL, Keelan P, Munger TM, et al. Clinical presentation, investigation, and management of pulmonary vein stenosis complicating ablation for atrial fibrillation. Circulation 2005; 111:546–54.
45 Alkadhi H, Wildermuth S, Plass A, et al. Aortic stenosis: comparative evaluation of 16-detector row CT and echocardiography. Radiology 2006; 240:47–55.
46 Tatli S, Lipton MJ. CT for intracardiac thrombi and tumors. Int J Cardiovasc Imag 2005; 21:115–31.
47 Grebenc ML, Rosado-de-Christenson ML, Green CE, Burke AP, Galvin JR. Cardiac myxoma: imaging features in 83 patients. Radiographics 2002; 22:673–89.
48 Juergens KU, Grude M, Maintz D, et al. Multi-detector row CT of left ventricular function with dedicated analysis software versus MR imaging: initial experience. Radiology 2004; 230:403–10.
49 Orakzai SH, Orakzai RH, Nasir K, Budoff MJ. Assessment of cardiac function using multidetector row computed tomography. J Comput Assist Tomogr 2006; 30:555–63.
50 Gerber BL, Belge B, Legros GJ, et al. Characterization of acute and chronic myocardial infarcts by multidetector computed tomography: comparison with contrast-enhanced magnetic resonance. Circulation 2006; 113:823–33.
51 Siegel MJ, Bhalla S, Gutierrez FR, Billadello JB. MDCT of postoperative anatomy and complications in adults with cyanotic heart disease. AJR Am J Roentgenol 2005; 184:241–7.
52 Flohr TG, McCollough CH, Bruder H, et al. First performance evaluation of a dual-source CT (DSCT) system. Eur Radiol 2006; 16:256–68.
53 Finn JP, Nael K, Deshpande V, Ratib O, Laub G. Cardiac MR imaging: state of the technology. Radiology 2006; 241:338–54.
54 Poustchi-Amin M, Gutierrez FR, Brown JJ, et al. How to plan and perform a cardiac MR imaging examination. Radiol Clin North Am 2004; 42:497–514.
55 Restrepo CS, Largoza A, Lemos DF, et al. CT and MR imaging findings of benign cardiac tumors. Curr Probl Diagn Radiol 2005; 34:12–21.
56 Rienmuller R, Groll R, Lipton MJ. CT and MR imaging of pericardial disease. Radiol Clin North Am 2004; 42:587–601.
57 Didier D. Assessment of valve disease: qualitative and quantitative. Magn Reson Imaging Clin N Am 2003; 11:115–34.
58 Soler R, Rodriguez E, Remuinan C, Bello MJ, Diaz A. Magnetic resonance imaging of primary cardiomyopathies. J Comput Assist Tomogr 2003; 27:724–34.
59 Bluemke DA, Krupinski EA, Ovitt T, et al. MR Imaging of arrhythmogenic right ventricular cardiomyopathy: morphologic findings and interobserver reliability. Cardiology 2003; 99:153–62.
60 Alfakih K, Reid S, Jones T, Sivananthan M. Assessment of ventricular function and mass by cardiac magnetic resonance imaging. Eur Radiol 2004; 14(10):1813–22.
61 Reddy GP, Higgins CB. Congenital heart disease: measuring physiology with MRI. Semin Roentgenol 1998; 33(3):228–38.
62 Wu KC, Lima JA. Noninvasive imaging of myocardial viability: current techniques and future developments. Circ Res 2003; 93:1146–1158.
63 Kim DH, Choi SI, Chang HJ, Choi DJ, Lim C, Park JH. Delayed hyperenhancement by contrast-enhanced magnetic resonance imaging: Clinical application for various cardiac diseases. J Comput Assist Tomogr 2006; 30:226–32.

7

Diagnosis of Pulmonary Embolus

Cesario Ciccotosto
U.O.C. Radiologia, Ospedale S. Donato, Arezzo, Italy

Lawrence R. Goodman
Departments of Diagnostic Radiology and Pulmonary Medicine and Critical Care, Section of Thoracic Imaging, Medical College of Wisconsin and Froedtert Memorial Lutheran Hospital, Milwaukee, Wisconsin, U.S.A.

Lacey Washington
Department of Radiology, Section of Thoracic Imaging, Duke University, Durham, North Carolina, U.S.A.

INTRODUCTION

Pulmonary embolus (PE) and deep venous thrombosis (DVT) are two interrelated components of pulmonary thromboembolic disease (PTE). Both are difficult to diagnose clinically and there are many competing tests, some clinical, some laboratory, and some imaging, used for PTE diagnosis. All have strengths and drawbacks. As imagers, it is our task to individualize these exams, or combination of exams, to fit the particular patient. A "one approach fits all" strategy is an inefficient use of resources.

A key component of the diagnostic workup for PE involves the use of blood tests. The diagnostic utility of plasma measurements of circulating D-dimer (a specific derivative of cross-linked fibrin) in patients with acute PE has been extensively evaluated (1). A normal D-dimer test seems to be sensitive in excluding PE, particularly when the clinical suspicion is moderate or low. The use of a reproducible D-dimer assay with a pretest clinical scoring model, like the Wells criteria, has a negative predictive value as high as 99.5% and can safely rule out PTE without subsequent imaging studies (2). A positive D-dimer test means that DVT or PE is possible, but it is by no means proof. Positive D-dimer is nonspecific, especially in inpatients with concomitant inflammatory diseases, in ICU patients, pregnant patients, or in patients after surgery and further testing is required.

Ventilation perfusion scanning (V/Q) has been the keystone imaging modality for the past 40 years. The multi-institutional Prospective Investigation of Pulmonary Embolism Diagnosis (PIOPED) Study (3) demonstrated that a normal ventilation perfusion scan has a 96% negative predictive value and provides sufficient evidence to withhold anticoagulation. Similarly, a high-probability scan coupled with a high-probability clinical suspicion has a 96% positive predictive value for PE. Unfortunately, even using the revised PIOPED criteria for V/Q interpretation, the majority of patients have low or indeterminate probability scans, which are inconclusive for PTE diagnosis and therefore usually require additional imaging (4).

In a patient population with good cardiopulmonary reserve, an inconclusive ventilation perfusion scan, and serial negative lower extremity, Doppler ultrasounds (LEUS) provide very strong evidence that anticoagulation can be withheld (5). However, as a single isolated study, a negative lower extremity study does not exclude PE. In fact, approximately one-half of PE patients have negative lower extremity studies.

A traditional approach indicates that in a high-risk patient with inconclusive scintigraphy, pulmonary angiography should follow. This was the gold standard but was often omitted because it is invasive and because of the perceived risks. A negative pulmonary angiogram indicates that anticoagulation can be safely withheld (6). Similarly, serial LEUS was not obtained in the majority of eligible patients. A decision to anticoagulate or not to anticoagulate patients was frequently based on inconclusive scintigraphy and perceived clinical probability, a sub-optimal situation (7).

Helical CT (CTA) pulmonary angiography provides a better, but not perfect, alternative to traditional PTE imaging. The current generation of multislice helical CT scanners provides high-quality axial images of the contrast-enhanced pulmonary vessels and lower extremity veins. As in angiography or venography, the clot is displayed directly as a filling defect in the contrast column. CT is also able to detect other pulmonary and lower extremity diseases that may mimic PTE or DVT. CT is not without its shortcomings. However, many studies have shown that CTA is approximately 75–95% sensitive for PE (8–16).

CT will often miss small clots in subsegmental vessels (8). These very small clots are the same clots, however, that result in inconclusive scintigraphy and a high rate of interobserver disagreement on pulmonary angiography. Respiratory motion also degrades the depiction of small vessels, resulting in suboptimal scans in 5–10% of patients (12). Despite these limitations, the clinical outcome for patients with negative CTAs who are not anticoagulated is very good. We recently reported a study of 198 CTA negative patients (42% of whom also had LEUS) and 350 scintigraphy negative or low-probability patients (22% of whom had LEUS) who were not anticoagulated. After 3 months of clinical follow-up, the rate of subsequent PE was 1% for negative CT, 0% for normal scintigraphy, and 3.4% for low-probability scintigraphy (17). Multiple other studies have confirmed that the incidence of PE within 3 months of a negative CT is similar to that after a negative angiogram (18,19).

For comparison, patients anticoagulated for PE have a 5% incidence of subsequent PE (20). CT is also expensive but is cost-effective relative to other strategies that require multiple imaging studies in the majority of patients.

With the advent of multislice CT (MDCT) scanners there is even better visualization of the small pulmonary arteries, particularly at the segmental, subsegmental, and smaller levels, due to shorter gantry rotation times, faster pitches, and thinner slices. Schoef et al. found that 75% of subsegmental pulmonary arteries are well visualized with 1.25 mm slices compared to 36% with 3-mm thick slices (21,22).

The use of MD-CTA further improves interobserver agreement about the presence or absence of emboli and facilitates visualization of peripheral arteries in patients with underlying pulmonary disease (23).

A recent addition to the CT armamentarium for PTE is CT venography (CTV). Axial or helical scans through the lower extremity veins to the knee are obtained 3 min after completion of the contrast injection for the pulmonary arterial CT (24–26). These studies are easy to perform and are easy to interpret. PIOPED II showed a 96% agreement between CTV and LEUS, which is similar to several smaller studies (13,14). PIOPED II showed almost no diagnostic benefit to imaging the inferior vena cava (IVC) and iliac veins. Imaging above the level of the femoral veins can be omitted when pelvic DVT is not likely (13).

Incorporating CTV with CTA assures that the pulmonary arteries and lower extremity veins are imaged in every patient. It is very time effective for both patient and referring physician to be able to complete the venous thromboembolism (VTE) work-up in one 20–30 min trip to the CT suite.

The addition of CTV has been somewhat controversial, as it adds expense and radiation; different authors disagree on whether the benefit from additional yield of CTV outweighs the disadvantages. PIOPED II showed a 7% increase in the diagnosis of venous thromboembolism from the addition of CTV to CTA alone (13). Other studies have shown a wide range of benefit, varying from 1% to 27% (14,27–29). A benefit may also be present in patients with known PE if knowing the residual lower extremity clot burden is helpful in making therapeutic decisions on IVC filter placement or clot lysis strategies

We believe that scintigraphy, lower extremity Doppler ultrasound, CT of the pulmonary arteries and veins, and pulmonary angiography can be used in a multi-arm, cost-effective algorithm that utilizes the strong points of each imaging modality and minimizes the weaknesses of each (8). The following list outlines our algorithm with its rationale.

1. V/Q scanning: Studies have shown that patients with a normal chest radiograph have a higher likelihood of a definitive scintigraphic answer (normal, very low probability, and high probability). Patients with a normal chest radiograph should start with a perfusion or V/Q. Inconclusive studies require further imaging, directed by the clinical situation.
2. Lower extremity Doppler ultrasound: Ultrasound is relatively inexpensive and is highly accurate for symptomatic DVT but is less accurate for asymptomatic (non-occlusive) DVT. Patients with symptoms of DVT should have a lower extremity Doppler ultrasound first. If positive, anticoagulation is indicated. It is up to the individual clinician to decide whether additional imaging for PE is required. A negative LEUS scan does not eliminate a PE.
3. Helical CTA and CTV: In patients with abnormal chest radiographs, and without signs and symptoms of DVT, CT evaluation of the chest and lower extremities should be performed. Inconclusive studies may lead to additional imaging.

BRONCHOVASCULAR ANATOMY

In interpreting CT pulmonary angiography, it is important to be comfortable with normal bronchovascular anatomy in order to communicate findings accurately and to facilitate comparison of serial studies. For the most part, an embolus is described and located by naming the artery in which it is found. Beyond the central vessels, the artery is called by the name of the adjacent bronchus. Standard nomenclature for the bronchial segments was established by Jackson and Huber in 1943 (30).

The most important aid to interpreting CT bronchovascular anatomy is the workstation. To interpret CT pulmonary angiography, it is necessary to distinguish pulmonary arteries from veins, and the workstation can greatly simplify this task. First, a workstation with scroll capabilities allows the reader to follow peripheral vessels centrally to either the main pulmonary arteries or to the left atrium. Second, switching between lung and soft-tissue windows shows the relationship of the vessel to a bronchus. Pulmonary arteries parallel the bronchi and pulmonary veins run independently [the main exceptions to this are the lingular artery and the artery to the posterior sub segment of the left upper lobe; their origins are somewhat remote from the associated bronchi over short distances (31)]. In central parts of the lung, where many vessels and bronchi are in close proximity, it is helpful to note that the upper lobe arteries are usually central to the associated bronchi, and the middle lobe, lower lobe, and lingular arteries are peripheral to the associated bronchi (32).

Beyond these general principles, it is very helpful to know that there is considerable variability in the vascular anatomy at the segmental level and beyond. Most of these variations are minor and can be appreciated at the workstation. Variations usually consist of early bifurcation or the presence of a common trunk or of a multiplicity of vessels in association with a single bronchus. Also, it is common for subsegmental arteries to cross-segmental planes. The classic treatise by Boyden (33) on segmental anatomy of the lung was used as a source for the discussion below, along with several articles on cross-sectional anatomy (32,34–36), although the Boyden numbering system was felt to be cumbersome and therefore not used. Boyden's system, however, is included for reference (Table 1) (33).

The main pulmonary artery originates at the pulmonary valve and extends superiorly and posteriorly where it bifurcates into the right and left pulmonary arteries.

Right Pulmonary Arteries

Right Upper Lobe

The first branch of the right pulmonary artery is called the truncus anterior; after the takeoff of this vessel, the descending portion of the pulmonary artery is called the interlobar artery, as it lies in the interlobar fissure, lateral to the bronchus intermedius. The truncus anterior usually begins as a single artery that courses superiorly and anteriorly to the right main bronchus. This most commonly divides into an anterior segmental branch and an upper branch. The upper branch usually divides into apical and posterior segmental branches. However, there is commonly a branch from the interlobar pulmonary artery to the posterior segment of the upper lobe and sometimes a branch to the apical segment.

The numbering system described above applies exactly only if the bronchi and the arteries are precisely parallel, an uncommon scenario. If segments are supplied by arteries that do not directly parallel the bronchi, each artery derives its name from the bronchial segment it supplies. So, for example, a right middle lobe artery may bifurcate into an artery that supplies only a portion of the lateral segment, B^4, and a second artery that supplies the remainder of the lateral segment and the medial segment, B^5. In this case, the first artery is called A^4a, and the second artery is called A^{5+4}b. The two major branches of a numbered artery are called a and b, for example, A^3a and A^3b.

Table 1 Boyden's Numbering System for Segmental Anatomy of the Lung

Boyden number	Name of right lung segmental artery	Name of left lung segmental artery
A^1	*Right upper lobe*	*Left upper lobe*
	Apical segment artery	Apical artery (to the apical-posterior segment)
A^2	Anterior segment artery	Anterior segment artery
A^3	Posterior segment artery	Posterior artery (to the apical-posterior segment)
A^4	*Right middle lobe*	
	Lateral segment artery	Superior segment lingular artery
A^5	Medial segment artery	Inferior segment lingular artery
A^6	*Right lower lobe*	*Left lower lobe*
A^{7+8}	Superior segment artery	Superior aegment artery
		Anteromedial basal segment
A^7		Anteromedial basal segment artery
A^8	Medial basal segment artery	Medial subsegment artery
A^9	Anterior basal segment artery	Anterior subsegment artery
A^{10}	Lateral basal segment artery	Lateral basal segment artery
	Posterior basal segment artery	Posterior basal segment artery

Right Middle Lobe

Approximately half of the time, two right middle lobe arteries arise from a common trunk from the right interlobar pulmonary artery, and about half of the time they arise as two separate branches of the interlobar artery. A branch of the medial segmental artery most frequently supplies the anterior aspect of the lateral segment.

Right Lower Lobe

Below the origin of the right middle lobe artery or arteries, the interlobar artery becomes the right lower lobe artery. It usually then gives off one or, occasionally, two posteriorly directed arteries to the superior segment of the right lower lobe. This is usually at the same level as, or slightly caudal to, the takeoff of the right middle lobe bronchus. The name of the artery beyond the origin of the superior segmental artery is the pars basalis or basal artery or trunk, and this gives off the basal segmental arteries. In slightly more than half of cases, the medial basal segmental artery arises first or arises first as a common trunk with the anterior segmental artery, this representing a very variable artery. Finally, the lateral basal and posterior basal arteries arise independently or bifurcate from a common trunk, again with significant variability.

Left Pulmonary Arteries

Unlike the right upper lobe, the left upper lobe artery arches over the top of the left upper lobe bronchus, which therefore is "hyparterial." Apart from this difference, the arterial branching pattern on the left is quite similar to that on the right. However, there tend to be more separate arteries on the left than the right, with "scattering of branches along the course of the main artery" (33).

Left Upper Lobe

Either single or multiple branches arising from the "pars anterior" of the left pulmonary artery supply the anterior segment of the left upper lobe. Additional branches may arise from this anterior portion and supply portions of the apical and/or lingular segments. Following these branches, apical and posterior arteries usually arise from the superior aspect of the arching left pulmonary artery and, unlike the apicoposterior segmental bronchus, which usually has a common origin, these two arteries most commonly arise separately.

Interlobar Segment

In contrast to the right side, on the left, the arterial supply to the superior segment of the lower lobe usually arises above the level of the lingular arteries. Both the superior segmental arteries and the lingular arteries may each arise as a single trunk or as two separate arteries.

Basal Segments

As on the right, the left pars basalis or basal trunk gives off arteries to the left lower basal segments. Just as there is usually a single left anteromedial basal segmental bronchus, there is usually a single left anteromedial segmental artery. However, in about half of cases, the artery to the lateral basal segment arises from a common trunk with this anteromedial branch, separate from a single branch to the posterior basal segment. In the other half of cases, the lateral basal segmental artery arises from a common trunk with the posterior basal segmental branch or in other configurations.

Subsegmental Arteries

As stated above, the subsegmental arteries are variable and may cross into adjacent segments. The Boyden system can be used to number subsegmental vessels, but because of the variability and complexity of the subsegmental arterial anatomy, we find it sufficient to identify an embolus as located in a subsegmental vessel arising from a particular segmental artery or located in a particular segment.

Venous Anatomy

As Boyden initially indicated, the naming of peripheral venous structures in the lungs is much more difficult than the naming of arteries, as the arteries can be named by the bronchi they correspond to, and thus by the segment they supply, while the veins are located remotely from the bronchi. Centrally, the left upper lobe veins drain into the superior pulmonary vein, and right and left lower lobe veins drain into the right and left inferior pulmonary veins. On the right, upper lobe veins usually form a common superior pulmonary vein that joins with middle lobe veins to form a common superior pulmonary venous confluence. The venous return from the right middle lobe sometimes enters the left atrium separately.

TECHNIQUE

The key to effective scanning for PE is careful attention to technique. Since 1992, when Remy-Jardin et al. (37) first reported helical CT for PE, helical scanners have become considerably faster and multidetector scanners have come on the market. This new equipment allows coverage of a larger volume of lung in a shorter period of time while obtaining thinner sections. By the time this chapter is published, further improvements will undoubtedly be in place. Therefore, we deal with the basic concepts of how to optimize technique with the understanding that you can modify the details as appropriate (31,38).

Anatomic Volume

Multidetector scanners permit the inclusion of the entire lung—apex to diaphragmin less than 10 s, well with—in the breath-hold of most patients.

Scan Direction

Caudal-to-cranial scanning assures that the lung bases, which are most susceptible to image degradation from respiratory motion, are scanned early in the breath-hold to minimize respiratory artifact. The direction becomes less important as the scanners become faster and apnea time becomes shorter.

Breathing

Minimizing respiratory motion is critical. Most patients can breath-hold for the required scan acquisition. Hyperventilation prior to scanning and nasal oxygen may help the marginal patient. In dyspneic patients, slow shallow breathing is usually sufficient to obtain adequate images of the central vessels. In patients on mechanical ventilation, the patient can often be held in apnea during the acquisition or, alternatively, the tidal volume and frequency can be minimized. Use of the highest-end scanners available will minimize respiratory motion.

Scan Parameters

Multiple studies have shown that the thinner the collimation, the better the depiction of the peripheral vessels. The choice of scan parameters varies with the available scanner equipment. Multislice scanners allow for 1.25- or 0.625-mm scans. Similarly, increasing pitch from 1 to 1.7 on helical CT or to 3 or 6 on multislice CT increases speed and decreases patient dose. Diminishing scan rotation time from 1 to 0.8 or 0.5 s increases speed further. Electron-beam CT allows for even more rapid acquisition. With each of these changes, there is a potential decrease in photon statistics and increased noise. This is especially detrimental in large patients, where scan parameters must be altered to increase the amount of radiation and thereby decrease noise (i.e., thicker slices, lower pitch, higher kVp and mAs).

Contrast Material

Intravenous contrast is best administered through an antecubital or central venous catheter. Most centers use nonionic contrast. There is no uniform agreement as to the best injection protocol. Most studies have shown that 100–120 cc of full strength nonionic contrast injected at 3–5 cc/s provides excellent vessel opacification. With the faster scanning protocols, 50–80 cc should suffice for diagnosis of PE alone.

As a general rule, the volume of contrast should be chosen so that scanning begins at an appropriate time delay from the initiation of contrast administration, and the injection does not continue after the scans have been completed. If the lower extremity veins are to be studied also, 120 cc is necessary to provide adequate opacification of the veins. With a larger bolus, timing is easier.

There is no universal agreement on the optimal time between onset of contrast injection and scanning. We utilize a preliminary time–density curve to determine the time of peak pulmonary artery enhancement. This utilizes 18 cc of contrast injected over 6 s while the pulmonary artery is being scanned every 3 s for 20 s. The contrast peak is then graphed and 5 s are arbitrarily added to determine scan delay time. In the vast majority of patients, the scan delay is 15–20 s. Many centers empirically use a 15- to 25-s delay without resorting to a time–density curve. In an occasional patient, a specific area is not adequately evaluated on the initial CT because of suboptimal contrast enhancement or respiratory motion. A repeat focal scan through that area can be done using a supplemental 50 cc of contrast and a revised delay based on the prior scan. Alternatively, bolus tracking with a cursor in the main pulmonary artery that triggers scanning at a preset threshold can be used. A timing method should be used in patients with suspected or known cardiac dysfunction because the optimum scan delay time can be 40 s or more.

Lower Extremity Venous Studies

Optimal scanning parameters have not been agreed on (25,39). A reasonable approach involves scanning from the femoral necks to the knees starting 3 min after completion of the IVC contrast injection for the pulmonary arteries. No additional contrast is necessary, although 100–120 cc total contrast dose appears to be necessary to obtain adequate enhancement of the veins to 80–100 HU. The ankles are placed together. At our center, 5-mm scans are obtained every 2 cm. Some centers scan continuously, obtaining complete imaging of the veins, but at the cost of increased radiation dose. PIOPED II and others have emphasized the low yield of IVC and iliac scanning and recommend femoral and popliteal scanning only (acetabula to knees) (13).

CT FINDINGS OF ACUTE PULMONARY EMBOLISM

A diagnosis of PE is made when the embolus is seen as an area of low attenuation in a contrast-enhanced pulmonary artery (38). Acute pulmonary emboli may be manifested as partial or complete filling defects in vessels, by the "railway track sign," or as mural defects.

A partial filling defect means that clot is seen within a vessel, surrounded by contrast (Fig. 1); a filling defect is complete when the entire artery fails to opacify due to a central filling defect. In the setting of acute embolus, vessels that are completely filled with clot may enlarge compared with similar vessels of the same generation. This is in contrast to the smaller diameter seen with chronic thromboembolic disease (31). The "railway track sign" is the demonstration of a clot floating within the vessel (Fig. 2), and a mural defect is defined as a clot that appears adherent to the wall of a vessel, with contrast not completely surrounding the clot. In acute thromboembolic disease, mural thrombi, seen on axial images, usually form acute angles with the vessel walls in vessels that are sufficiently large to examine for this finding (31).

There should be a sharp interface between the filling defect of a PE and adjacent contrast, and the filling defect should be seen on more than one image. Looking for these findings should prevent the misdiagnosis of minor mixing inhomogeneity or other artifacts as emboli. The failure to visualize a vessel should not lead to a diagnosis of PE.

PE may rarely be visible on unenhanced CT (Figs. 3 and 4), as either hyperattenuating areas or hypoattenuating areas of intraluminal thrombus in the central pulmonary arteries (40). Massive PE may cause right ventricular dysfunction and reduced cardiac output (41). Right ventricular enlargement may be visible on CT, with displacement of the interventricular septum toward the left ventricle (Fig. 5). Evaluation of right heart enlargement in patients with a positive CT PE protocol is a promising risk stratification tool (28,42,43).

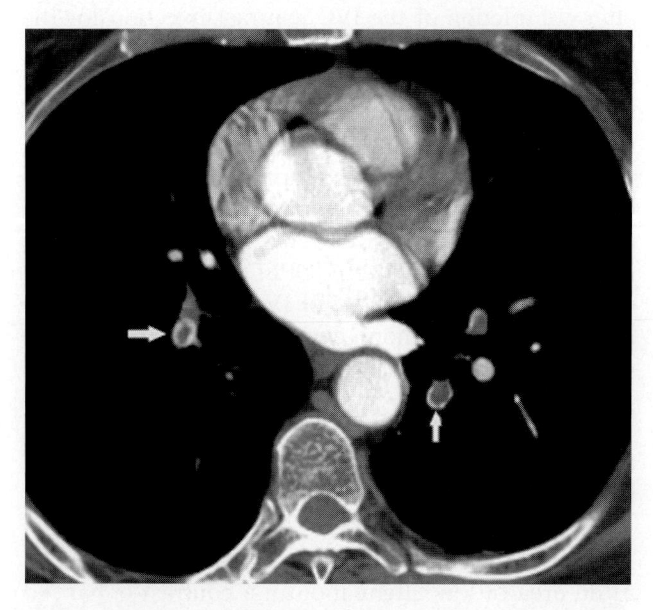

Figure 1 Acute pulmonary embolus (PE). A partial-filling defect is seen in a right lower lobe (RLL) artery, with central low attenuation surrounded by high-attenuation contrast (*arrow*). On the left there are segmental pul-monary emboli in left lower lobe (LLL) that result in an eccentrically positioned partial filling defect (*arrow*), which is surrounded by contrast material and forms acute angle with the arterial wall.

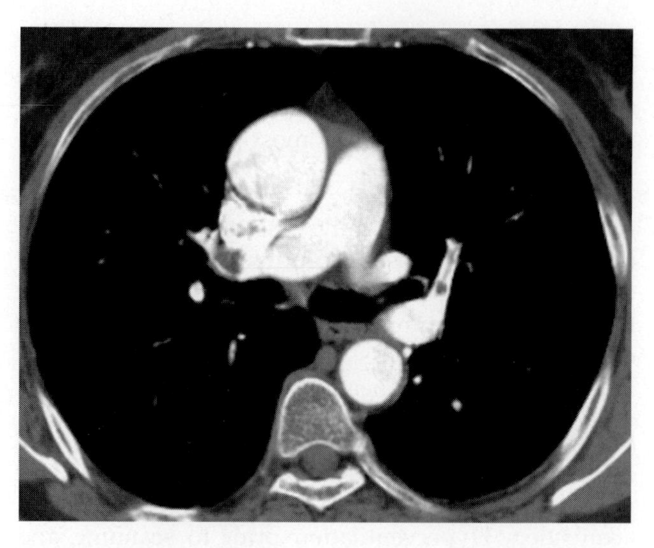

Figure 2 Acute pulmonary embolus (PE). "Railway track sign" of clot floating in the anterior segmental left upper lobe (LUL) artery. A mural thrombus forming acute angles with the vessel wall is present in the RUL artery.

Reflux of contrast material into the IVC may also be encountered, as a sign of elevated right heart pressures, although some contrast reflux may be normal at faster injection speeds of 4–5 s (44). The main pulmonary artery may enlarge to >28 mm and the left and right arteries to >18 mm, as pulmonary artery pressures increase (43,45).

Peripheral wedge-shaped areas of hypoattenuation that may represent infarcts, along with linear bands, have been demonstrated to be statistically significant ancillary findings associated with acute PE (Fig. 6) (46). However, these radiologic features are not specific for PE.

POSTPROCESSING TECHNIQUES

Postprocessing techniques [multiplanar reformation (MPR), maximum intensity projection (MIP), and virtual angioscopy] are not used routinely in the diagnosis of PE. When transverse sections provide a confident analysis of all the pulmonary arteries, 2D and 3D reformations provide no additional information. Sometimes an in-plane or oblique arterial branch or an area of linear perivascular soft tissue may generate an area of low density that may be confused with PE in the axial plane. This artifact is due to partial volume effect between lung parenchyma or perivascular lymphatic tissue and the contrast-enhanced pulmonary artery. The vessels that most often run in the axial plane are the right middle lobe and lingular arteries, the anterior segmental arteries of the upper lobes, and the superior segmental arteries of

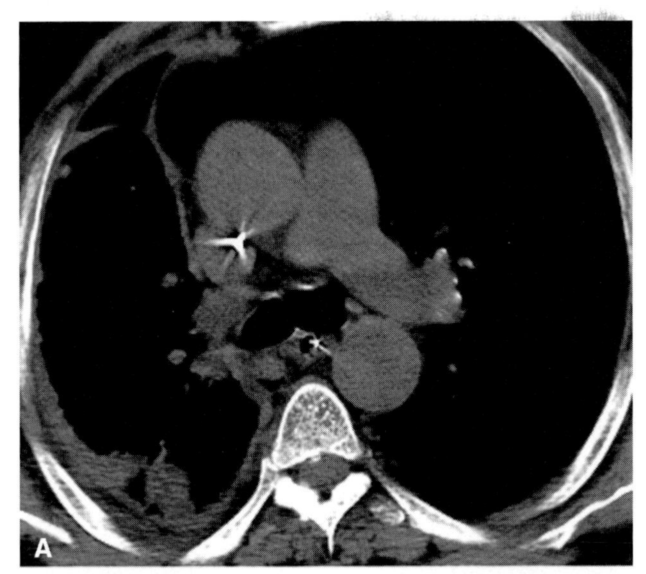

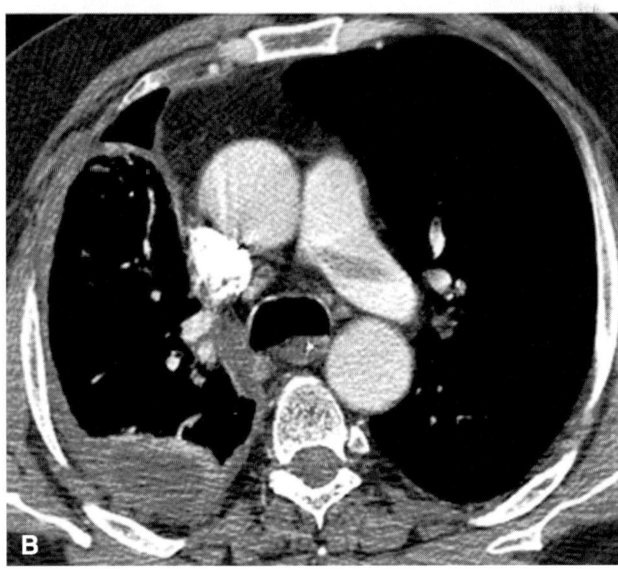

Figure 3 Acute PE in patient with right mesothelioma. Unenhanced CT scan (**A**) shows central hypoattenuating clot in the left main pulmonary artery. Enhanced CT scan (**B**) confirms presence of embolus.

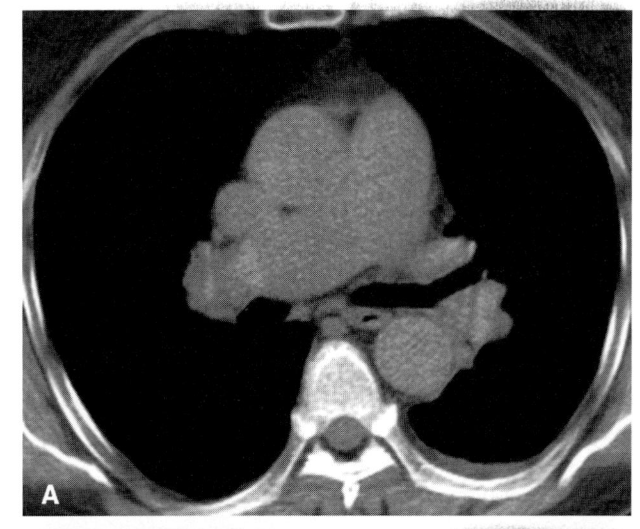

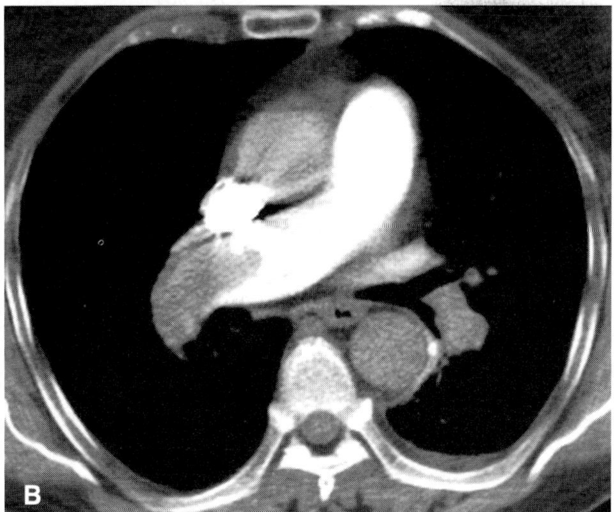

Figure 4 Acute central pulmonary embolus (PE) in a 42-year-old man who presented with chest pain and severe dyspnea. Unenhanced CT scan (**A**) reveals the presence of central hyperattenuating clot in the right main pulmonary artery. Enhanced CT scan (**B**) confirms presence of embolus.

the lower lobes (47,48). In these cases, the vessels are displayed better by high-quality MPRs that use data obtained from a contiguous helical thin section data set available from high-end MDCT scanners. The images may be reformatted in any anatomical plane (coronal, sagittal, oblique, or curvilinear view). Sliding thin-slab MIP are an excellent tool for evaluating the peripheral pulmonary arteries, and should be applied if no central embolus is found on axial images (Figs. 7 and 8). They have been shown to considerably improve the detection of small peripheral emboli (49). Virtual endoscopy provides a direct view of the intraluminal clot. Its clinical utility has yet to be determined.

Another potential application of MPRs is the evaluation of chronic thromboembolic disease. The creation of MPRs through the longitudinal axis of obliquely oriented vessels can overcome some of the difficulties encountered with axial images in the identification of focal arterial stenoses and webs or in separating eccentric, adherent thrombus from adjacent lymphatic tissue (50).

Computer-assisted diagnosis may be applicable to PE in the near future.

PITFALLS IN DIAGNOSES

There are many pitfalls in the interpretation of PE, even for the experienced reader (26,36). The three most important strategies for avoiding pitfalls were

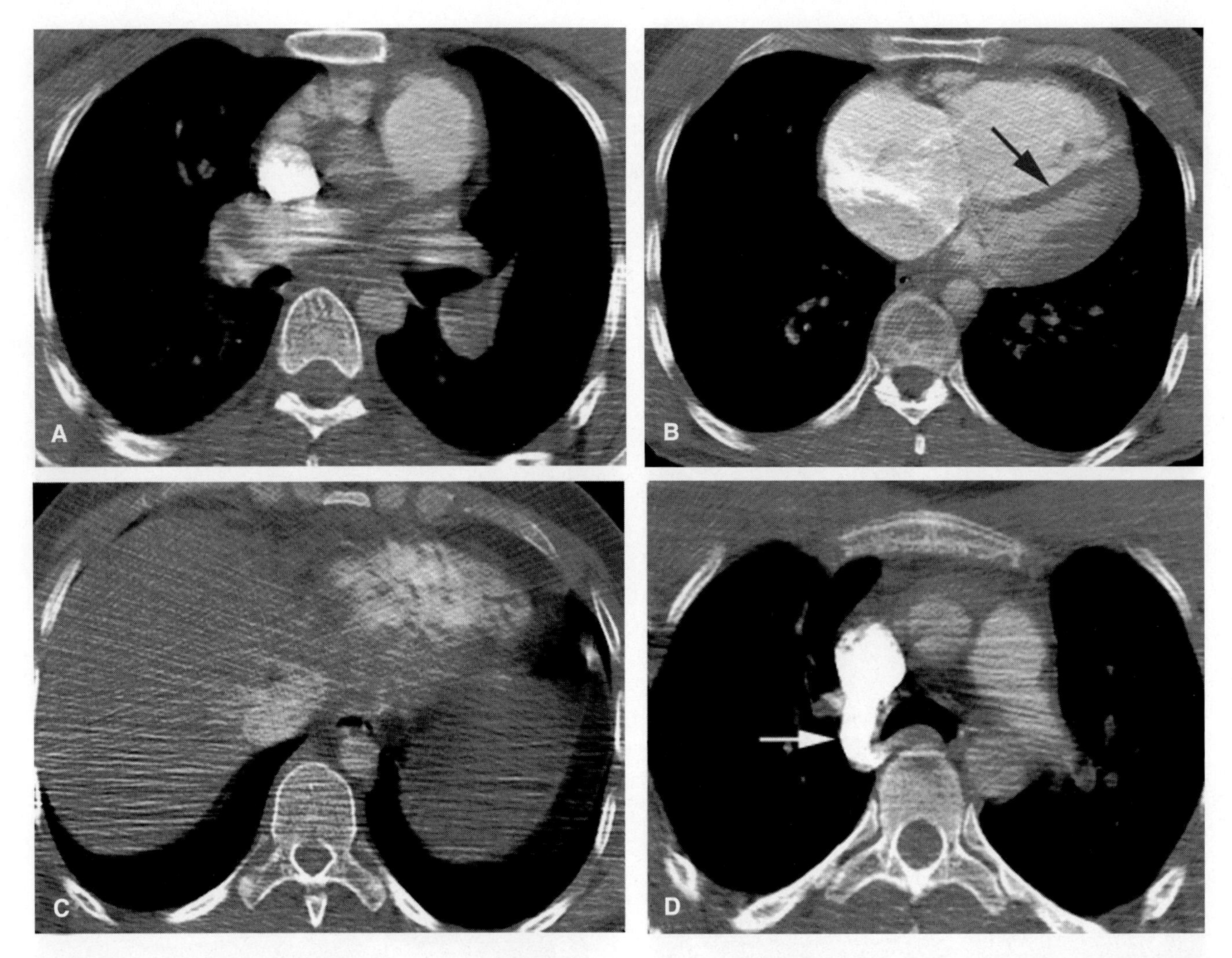

Figure 5 Acute central pulmonary embolus (PE) in a 39-year-old man presenting with acute onset of dyspnea. CT scan (**A**) shows multiple endoluminal clots on both sides responsible for complete filling defects at the level of central pulmonary arteries; the main pulmonary artery is enlarged compared with adjacent aorta. Axial CT pulmonary angiogram obtained at the level of the heart (**B**) shows other signs of pulmonary hypertension: note the severe dilatation of the right ventricle and the compression of the left ventricle; also note the left ward bowing of the inter-ventricular septum (*arrow*). Reflux of contrast medium into the hepatic veins are present (**C**) and the azygos vein (*arrow*) is enlarged (**D**).

discussed above: meticulous technique, understanding of normal anatomy and common variants, and interpretation on a workstation. The remaining major impediments to reading include technical problems that thwart diagnosis and anatomical or disease entities that mimic PE.

Technical Problems

Respiratory Motion

Vessel motion will often cause the pulmonary arteries to appear less dense. If the vessels on adjacent images appear normal, and the lung windows reveal respiratory motion in the slice in question, it is almost certainly a respiratory artifact. As a general strategy, PE should be visible on two or more images for confident diagnosis.

Streak Artifacts

Linear artifacts arising from high-density structures, such as the contrast-enhanced superior vena cava, calcified lymph nodes, or surgical clips, can cause apparent lucencies in a contrast-enhanced pulmonary artery. The artifact source is usually readily apparent and the defect is linear in the axial plane.

Hyperdense Vessels

Small nonocclusive clots may not be visible in densely enhanced larger pulmonary arteries. After routine reading on soft tissue windows, one should reread the images of the proximal arteries at a wider window and higher level. A window width and level of 700/100 HU is applicable to most patients. Caution should be used in altering window and level because this accentuates artifacts such as inhomogeneous

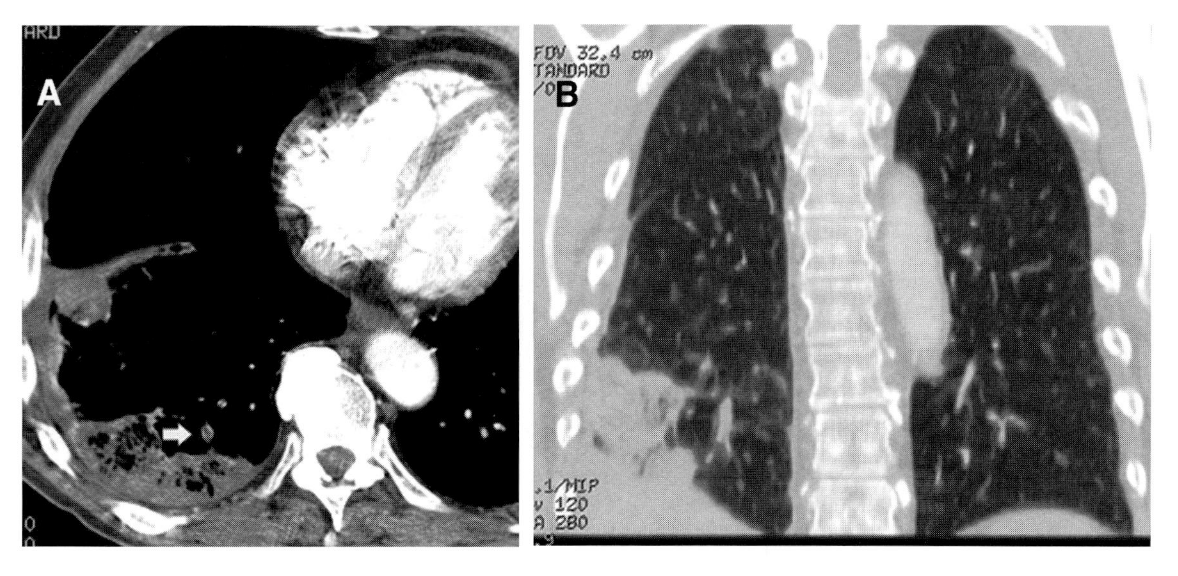

Figure 6 Acute pulmonary embolus (PE) in a 59-year-old man who presented with chest pain and dyspnea. CT scan (**A**) shows a pulmonary embolus within the postero-basal subsegmental of the right lower lobe artery (*arrow*). The artery is enlarged compared with adjacent patent vessels. Coronal maximum intensity projection (**B**) shows a wedge-shaped non enhancing soft tissue with small irregular air inclusions in the corresponding right lower lobe, consistent with pulmonary infarct, the CT version of "Hampton's hump."

contrast mixing. In general the margins of flow defects are less distinct than the margins of a PE.

Underenhanced Vessels

If all the vessels are not well enhanced, either the timing of injection was faulty or there was a mechanical problem with the injection, the catheter, or the veins leading to the right heart. Right heart failure may also delay pulmonary artery opacification. With faster scanning protocols, it is possible to enhance the pulmonary arteries well before contrast reaches the veins on the initial images. This may simulate a PE. Valsalva maneuver may alter hemodynamics and result in suboptimal opacification in some areas, simulating PE.

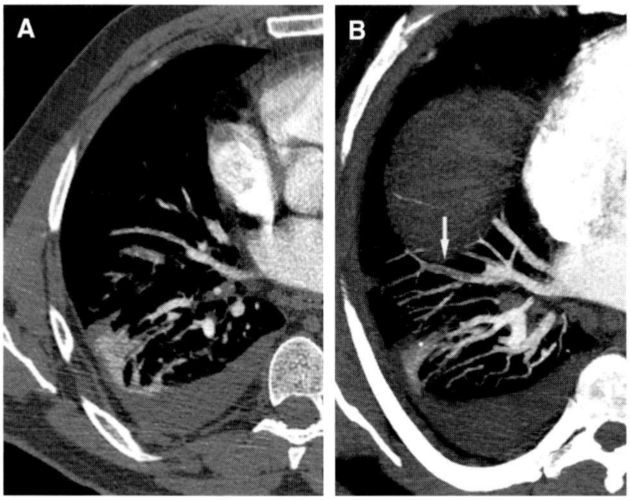

Figure 7 Post-processing techniques. Small subsegmental embolus that was primarily missed on axial section (**A**) but picked up on axial thin-slab maximum intensity projection (*arrow*) (**B**). On the right there are also small pleural effusion and pulmonary infarct.

Edge Enhancement

Avoid edge enhancement as used in high-resolution lung algorithms. Edge enhancement causes the margins of the vessels to appear dense. By comparison, the center of the vessel appears more lucent and may be misinterpreted as a PE. A "smooth" or "low-spatial frequency" reconstruction algorithm should always be used.

Noisy Images

To avoid excessive noise in large patients, especially at the shoulder and hips, kVp and mAs should be increased, the pitch decreased, and thicker images viewed.

Anatomical Problems

Vessel Bifurcation

Axial images through the bifurcation of a pulmonary artery often produce the appearance of a central lucency. Workstation paging, above and below, easily identifies these as branch points (Fig. 9).

In-Plane Vessels

Segmental vessels of the middle lobe, the lingula, the superior segments of the lower lobes, and the anterior segments of the upper lobes tend to undulate in and out of the plane or across the plane obliquely, causing pseudofilling defects. Again, cine viewing on a workstation overcomes this problem. If the contrast

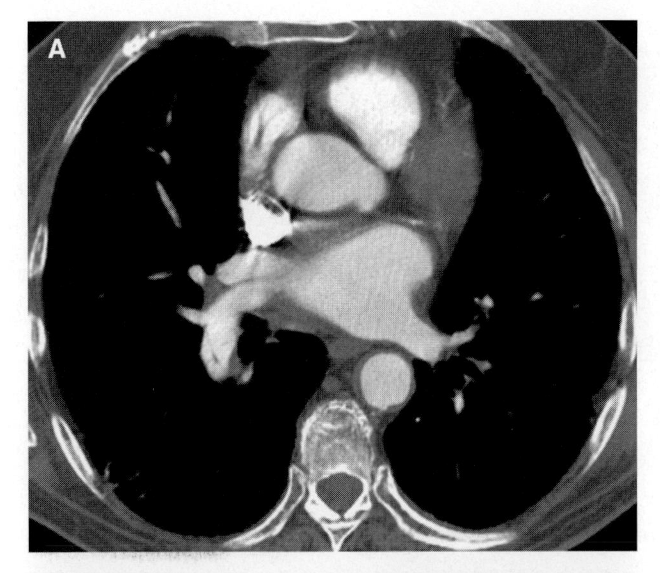

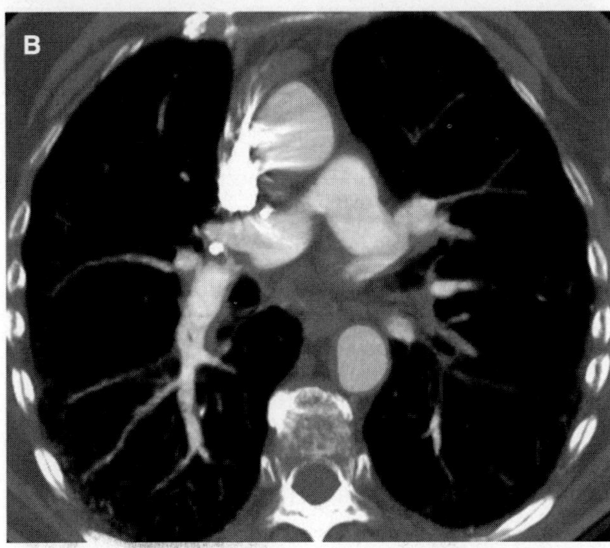

Figure 8 Chronic PE in a patient with idiopatic pulmonary fibrosis. CT scan (**A**) and axial oblique MIP image (**B**) depict a linear web (arrows) in the right interlobar pulmonary artery and left pulmonary artery cut-off.

column ends in a sharp meniscus, a PE is likely to be present; if it tails off gradually, it is more likely an artifact. Multiplanar reconstructions are often helpful.

Lymphatic and Connective Tissue

Even in normal patients, there is frequently amorphous lymphatic tissue adjacent to the main, lobar, and proximal segmental vessels. These are often not well-defined "nodes." Lymphatic tissue parallel to the arteries may be volume averaged "into" the adjacent contrast-filled vessel. This is an especially difficult problem at the bifurcation of the right pulmonary artery into the truncus anterior and the interlobar artery and at the origin of the left upper lobe arteries. The lymphatic tissue is usually present over many images and workstation paging usually resolves these issues. It may be especially difficult to distinguish the parallel lymphatic tissue from the wall thickening of chronic PE. Multiplanar reconstructions are especially helpful in solving this problem.

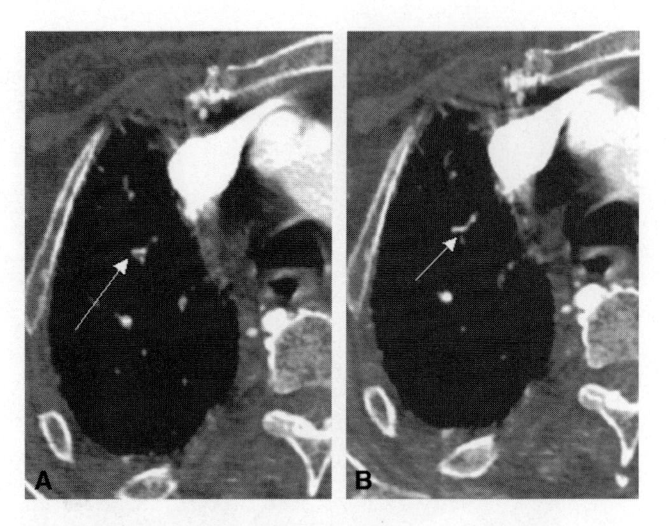

Figure 9 Vessel bifurcation. (**A**) There appears to be a small lucency in a subsegmental vessel in the right upper lobe (arrow). (**B**) Shows vessel bifurcation at this site.

Mucous Plugs

Mucous filled small- and medium-sized bronchi appear as low-density cylindrical structures, coursing through the lung in exactly the same planes as the pulmonary arteries. These are easily misinterpreted as occluded pulmonary arteries. On mediastinal windows, a contrast-enhanced vessel runs directly adjacent to each of these structures and, on lung windows, no air is visible in the expected location of the bronchus (Fig. 10).

Parenchymal Disease

Atelectasis, pneumonia, emphysema, and so on often distort pulmonary arteries. In general, with cine paging, one can follow the distorted vessels into the periphery of the lung. In emphysema, the peripheral vessels are markedly attenuated. The failure to visualize enhanced peripheral vessels, without a demonstrable, central-filling defect, should not be interpreted as a sign of PE.

DEEP VENOUS THROMBOSIS OF THE LOWER EXTREMITY

Findings that indicate the diagnosis of acute DVT on CTV include an intravascular filling defect of low density or total lack of enhancement of a venous region (Fig. 11) (24,51,52). Ancillary findings of DVT are enlargement of the thrombosed vein, wall enhancement, and perivenous edema. With acute occlusive thrombosis, the vein enlarges, sometimes to twice the size of the accompanying artery. The vein wall may enhance to a density equal to or higher than

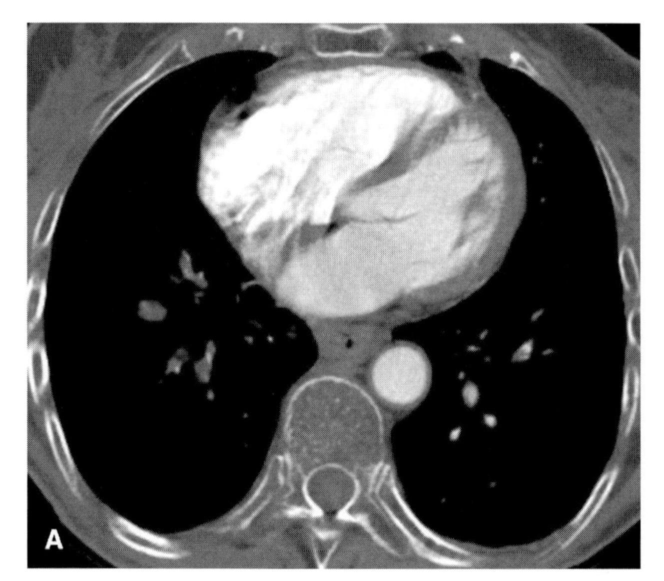

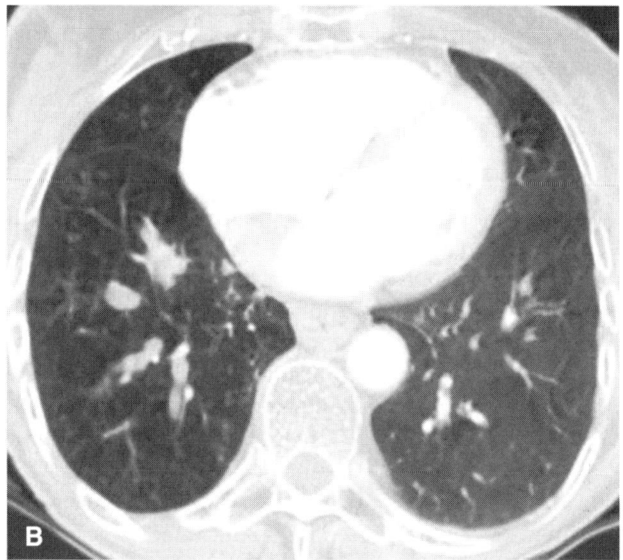

Figure 10 Mucous plug. (**A**) There is a branching soft tissue density (mucoid impaction) supplying the basal segments of the right lower lobe (RLL). It has the appearance of a clot-filled vessel. However, the contrast-filled pulmonary artery is immediately medial to this area. (**B**) On the lung windows, there is no air-filled bronchus in basal segments of the right lower lobe. Decreased lung opacity in the RLL is caused by airway disease.

muscle density. An additional finding seen in DVT is a focal perivenous soft-tissue infiltration that is probably due to local edema. This finding, not specific for DVT, is most easily detectable in the thigh and popliteal regions where fat surrounds the veins.

For the diagnosis of chronic DVT on CTV, we have used criteria analogous to criteria used in venography to identify chronic thrombus. In chronic disease, the vein is often smaller than the accompanying artery (Fig. 12), may be calcified, and may not carry contrast-enhanced blood. In addition, extensive collateral veins are an indication that chronic disease

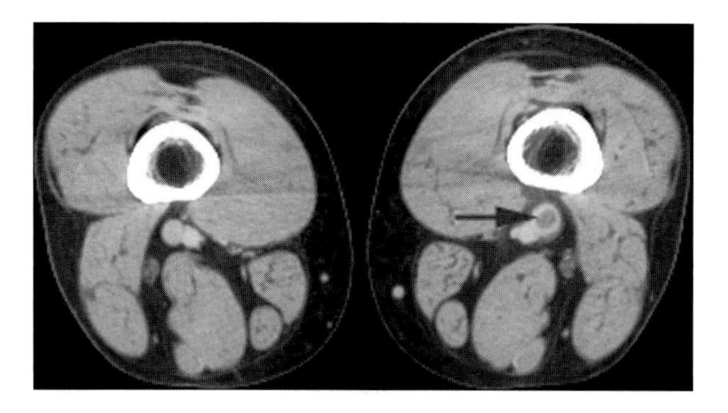

Figure 11 Acute deep venous thrombosis. CT venography image of the mid-thigh shows a clot in the left superficial femoral vein (*arrow*). The vein is enlarged. Note the enhanced thick wall, and the perivenous edema of the left superficial femoral vein. Compare with that of a normal left superficial femoral vein.

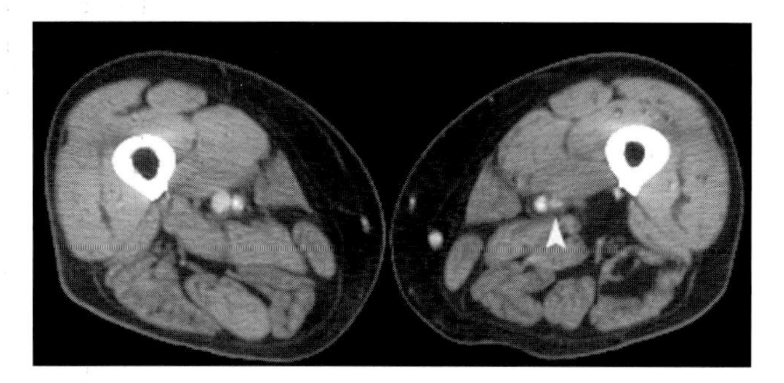

Figure 12 CT venography image in patient with chronic deep venous thrombosis (DVT). The left superficial femoral vein (*arrowhead*) is small; compare with that of the normal right superficial femoral vein.

is present. Their presence, however, does not rule out acute clot superimposed on chronic clot.

CTV can define additional disease (e.g., focal venous aneurysm, abdominal tumor, muscle hematoma, bone fractures, and arterial thrombosis) that may alter on patient management (50). Occasionally, incidental findings that will not necessarily affect patient management are revealed, such as a Baker's cyst, or suprapatellar effusions (51,52).

CHRONIC PULMONARY EMBOLISM

After an event of acute PE, the thrombi usually undergo complete resolution through the process of fibrinolysis, which takes weeks to months (53–55), to reestablish normal pulmonary hemodynamics. With large thrombi, this may take longer. In a study of patients with massive acute PE, despite adequate treatment, some abnormal findings were found at posttherapeutic CTs in 32 patients (52%) after a mean of 11 months (53). However, for reasons as yet unclear, a small fraction of patients do not experience normal clot lysis. Instead, clots in these patients undergo

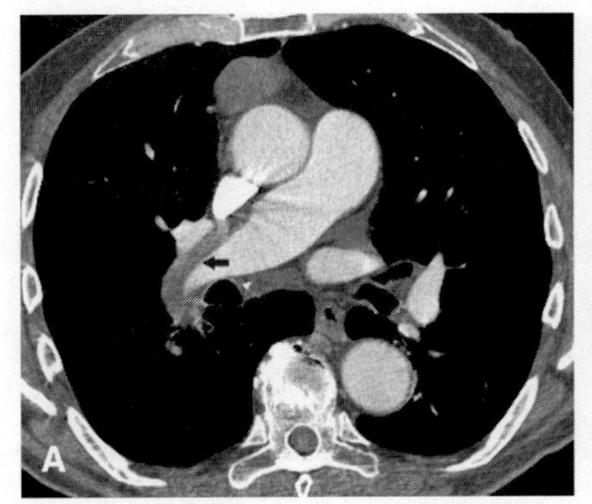

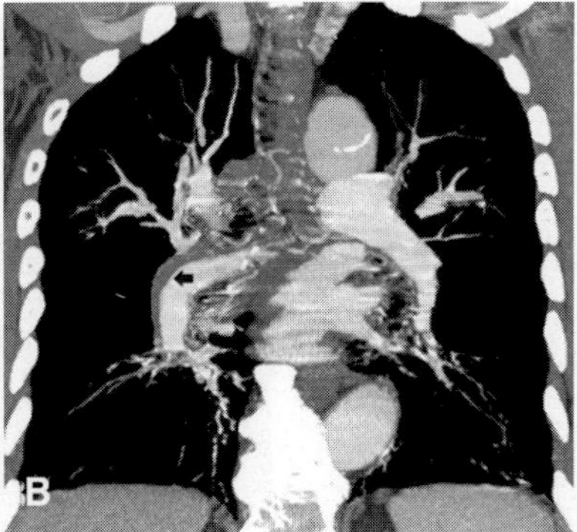

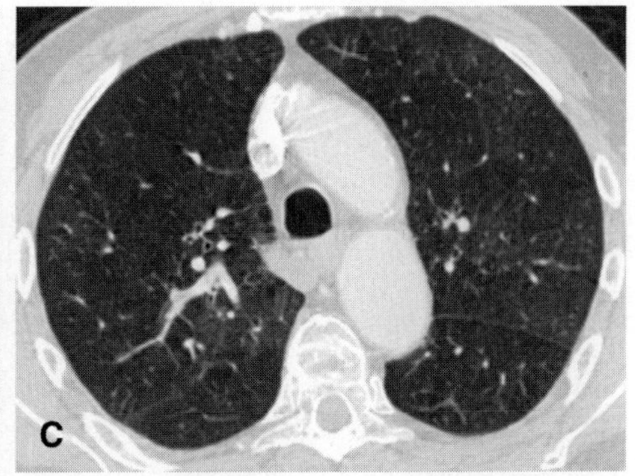

Figure 13 Chronic pulmonary embolus (PE). CT scan (**A**) and coronal maximum intensity projection (MIP) (**B**) show an eccentric thrombus (*arrows*) in the right main pulmonary artery. Lung window (**C**) demonstrates a mosaic perfusion pattern. The dark regions of underperfused lung are seen to contain vessels that are smaller than the adjacent patent vessels in the normally perfused lung. Incidental thymoma is present in the anterior mediastinum (**A**).

variable degrees of organization, recanalization, and retraction. The residual strictures, webs, and membranous occlusions cause vascular stenosis. Substantial burdens of chronic pulmonary artery embolism may cause pulmonary artery hypertension (PAH) refractory to medical treatment (54,56).

It is important to recognize chronic pulmonary thromboembolism (CPTE) in order to distinguish it from acute PE, since PAH due to CPTE can potentially be cured by thromboendarterectomy. Diagnostic procedures in these patients may confirm the diagnosis, demonstrate operative feasibility, and possibly document surgical success. Spiral CTA may help us understand changes within the central pulmonary arteries after PE and see morphologic and endoluminal changes due to chronic PE. Results of several studies confirm the value of CT in the diagnosis of CPTE (53,57–61). Both pulmonary vascular and lung parenchymal abnormalities have been noted.

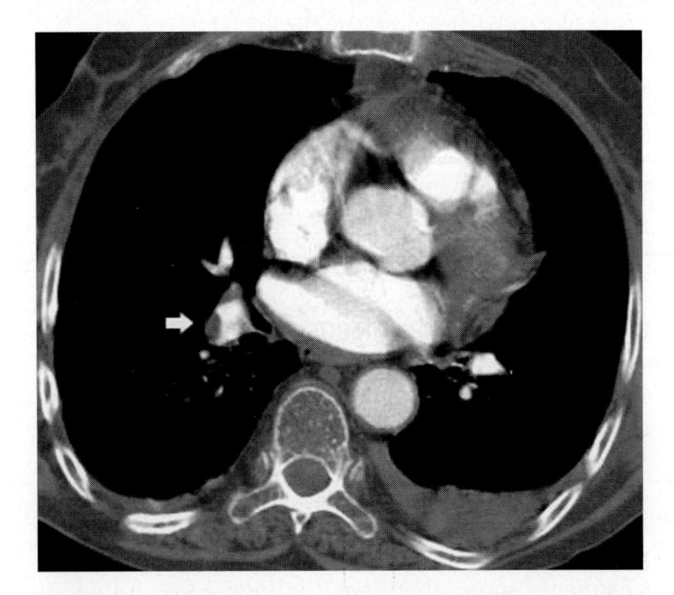

Figure 14 Chronic pulmonary embolus (PE). CT scan of 50-year-old man with chronic pulmonary thromboembolism. Mediastinal window through midzone reveals marginated mural thrombus in the right inferior lobar pulmonary artery (*arrow*). Bilateral pleural effusions are present.

Vascular Abnormalities

Pulmonary angiography is the most widely used technique to diagnose CPTE and to define the location and proximal extent of disease. Pulmonary angiograms usually reveal intimal irregularities, webs, abrupt narrowing, poststenotic dilatation, and tortuous vessels (62). Residual mural thromboemboli that thicken the wall but do not deform the endovascular contour may be missed at catheter angiography.

CT may show direct and indirect signs of CPTE. The direct CT findings are visualization of complete obstruction or adherent thrombotic clot (sometimes calcified) (Figs. 13 and 14). Adherent clot causes the vessel wall to appear eccentrically thickened. There may also be evidence of recanalization within the intraluminal defect and arterial stenosis or webs (Fig. 8) (61). The indirect CT findings are mural irregularities in central and peripheral pulmonary branches, abrupt narrowing of the vessel diameter, and abrupt cutoff of distal lobar or segmental artery branches (61). CT scans also depict changes of the systemic arterial circulation. In CPTE, the bronchial circulation is increased because peripheral bronchopulmonary anastomoses help maintain the pulmonary circulation. In one study, dilatation and tortuosity of bronchial arteries were seen in 77% of 39 patients with CPTE, and the authors suggested that the presence of visible bronchial arteries on CT is a significant criterion to suggest CPTE (63).

The morphology and shape of the central pulmonary arteries and the heart may be helpful for the diagnosis of CPTE. Additional diagnostic findings include enlargement of the central pulmonary

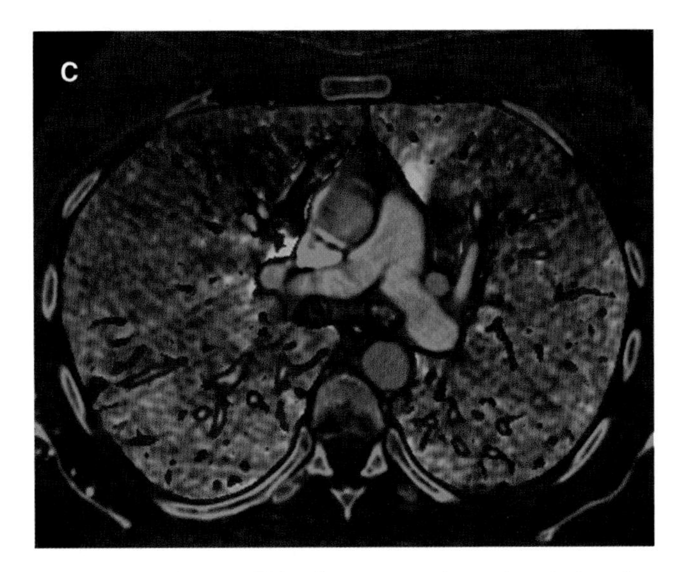

Figure 1.2 Normal CT pulmonary angiography study using single acquisition dual-energy technique. (**C**) CT perfusion imaging. Conventional image fused with color-coded calculated map of iodine distribution in the lung parenchyma. (*For* Figure 1.2 **A**, **B**, *and* **D** *and complete caption, see page 4.*)

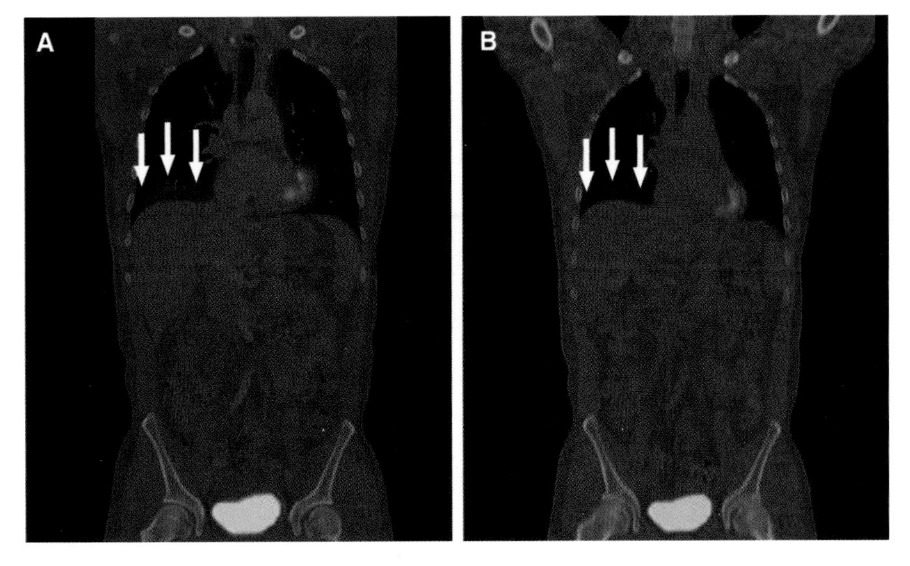

Figure 2.1 Dual PET-CT examinations of a 63-year-old male with history of non–small cell lung cancer. (*For complete caption, see page 12.*)

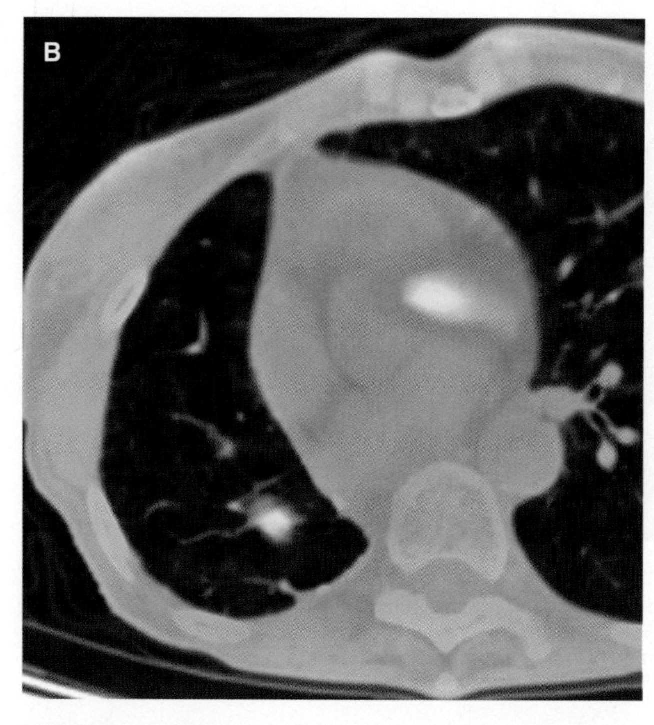

Figure 2.2 Evaluation of a pulmonary nodule in a 69-year-old woman. (**B**) Fused image from a dual PET-CT examination clearly demonstrates focal intense FDG uptake, with the nodule indicative of malignancy. (*For* Figure 2.2 **A** *and complete caption, see page 13.*)

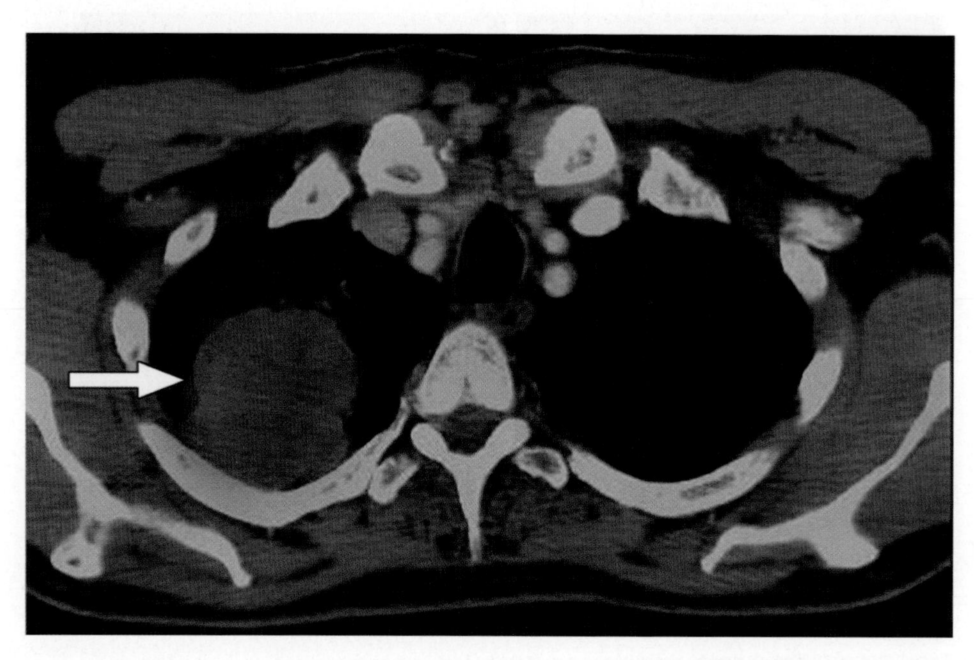

Figure 2.3 Dual PET-CT in a 61-year-old for initial staging of lung cancer. (*For complete caption, see page 13.*)

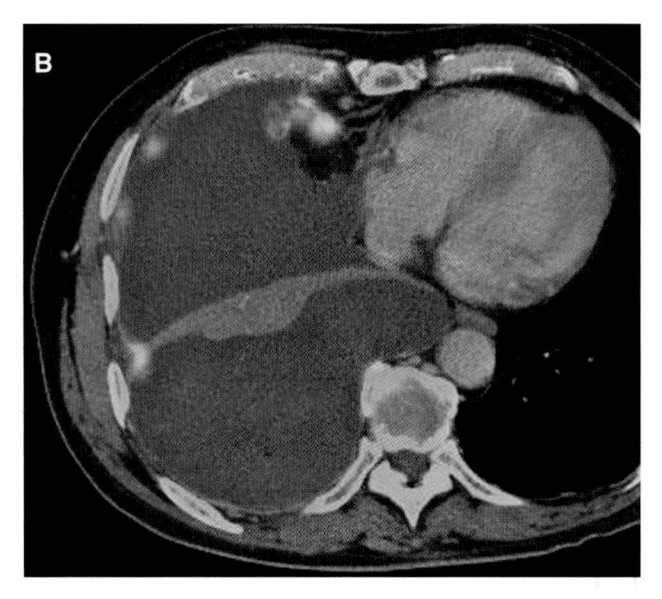

Figure 2.5 Dual PET-CT in a 79-year-old male with non–small cell lung cancer. (**B**) Fused dual PET-CT images demonstrate foci of intense pleural FDG uptake, confirming pleural involvement. (*For* Figure 2.5 **A** *and complete caption, see page 15.*)

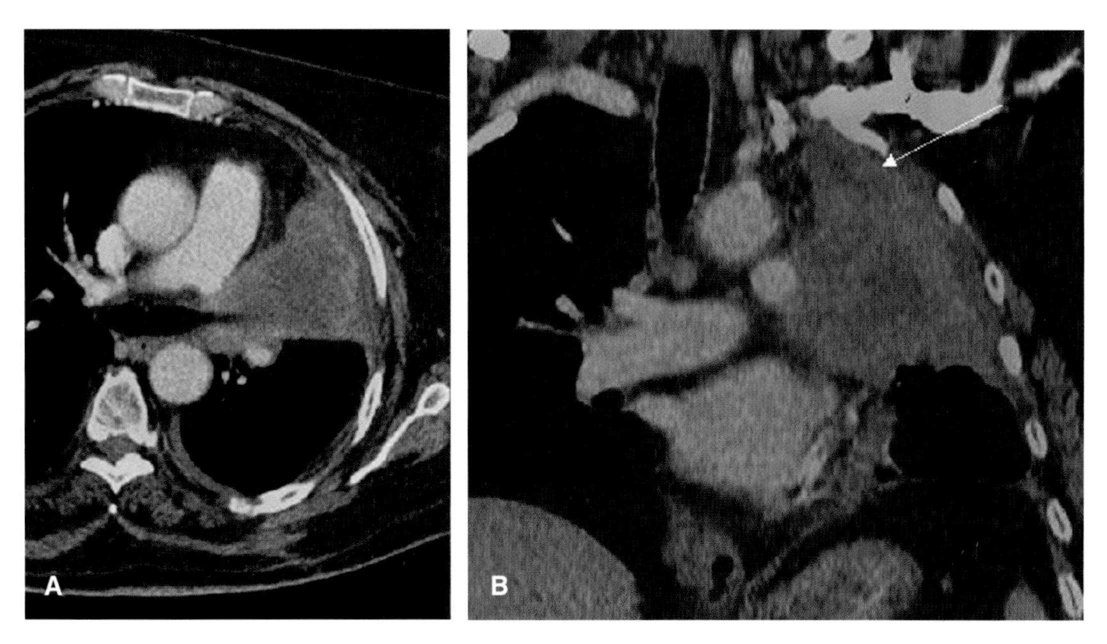

Figure 2.6 Dual PET-CT in a 64-year-old with non small-cell lung cancer. (*For complete caption, see page 15.*)

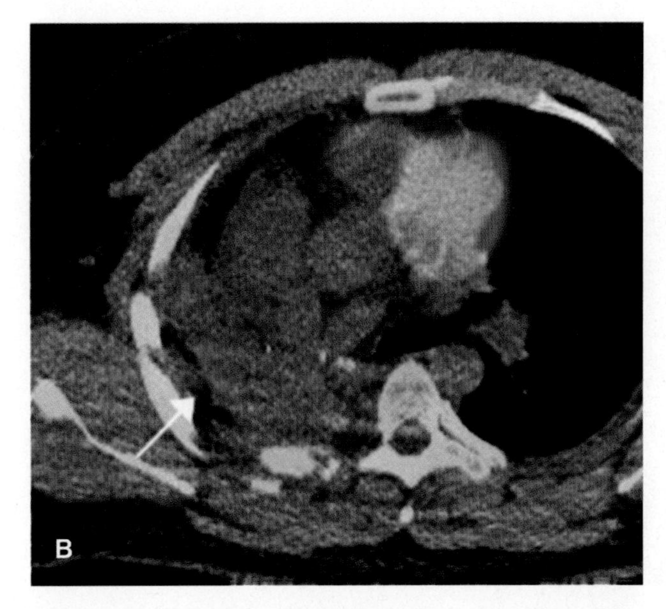

Figure 2.7 Dual PET-CT examination in a 43-year-old male, two years after a right pneumonectomy for non–small cell lung cancer. (**B**) Dual PET-CT image demonstrates an area of pleural thickening with intense FDG uptake that likely represents recurrent disease. (*For* Figure 2.7 **A** *and complete caption, see page 17.*)

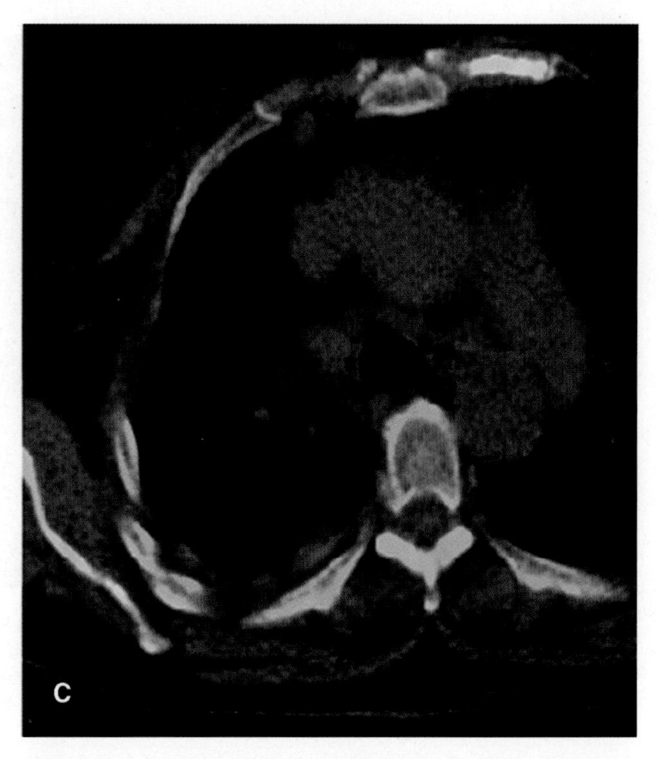

Figure 2.8 Images from a dual PET-CT in a 74-year-old woman with non–small cell lung cancer status post talc pleurodesis. (**C**) Fused dual PET-CT image demonstrates the foci of intense FDG uptake corresponding to the high-density talc. (*For* Figure 2.8 **A** *and* **B** *and complete caption, see page 18.*)

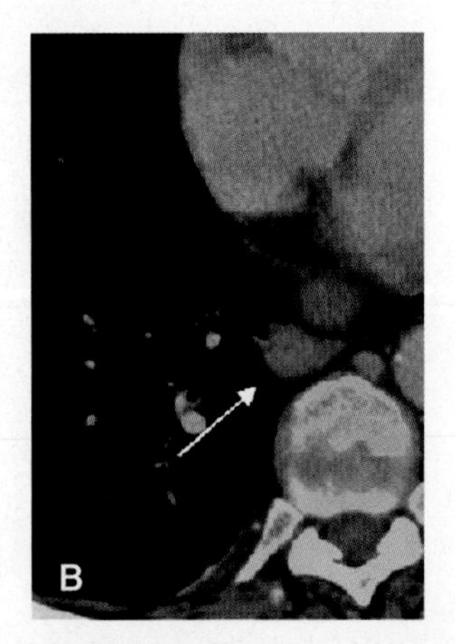

Figure 2.9 Dual PET-CT for restaging in a patient with non–small cell lung cancer. (**B**) Fused dual PET-CT image demonstrates that the focus of FDG uptake corresponds to the esophagus rather than an abnormal lymph node. (*For* Figure 2.9 **A** *and complete caption, see page 18.*)

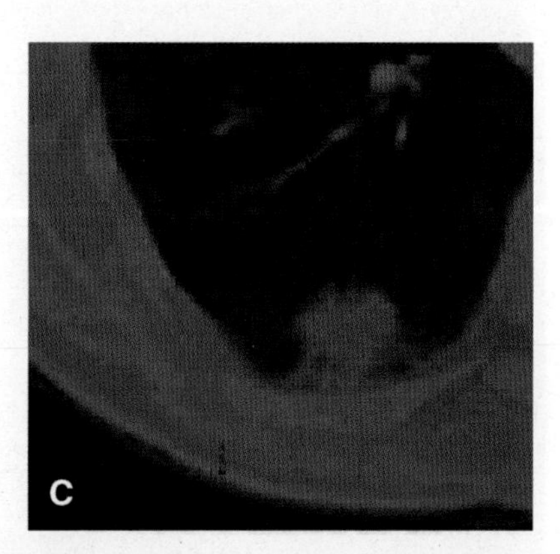

Figure 2.10 Dual PET-CT in a 63-year-old female with suspected lung cancer. (**C**) Fused images demonstrate FDG uptake corresponding to the right lower lobe nodule. (*For* Figure 2.10 **A** *and* **B** *and complete caption, see page 19.*)

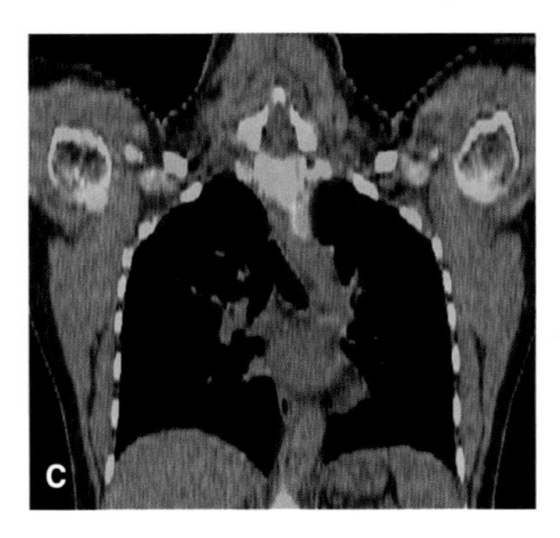

Figure 2.11 Dual PET-CT in a 32-year-old woman with thyroid cancer. (**C**) Fused dual PET-CT image demonstrates localization of the intense supraclavicular uptake to regions of fat, consistent with uptake within brown adipose tissue. (*For* Figure 2.11 **A** *and* **B** *and complete caption, see page 20.*)

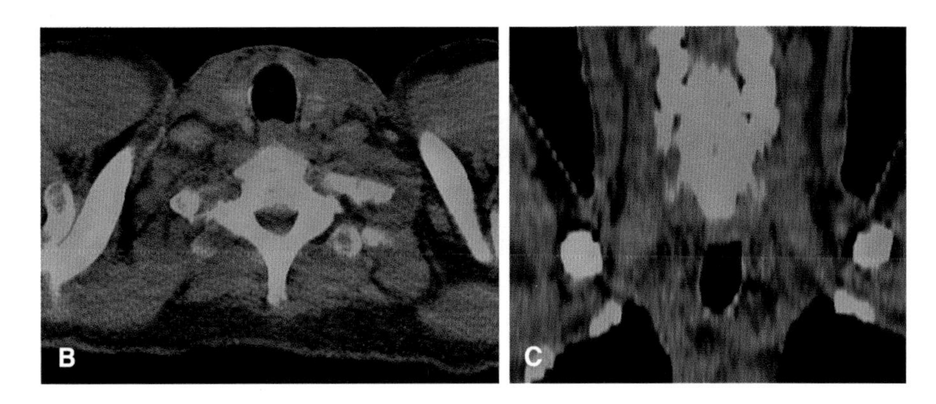

Figure 2.12 A 53-year-old male with a history of lymphoma. (**B**,**C**) Axial and coronal fused images from the dual PET-CT demonstrate that the linear, symmetric, bilateral FDG uptake corresponds to the anterior scalene muscles bilaterally. (*For* Figure 2.12 **A** *and complete caption, see page 21.*)

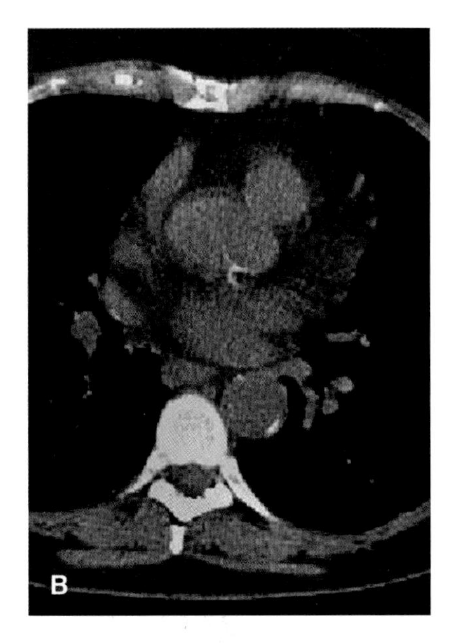

Figure 2.13 Dual PET-CT examination for staging in a 63-year-old man with a gastrointestinal stromal tumor. (**B**) Fused dual PET-CT images demonstrate the focus of FDG uptake corresponding to a focus of fat in the interatrial septum. (*For* Figure 2.13 **A** *and complete caption, see page 21.*)

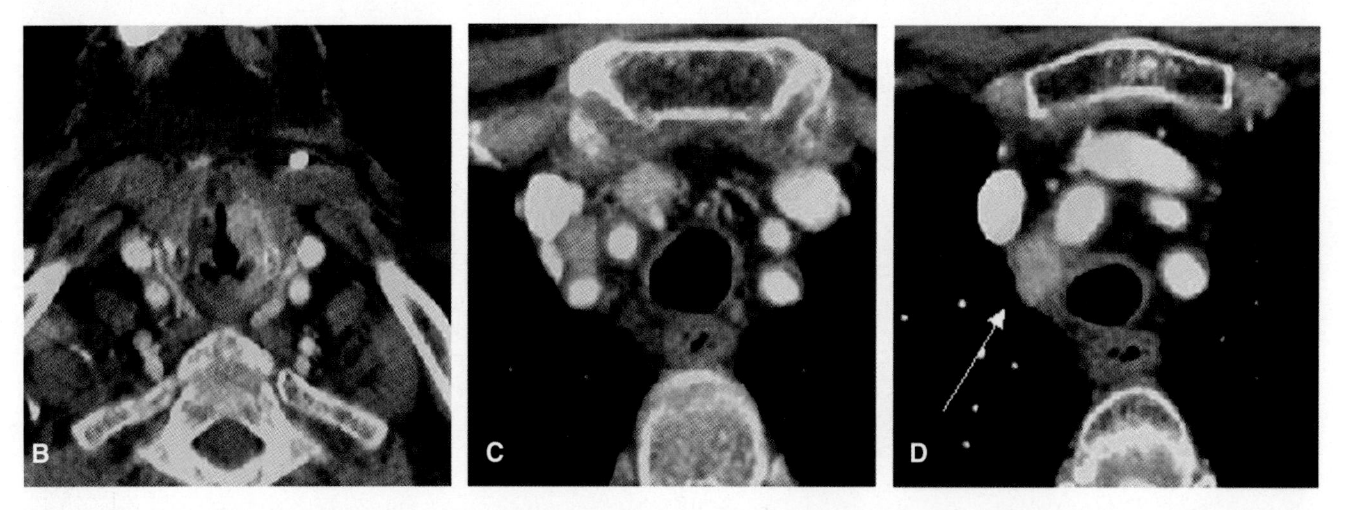

Figure 2.14 Restaging dual PET-CT in a 63-year-old female with non–small cell lung cancer. (**B**) Fused dual PET-CT images demonstrate intense FDG uptake in the region of the normal, nonparalyzed, left vocal cord. (**C**,**D**) Dual PET-CT images demonstrate FDG-avid, right, high, paratracheal lymphadenopathy in the region of the right recurrent laryngeal nerve. (*For* Figure 2.14 **A** *and complete caption, see page 22.*)

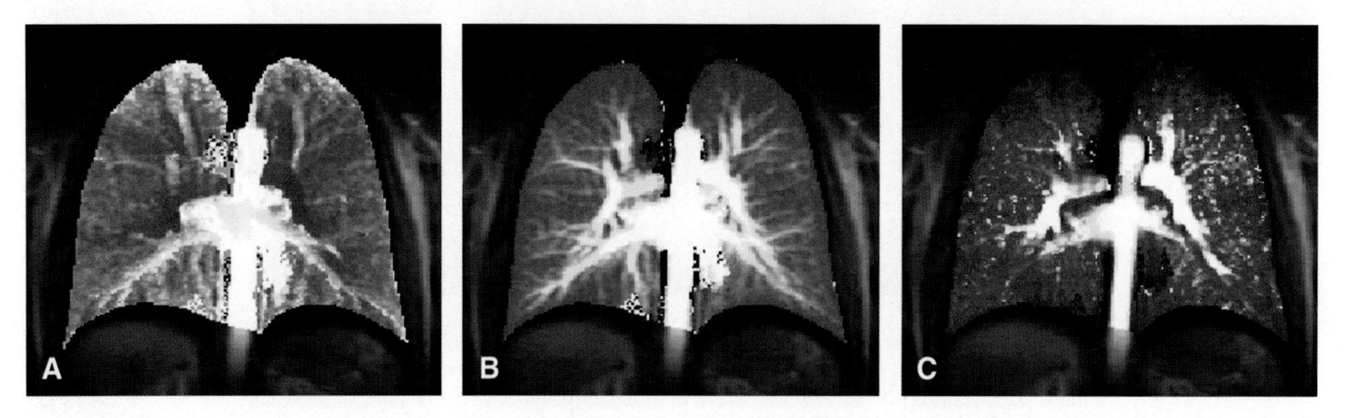

Figure 3.4 Parametric maps of transit time (**A**), blood volume (**B**), and blood flow (**C**). (*For complete caption, see page 27.*)

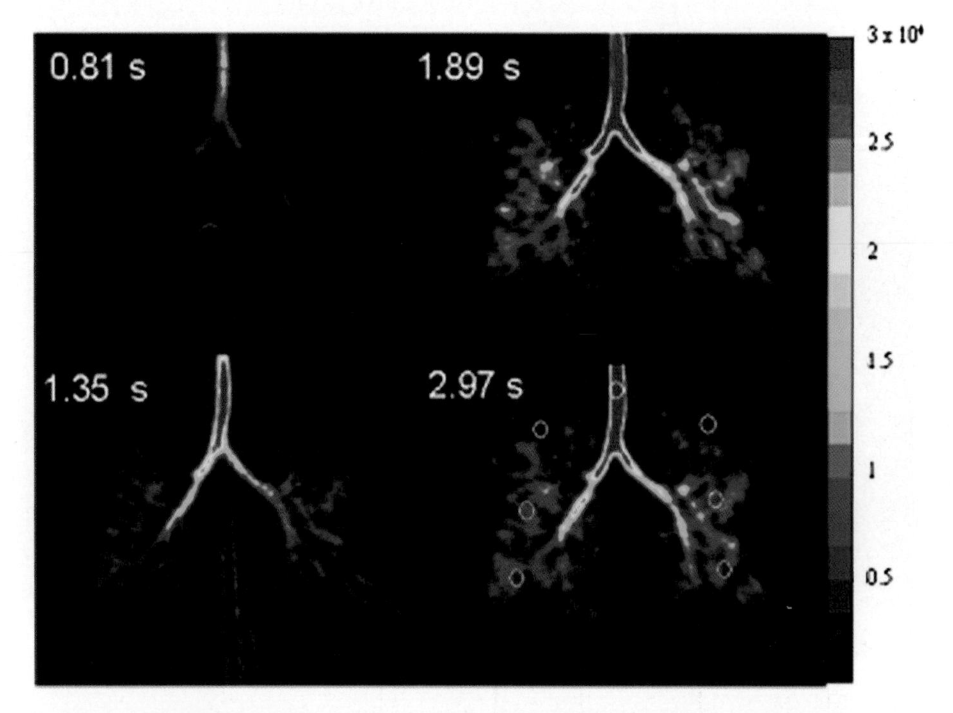

Figure 3.7 Dynamic coronal hyperpolarized helium MR ventilation images from a patient with cystic fibrosis showing inhomogeneity of ventilation. (*For complete caption, see page 30.*)

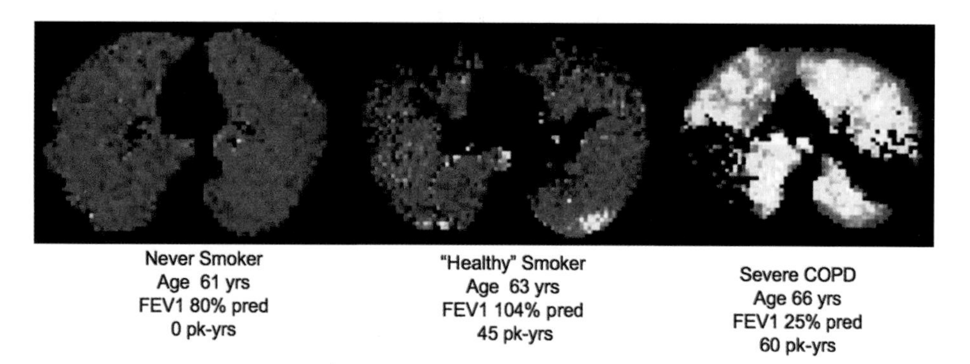

Figure 3.10 Axial hyperpolarized helium MR apparent diffusion coefficient (ADC) maps in a subject who never smoked, a healthy smoker, and a patient with chronic obstructive pulmonary disease (COPD). (*For complete caption, see page 32.*)

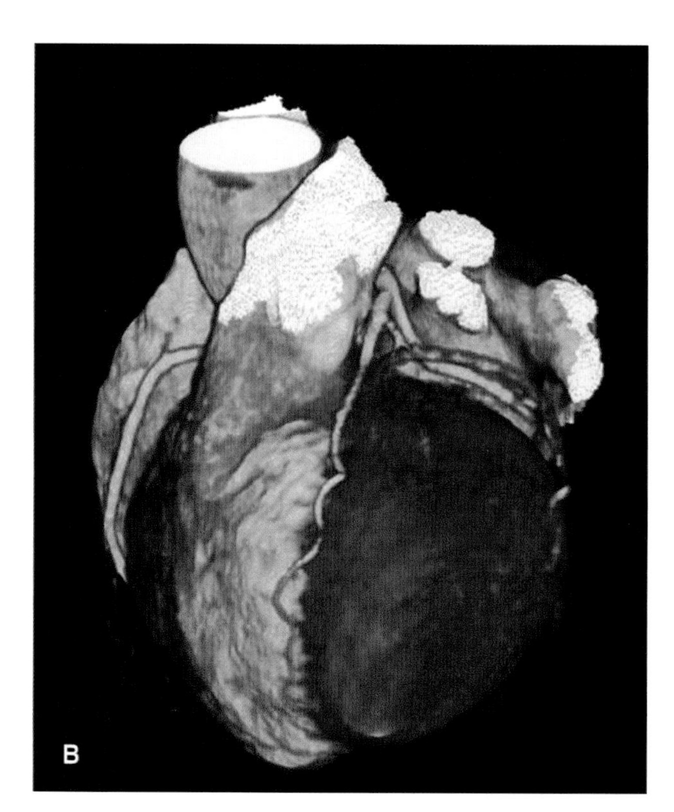

Figure 6.2 48-year-old man with atypical chest pain. (**B**) Volumetric rendering from a normal coronary artery study. (*For* Figure 6.2 **A** *and complete caption, see page 75.*)

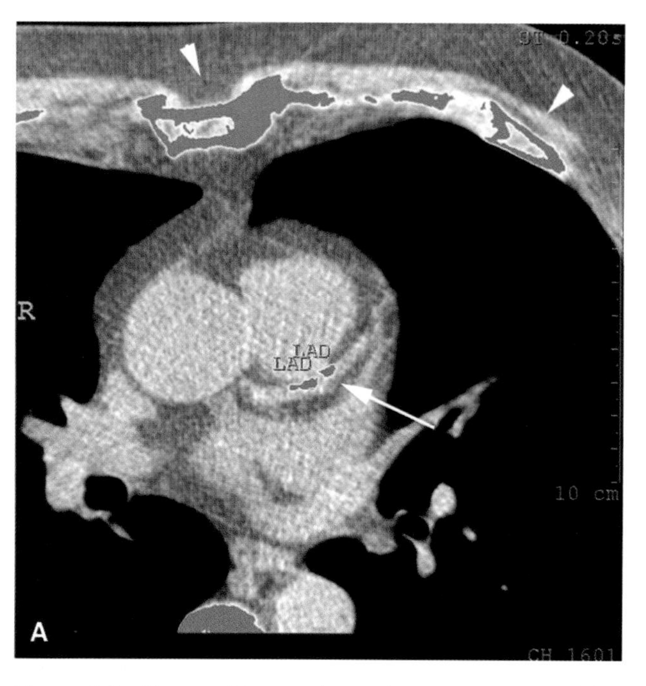

Figure 6.3 60-year-old man who underwent coronary calcium scoring as part of a clinical study. (**A**) The calcium scoring software in this unenhanced, prospectively ECG-gated, cardiac CT automatically highlights areas with Hounsfield Unit values greater than 130 with pink shading (*arrowheads*). The operator circles highlighted areas corresponding to the coronary artery, which are then re-shaded blue (*arrow*). (*For* Figure 6.3 **B** *and complete caption, see page 75.*)

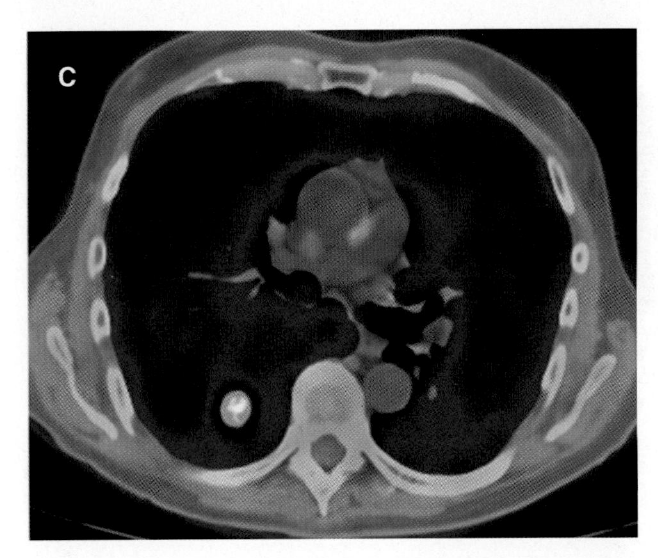

Figure 9.23 Non–small cell lung cancer manifesting as hypermetabolic nodule. (**C**) Integrated CT-PET shows increased uptake of FDG in spiculated right lung nodule. (*For* Figure 9.23 **A** *and* **B** *and complete caption, see page 138.*)

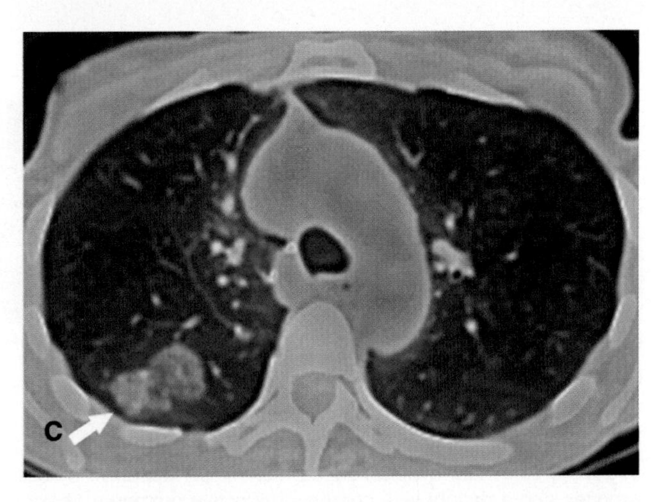

Figure 9.24 Bronchioloalveolar cell cancer manifesting as hypometabolic nodule. (**C**) Integrated CT-PET shows bilobed, partially solid nodule (ground-glass nodule with small solid soft tissue component) with minimal FDG-uptake when compared to mediastinum (*arrow*). (*For* Figure 9.24 **A** *and* **B** *and complete caption, see page 138.*)

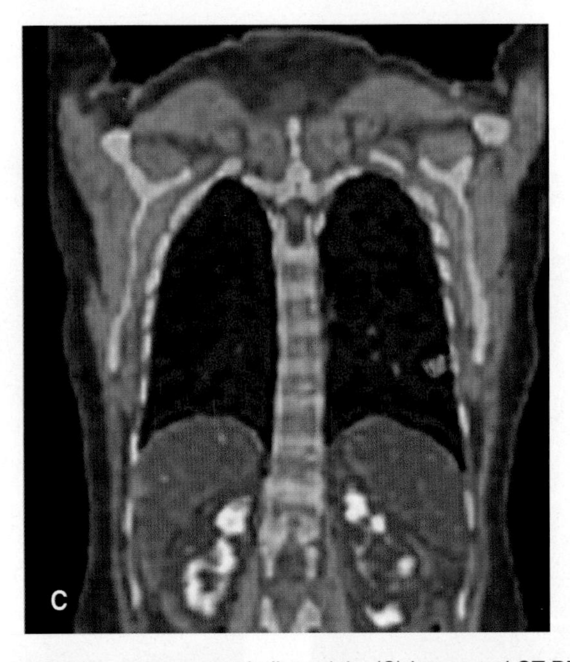

Figure 9.25 Necrotizing granuloma manifesting as hypermetabolic nodule. (**C**) Integrated CT-PET shows nodule in left lower lobe with increased FDG uptake within nodule. (*For* Figure 9.25 **A** *and* **B** *and complete caption, see page 139.*)

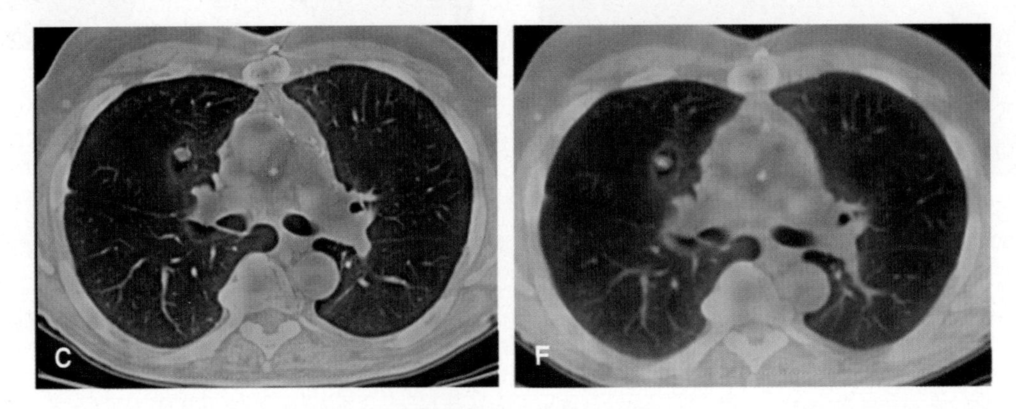

Figure 9.26 A 73-year-old man with lung cancer and inaccurate quantification of FDG uptake on integrated CT-PET scan due to respiratory motion. (**C**) Shows hypermetabolic right upper lobe nodule. (**F**) Shows visual increase in FDG uptake by nodule. (*For* Figure 9.26 **A**, **B**, **D**, *and* **E** *and complete caption, see page 139.*)

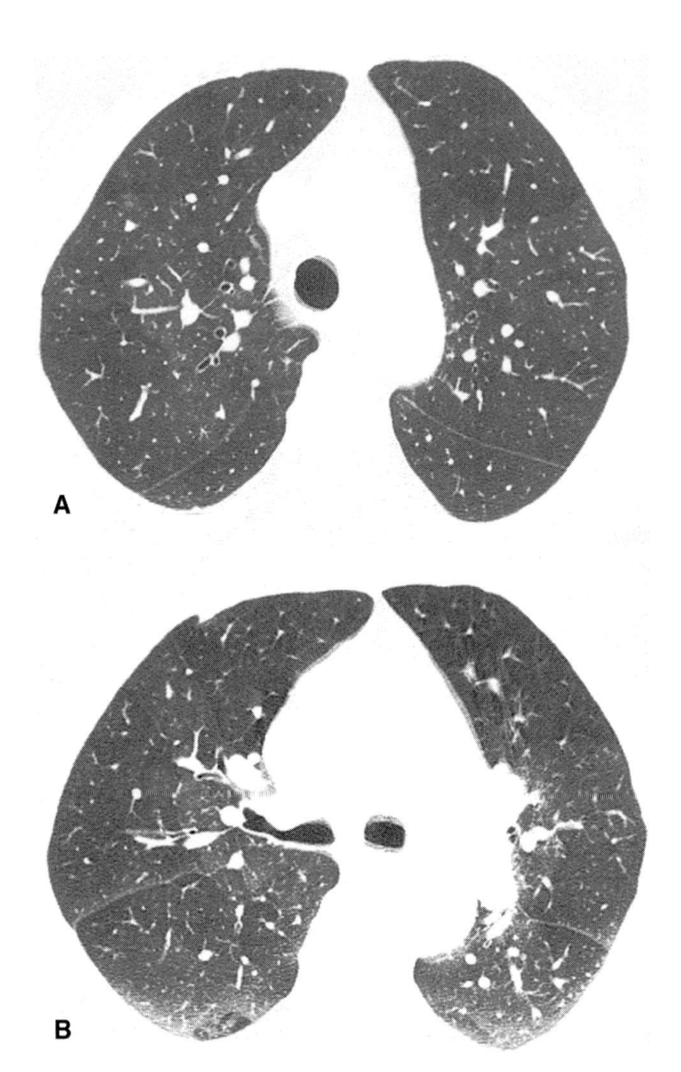

Figure 15 Mosaic perfusion in a patient with chronic pulmonary embolus (PE). High-resolution CT through the upper lobes (**A**) shows areas of reduced attenuation caused by vascular obstruction (i.e., mosaic perfusion). Vessels within the hypoperfused regions are reduced in size and thick vessels are seen within the hyperperfused regions. There is no air-trapping on expiratory scan (**B**).

arteries, which are frequently greater in diameter than the aorta. The CT scan is an important tool for detection of PAH: a main pulmonary artery diameter 29 mm and an increased ratio between the diameter of segmental arteries and corresponding bronchi have high specificity (100%) for predicting the presence of PAH (64). Patients with CPTE develop right ventricular hypertrophy in response to significant elevation of pulmonary vascular resistance. Over time, right ventricular function deteriorates, even in the absence of recurrent PE, presumably because of the development of hypertensive vascular lesions in the non-obstructed pulmonary artery bed. The right heart dilates (65). Bronchial arteries also increase in size in chronic PE with hypertension (66).

Parenchymal Abnormalities

A mosaic pattern of attenuation, with localized areas of decreased and increased attenuation, is a non-specific finding of CPTE that may be seen on high-resolution CT (HRCT) in various infiltrative lung, airway, or vascular diseases. In CPTE, there are often patchy areas of decreased attenuation and vascularity that correspond to areas of chronically decreased perfusion (Fig. 13C). They are sharply marginated from adjacent areas with increased or normal attenuation and vessel size that correspond to areas of normal or hyperperfusion (Fig. 15A) (67–69). Expiratory images may help distinguish the mosaic perfusion of CPTE from that caused by small airways disease (Fig. 15B). In a study of parenchymal abnormalities in 75 patients with CPTE, 58 patients (77.3%) showed mosaic perfusion with normal or dilated pulmonary arteries in areas of relatively increased attenuation (61). Residual scars from prior pulmonary infarction and cylindrical bronchiectasis are common (70,71). In low attenuation areas of diminished perfusion, there may be no visible vessel adjacent to the bronchus.

POSTEMBOLECTOMY FINDINGS

Pulmonary hypertension related to chronic thromboembolic disease may be treated in selected patients with thromboendarterectomy. In this procedure, as described by Jamieson, an endarterectomy of the entire pulmonary vascular bed is performed from the central through subsegmental arteries, while the patient is under circulatory arrest (72). However, despite the fact that surgical description involves removal of very distal clot from peripheral arteries, according to Bergin et al., preoperative CT angiographic features of patients with good response to surgery include the presence of central pulmonary emboli and limited evidence of small vessel disease (73). For this reason, CT, which better evaluates the central vessels, can be expected to show dramatic changes after successful surgery.

There is very little literature on the postoperative CT findings after pulmonary thromboendarterectomy. Increased enhancement of pulmonary vessels and improved lung perfusion have been described on MR imaging in a patient who underwent thromboendarterectomy (74). In our limited experience, as expected, CT demonstrates that the narrowed vessel lumen returns toward normal with enhancement of vessels that previously contained emboli. The "thick wall" of the vessels often returns to normal, or near normal, and the mosaic perfusion of the parenchyma regresses considerably, but incompletely. CT may therefore be an additional tool in evaluating surgical success, to be used with clinical parameters and well-described echocardiographic findings such as right ventricular remodeling and reversal of tricuspid regurgitation.

REFERENCES

1 Ahearn GS, Bounameaux H. The role of the D-dimer in the diagnosis of venous thromboembolism. Semin Respir Crit Care Med 2000; 21:521–36.
2 Wells PS, Anderson DR, Rodger M, et al. Excluding pulmonary embolism at the bedside without diagnostic imaging: management of patients with suspected pulmonary embolism presenting to the emergency department by using a simple clinical model and D-dimer. Ann Intern Med 2001; 135:98–107.
3 PIOPED Investigators. Value of the ventilation/perfusion scan in acute pulmonary embolism: results of the prospective investigation of pulmonary embolism diagnosis (PIOPED). J Am Med Assoc 1990; 263:2753–9.
4 Goodman L, Lipchik RJ. Diagnosis of acute pulmonary embolism: time for a new approach. Radiology 1996; 199:25–7.
5 Hull R, Raskob G, Panjuu A, Gill G. A new noninvasive management strategy for patients with suspected pulmonary embolism. Arch Intern Med 1989; 149: 2459–555.
6 Novelline R, Baltarowich O, Athanasoulis C, Waltman A, Greenfield A. The clinical course of patients with suspected pulmonary embolism and a negative pulmonary arteriogram. Radiology 1978; 126:561–67.
7 Khorasani R, Gudas T, Hikpoor N, Polak J. Treatment of patients with suspected pulmonary embolism and intermediate-probability lung scans: is diagnostic imaging underused? Am J Radiol 1997; 169: 1355–7.
8 Goodman L, Curtin J, Mewissen M, et al. Detection of pulmonary embolism in patients with unresolved clinical and scintigraphic diagnosis: helical CT versus angiography. Am J Radiol 1995; 164:1369–74.
9 Mayo J, Remy-Jardin M, Miiller N, et al. Pulmonary embolism; prospective comparison of spiral helical CT with ventilation-perfusion scintigraphy. Radiology 1997; 205:447–52.
10 Blachere H, Latrabe V, Montaudon M, et al. Pulmonary embolism revealed on helical CT angiography: comparison with ventilation-perfusion radionuclide lung scanning. Am J Radiol 2000; 174:1041–7.
11 Garg K, Sieler H, Welsh C, Johnston R, Russ P. Clinical validity of helical CT being interpreted as negative for pulmonary embolism: implications for patient treatment. Am J Radiol 1999; 172:1627–31.
12 Remy-Jardin M, Remy J, Baghaie F, Fribourg M, Artaud D, Duhamel A. Clinical value of thin collimation in the diagnostic workup of pulmonary embolism. Am J Radiol 2000; 175:407–11.
13 Stein PD, Fowler SE, Goodman LR, Gottschalk A, Hales CA, Hull RD. Multidetector computed tomography for acute pulmonary embolism. PIOPED II N Engl J Med 2006; 354:2317–27.
14 Perrier A, Roy P-M, Sanchez O, et al. Multidetector-row computed tomography in suspected pulmonary embolism. N Engl J Med 2005; 352:1760–8.
15 Blachere H, Latrabe V, Montaudon M, et al. Pulmonary embolism revealed on helical CT angiography: comparison with ventilation-perfusion radionuclide lung scanning. Am J Radiol 2000; 174:1041–7.
16 Qanadli SD, Hajjam ME, Mesurolle B, et al. Pulmonary embolism detection: prospective evaluation of dual-section helical CT versus selective pulmonary arteriography in 157 patients [comment]. Radiology 2000; 217:447–55.
17 Goodman L, Lipchik R, Kuzo R, Liu Y, McAuliffe T, O'Brien D. Subsequent pulmonary embolism: risk after a negative helical CT pulmonary angiogram—prospective comparison with scintigraphy. Radiology 2000; 215(2): 535–42.
18 Tillie-Leblond I, Mastora I, Radenne F, et al. Risk of pulmonary embolism after a negative spiral CT angiogram in patients with pulmonary disease: 1-year clinical follow-up study. Radiology 2002; 223:461–7.
19 Quiroz R, Kucher N, Zou KH, et al. Clinical validity of a negative computed tomography scan in patients with suspected pulmonary embolism: a systematic review. JAMA 2005; 293:2012–7.
20 Hirsh J. Low-molecular-weight heparin: a review of the results of recent studies of the treatment of venous thromboembolism and unstable angina. Circulation 1998; 98:1575–82.
21 Coche E, Verschuren N, Keyeux A, et al. Diagnosis of acute pulmonary embolism in outpatients: comparison of thin collimation multi-detector row spiral CT and planar ventilation-perfusion scintigraphy. Radiology 2003; 229:757–65.
22 Schoef UJ, Holzknecht N, Helmberger TK, et al. Subsegmental pulmonary emboli: improved detection with thin collimation multi-detector row spiral CT. Radiology 2002; 222:483–90.
23 Patel S, Kazerooni EA, Cascade PN. Pulmonary embolism: optimization of small pulmonary artery visualization at multi-detector row CT. Radiology 2003; 227:455–60.
24 Loud P, Katz D, Klippenstein D, Shah R, Grossman Z. Combined CT venography and pulmonary angiography in suspected thromboembolic disease: diagnostic accuracy for deep venous evaluation. Am J Radiol 2000; 174:61–5.
25 Loud PA, Katz DS, Bruce DA, Klippenstein DL, Grossman ZD. Deep venous thrombosis with suspected pulmonary embolism: detection with combined CT venography and pulmonary angiography. Radiology 2001; 219(2):498–502.
26 Coche EE, Hamoir XL, Hammer FD, et al. Using dual-detector helical CT angiography to detect deep venous thrombosis in patients with suspicion of pulmonary embolism: diagnostic value and additional findings. Am J Radiol 2001; 176:1035–8.
27 Cosmic MS, Goodman LR, Lipchik RJ, Washington L. Detection of deep venous thrombosis with combined helical CT scan of the chest and CT venography in unselected cases of suspected pulmonary embolism.

Presented at the American Thoracic Society. Atlanta, Georgia, 2002.
28 Ghaye B, Nchimi A, Noukoua CT, Dondelinger RF. Does multi-detector row CT pulmonary angiography reduce the incremental value of indirect CT venography compared with single-detector row CT pulmonary angiography? Radiology 2006; 240(1): 256–62.
29 Ghaye B, Ghuysen A, Willems V, Lambermont B, Gerard P, D'Orio V, et al. Severe pulmonary embolism: pulmonary artery clot load scores and cardiovascular parameters as predictors of mortality. Radiology 2006; 239:884–91.
30 Jackson C, Huber J. Correlated applied anatomy of the bronchial tree and lungs with a system of nomenclature. Dis Chest 1943; 9:319–26.
31 Kuzo R, Goodman L. CT evaluation of pulmonary embolism: technique and interpretation. Am J Radiol 1997; 169(4):959–65.
32 Jardin M, Remy J. Segmental bronchovascular anatomy of the lower lobes: CT analysis. Am J Radiol 1985; 147:457–68.
33 Boyden E. Segmental Anatomy of the Lungs. New York: McGraw-Hill, 1955.
34 Lee K, Bae W, Lee B, Kim I, Choi E, Lee B. Bronchovascular anatomy of the upper lobes: evaluation with thin-section CT. Radiology 1991; 181:765–72.
35 Lee K, Im J, Kim Y, Jung S, Lee B, Han M, et al. CT anatomy of the lingular segmental bronchi. J Comput Assist Tomogr 1991; 15:86–91.
36 Naidich D, Zinn W, Ettenger N, McCauley D, Garay S. Basilar segmental bronchi: thin-section CT evaluation. Radiology 1988; 169:11–6.
37 Remy-Jardin M, Remy J, Wattinne L, Giraud F. Central pulmonary thromboem-bolism: diagnosis with spiral volumetric CT with the single-breath-hold technique—comparison with pulmonary angiography. Radiology 1992; 185:381–7.
38 Remy-Jardin M, Remy J, Artaud D, Deschildre F, Fribourg M, Beregi J. Spiral CT of pulmonary embolism: technical considerations and interpretive pitfalls. J Thorac Imaging 1997; 12:103–17.
39 Ghaye B, Dondelinger RF. Non-traumatic thoracic emergencies: CT venography in an integrated diagnostic strategy of acute pulmonary embolism and venous thrombosis. European Radiology 2002; 12:1906–21.
40 Cobelli R, Zompatori M, De Luca G, Chiari G, Bresciani P, Marcato C. Clinical usefulness of computed tomography study without contrast injection in the evaluation of acute pulmonary embolism. J Comput Assist Tomogr 2005; 29:6–12.
41 Oliver TB, Reid JH, Murchison JT. Interventricular septal shift due to massive pulmonary embolism shown by CT pulmonary angiography: an old sign revisited. Thorax 1998; 53:1092–4.
42 Schoef UJ, Kucher N, Kipfmueller F, Quiroz R, Costello P, Golhaber SZ. Right ventricular enlargement on chest computed tomography: a predictor of early death in acute pulmonary embolism. Circulation 2004; 110:3276–80.
43 Ghaye B, Ghuysen A, Willems V, et al. Severe pulmonary embolism: pulmonary artery clot load scores and cardiovascular parameters as predictors of mortality. Radiology 2006; 239:884–91.
44 Yeh BM, Kurzman P, Foster E, Qayyum A, Joe B, Coakley F. Clinical relevance of retrograde inferior vena cava or hepatic vein opacification during contrast-enhanced CT. [see comment]. Am J Radiol 2004; 183:1227–32.
45 Tan RT, Kuzo R, Goodman LR, Siegel R, Haasler GB, Presberg KW. Utility of CT scan evaluation for predicting pulmonary hypertension in patients with parenchymal lung disease. Medical College Chest 1998; 113:1250–6.
46 Coche EE, Mller NL, Kim K, et al. Acute pulmonary embolism: ancillary findings at spiral CY. Radiology 1998; 207:753–8.
47 Remy-Jardin M, Remy J, Cauvain O, Petyt L, Wannebroucq J, Beregi J.-P. Diagnosis of central pulmonary embolism with helical CT: role of two-dimensional multiplanar reformations. Am J Radiol 1995; 165:1131–8.
48 Simon M, Boiselle PM, Choi JR, Rosen MP, Reynolds K, Raptopoulos V. Paddle-wheel CT display of pulmonary arteries and other lung structures: a new imaging approach. Am J Radiol 2001; 177:195–8.
49 Jeong YJ, Lee KS, Yoon YC, et al. Evaluation of small pulmonary arteries by 16-slice multidetector computed tomography: optimum slab thickness in condensing transaxial images converted into maximum intensity projections images. J Comput Assist Tomogr 2004; 28:195–203.
50 Remy-Jardin M, Remy J. Spiral CT angiography of the pulmonary circulation. Radiology 1999; 212:615–36.
51 Katz D, Loud P, Klippenstein D, Shah R, Grossman Z. Extra-thoracic findings on the venous phase of combined computed tomography venography and pulmonary angiography. Clin Radiol 2000; 55:177–81.
52 Baldt M, Zontsich T, Kainberger F, Fleischmann G, Mostbeck G. Spiral CT evaluation of deep venous thrombosis. Semin US Comput Tomogr Mag Reson 1997; 18:369–75.
53 Remy-Jardin M, Louvegny S, Remy J, et al. Acute central thromboembolic disease: posttherapeutic follow-up with spiral CT angiography. Radiology 1997; 203:173–80.
54 Benotti J, Dalen J. The natural history of pulmonary embolism. Clin Chest Med 1969; 5:403–10.
55 Banas J, Brooks H, Evans G, Paraskas J, Dexter L. Resolution rate of acute pulmonary embolism in man. N Engl J Med 1969; 280:1194–9.
56 Moser K, Auger W, Fedullo P. Chronic major-vessel thromboembolic pulmonary hypertension. Circulation 1990; 81:1735–1743.
57 Bergin C, Sirlin C, Hauschildt J, et al. Chronic pulmonary thromboembolism: diagnosis with helical CT and MR imaging with angiographic and surgical correlation. Radiology 1997; 204:695–702.
58 Falaschi F, Palla A, Formichi B, et al. CT evaluation of chronic thromboembolic pulmonary hypertension. J Comput Assist Tomogr 1992; 6:897–903.
59 Tardivon A, Musset D, Maitre S, et al. Role of CT in chronic pulmonary embolism: comparison with pulmonary angiography. J Comput Assist Tomogr 1993; 17 (3):345–351.

60 Roberts H, Kauczor H.-U, Schweden F, Thelen M. Spiral CT of pulmonary hypertension and chronic thromboembolism. J Thorac Imag 1997; 12:118–27.
61 Schwickert HC, Schweden F, Schild HH, et al. Pulmonary arteries and lung parenchyma in chronic pulmonary embolism: preoperative and postoperative CT findings. Radiology 1994; 191:351–7.
62 Auger W, Fedullo P, Moser K, Buchbinder M, Peterson K. Chronic major-vessel thromboembolic pulmonary artery obstruction: appearance at angiography. Radiology 1992; 182:393–8.
63 Kauczor H.-U, Schwickert H, Mayer E, Schweden F, Schild H, Thelen M. Spiral CT of bronchial arteries in chronic thromboembolism. J Comput Assist Tomogr 1994; 18:855–61.
64 Tan R, Kuzo R, Goodman L, Siegel R, Haasler G, Presberg K. Utility of CT scan evaluation for predicting pulmonary hypertension in patients with parenchymal lung disease. Chest 1998; 113:1250–56.
65 Moser K, Bloor C. Pulmonary vascular lesions occurring in patients with chronic major vessel thromboembolic pulmonary hypertension. Chest 1993; 103: 685–92.
66 Remy-Jardin M, Duhamel A, Deken V, Bonaziz N, Dumont P, Remy J. Systemic collateral supply in patients with chronic embolic and primary pulmonary artery hypertension: assessment with multidetector row helical CT angiography. Radiology 2005; 235274–81.
67 Worthy S, Miiller N, Hartman T, Swensen S, Padley S, Hansell D. Mosaic attenuation pattern on thin-section CT scans of the lung: differentiation among infiltrative of the lung, airway, and vascular diseases as a cause. Radiology 1997; 205: 465–70.
68 Sherrick A, Swensen S, Hartman T. Mosaic pattern of lung attenuation on CT scans: frequency among patients with pulmonary artery hypertension of different causes. Am J Radiol 1997; 169:79–82.
69 King M, Bergin C, Yeung D, et al. Chronic pulmonary thromboembolism: detection of regional hypoperfusion with CT. Radiology 1994; 191:359–63.
70 Bergin C, Rios G, King M, Belezzuoli E, Luna J, Auger W. Accuracy of high-resolution CT in identifying chronic pulmonary thromboembolic disease. Am J Radiol 1996; 166:1371–7.
71 Remy-Jardin M, Remy J, Louvegny S, Artaud D, Deschildre F, Duhamel A. Airway changes in chronic pulmonary embolism: CT findings in 33 patients. Radiology 1997; 203:355–60.
72 Jamieson S. Pulmonary thromboendarterectomy. Heart 1998; 79(2):118–20.
73 Bergin C, Sirlin C, Deutsch R, et al. Predictors of patient response to pulmonary thromboendarterectomy. Am J Radiol 2000; 174(2):509–15.
74 Kreitner K.-F, Mayer E, Voigtlaender T, Thelen M, Oelert H. Three-dimensional contrast-enhanced magnetic resonance angiography in a patient with chronic thromboembolic pulmonary hypertension before and after thromboendarterectomy. Circulation 1999; 99:1101.

8

Multidetector Row CT Angiography of the Thoracic Aorta

Curtis E. Green and Jeffrey S. Klein
Department of Radiology, Section of Cardiothoracic Radiology, University of Vermont College of Medicine, Fletcher Allen Health Care, Burlington, Vermont, U.S.A.

INTRODUCTION

In recent years, advances in CT technology have led to an increasing role for CT angiography in the evaluation of a variety of aortic abnormalities. In this chapter, we review the role of multidetector row CT (MDCT) angiography in the assessment of congenital and acquired aortic abnormalities and compare this technique to other imaging modalities, including conventional aortography, MRI, and transesophageal echocardiography (TEE).

TECHNIQUE OF MULTIDETECTOR ROW THORACIC CT ANGIOGRAPHY

While the specific acquisition parameters will vary slightly on MDCT scanners with varying detector arrays, certain principles of MDCT thoracic aortography are constant across various platforms (Table 1):

1. Maximum detector array should be utilized.
2. Bolus timing software optimizes contrast delivery and luminal opacification.
3. Thin-section acquisition (<2 mm) with overlapping reconstructions improves both in-plane resolution (particularly important for subtle aortic injuries) and multiplanar and three-dimensional reconstructions.
4. Retrospective ECG gating to mid-to-late diastole should be employed to reduce motion artifacts in the ascending aorta, particularly in patients with suspected traumatic aortic injury (TAI) or acute aortic dissection or its variants.
5. Dense nonionic contrast injected at rapid infusion rates (>3 mL/s) for a volume of at least 100 mL is necessary for consistent high-quality aortic studies.
6. Unenhanced scans should precede a contrast-enhanced acquisition to allow detection of intramural hematomas (IMH).
7. Postprocessing of the MDCT data set with the generation of two- and three-dimensional reconstructions aids in lesion depiction and communication with the referring physicians.

CONGENITAL ANOMALIES OF THE AORTA

Embryology

It is not necessary to thoroughly understand the embryological development of the aorta to diagnose the various arch anomalies, but it is useful to have a basic idea about how anomalies arise, as it makes the imaging findings easier to understand. In the classic theoretical embryological double arch proposed by Edwards (Fig. 1), there are right and left aortic arches that connect the ascending and descending portions of the aorta (1). Each gives rise to a carotid and a subclavian artery. In normal development, the left arch persists and the part of the right arch distal to the origin of the right subclavian artery becomes atretic. This results in three great vessels arising from the arch: a right brachiocephalic artery composed of the proximal remnant of the right arch and the right carotid and subclavian arteries; a left common carotid artery; and a left subclavian artery. The remnant of the ductus arteriosus, the ligamentum arteriosum, connects the bottom of the transverse arch to the proximal left pulmonary artery. Essentially all of the developmental anomalies of the aortic arch branches can be explained by variations in which part of the embryological double arch becomes atretic.

Diagnosis of Congenital Aortic Anomalies and Vascular Rings

A vascular ring results from encircling of the trachea by a combination of the aorta and its branches and the ligamentum arteriosum. If the ring is tight enough, tracheal compression and respiratory compromise may result. It is important to remember that the mere presence of an arch anomaly does not mean that there is a vascular ring. The diagnosis of ring should be made on the basis of symptoms and anatomy, not anatomy alone. When presented with a patient with stridor, the evaluation should begin with a frontal and lateral chest radiographs and a barium esophagram. If these confirm the presence of airway compromise and suggest a vascular cause, further evaluation with cross-sectional imaging can be pursued. In this day

Table 1 MDCT Scanning Protocol for Thoracic Aortic Disease on 64-Detector CT

Procedural element	Protocol
Anatomic cephalocaudal extent of scan	Apex → base (trauma, aneurysm, follow-up) Apex → aortoiliac bifurcation (acute dissection or variant)
Kilovolt peak settings (kVp)	120
Gantry rotation time (s)	0.4
Pitch	0.2
ECG gating	Retrospective to 75% of R-R interval
Collimation	64 x 0.625 detector array
Reconstruction thickness/interval	Prospective 2.5 mm at 2 mm intervals Retrospective 0.9 mm at 0.45 mm intervals
Display field of view	Widest rib → widest rib from AP scout
Patient instructions during scanning	Single breath-hold after three maximal breaths
Precontrast scans	None (trauma, aneurysm, congenital lesion, follow-up) Apex → base (dissection or variant)
Contrast type/concentration/volume	Nonionic 370 mg% and 2 mL/kg (infants and children), 100–120 mL (adults)
Contrast injection rate	4 cc/s (adult) 1–2 cc/s (child)
Acquisition delay from start of injection to scan	Bolus tracking at proximal descending aorta, threshold of 125 H.
Reconstruction algorithm	Standard (soft tissue)

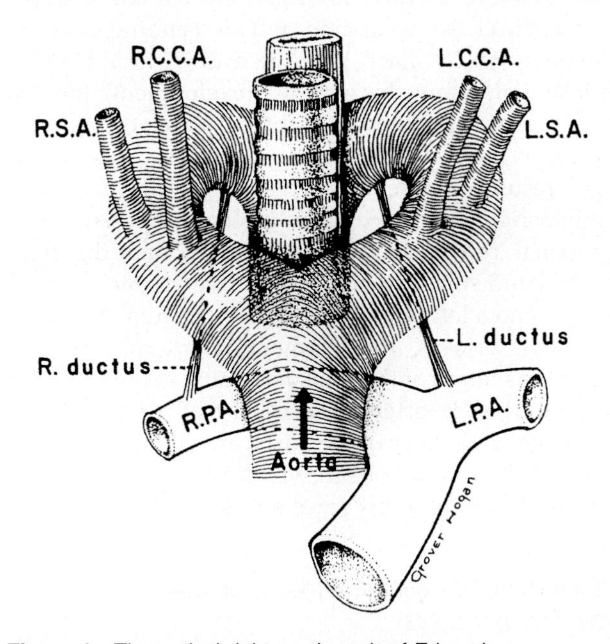

Figure 1 Theoretical right aortic arch of Edwards.

and age, there is little, if any, indication for angiographic evaluation of vascular anomalies.

MRI using spin-echo (black blood) techniques is an elegant method of delineating the mediastinal vascular anatomy in infants, children, and adults with suspected congenital aortic anomalies, particularly vascular rings and aortic coarctation (2). The lack of need for intravenous contrast and the ability to obtain two- and three-dimensional reformatted images to optimize display of aortic and branch anomalies make MRI the modality of choice in infants and children.

Rapid scanning with contrast-enhanced helical CT, particularly the recent advent of multidetector row scanners capable of very rapid scanning with thin collimation and minimal respiratory motion artifact, and the ability to retrospectively gate scan acquisition data to a consistent phase of the cardiac cycle in order to reduce aortic pulsation artifacts, provides information analogous to MRI (3). The scanning parameters and contrast administration used for MDCT aortography in infants and children are tailored to the individual examination, but follow the basic principles of CT aortography as outlined in Table 1. In neonates and children, however, a lower exposure technique is utilized to limit radiation dosage and the volume and rate of contrast administration is based on patient weight (2 mL/kg of 370 mg % nonionic contrast injected at 1–2 mL/s).

Double Aortic Arch

Persistence of both aortic arches is an uncommon anomaly that frequently results in tracheal compression. Most patients present early in life although double arch may present as an incidental finding in an asymptomatic patient or as a "mediastinal mass." In the majority of patients the right-sided arch is dominant, being larger, higher, and more anterior than the left-sided arch (Fig. 2). Each arch gives rise to a carotid and a subclavian artery. In some patients the left arch is atretic. In this case, double arch cannot readily be distinguished from right arch with aberrant left subclavian artery and a left ligamentum. Surgical repair consists of division of the nondominant arch and ligamentum.

Right Aortic Arch

Persistence of the right aortic arch with atresia of the left occurs in approximately 1/2200 persons without congenital heart disease. The incidence in certain congenital anomalies such as Tetralogy of Fallot and persistent truncus arteriosus can be as high as 50%.

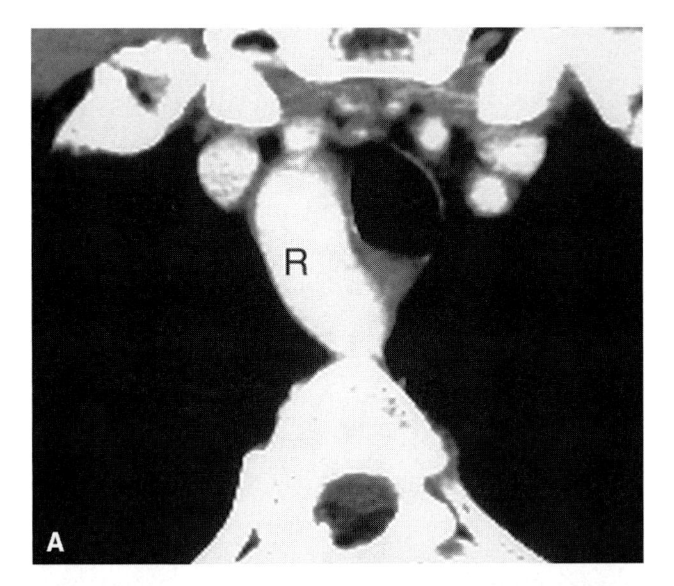

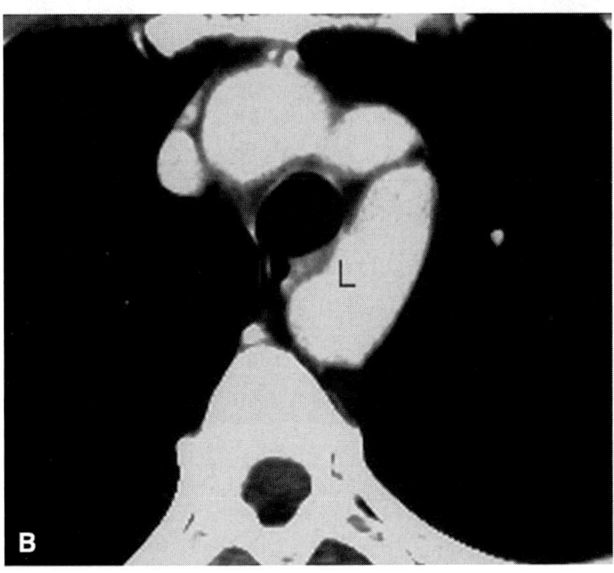

Figure 2 Double aortic arch in an asymptomatic 32-year-old man with lymphoma. (**A** and **B**) The right arch (R) is higher than the left (L). Usually it is larger, although not in this instance. The trachea is not compressed.

Most persons with right aortic arch are completely asymptomatic and come to medical attention because the right arch is misdiagnosed on chest radiographs as a mediastinal mass. There are two common types of right arch: those with mirror-image branching of the great vessels (Type 1) and those with aberrant origin of the left subclavian artery (Type 2).

In the Type 1 right arch, the first vessel arising from the arch is a left brachiocephalic artery, followed in order by the right common carotid artery and the right subclavian artery. This anomaly results from atresia of the embryonic double arch distal to the left subclavian artery. The CT appearance of the Type 1 arch is the exact mirror image of the typical left arch. (Fig. 3). These rarely cause symptoms of any kind, but are almost always associated with congenital heart disease.

In the Type 2 arch, the order of origination of the great vessels is left common carotid, right common carotid, right subclavian artery, and left subclavian artery. In this case the left subclavian artery arises from the proximal portion of the descending aorta, just below the origin of the ductus arteriosus. Because the ligamentum is almost always left-sided, there is the potential for a vascular ring, although it is uncommon for it to be clinically significant. With Type 2 right arch, the first branch of the aorta, the left common carotid, tends to be smaller than the typical brachiocephalic artery. The aberrant left subclavian artery arises from the aorta, just below the arch, and courses posterior to the esophagus before ascending to resume its normal course (Fig. 4).

With both types of right arch, the arch (by definition) passes to the right side of the trachea. In most cases the descending aorta is also on the right, not crossing over to the diaphragmatic hiatus until just above the diaphragm. Occasionally the arch will cross behind the esophagus at the level of the transverse arch, resulting in the so-called retroesophageal right arch (Fig. 5). These patients usually have an aberrant left subclavian artery and may be

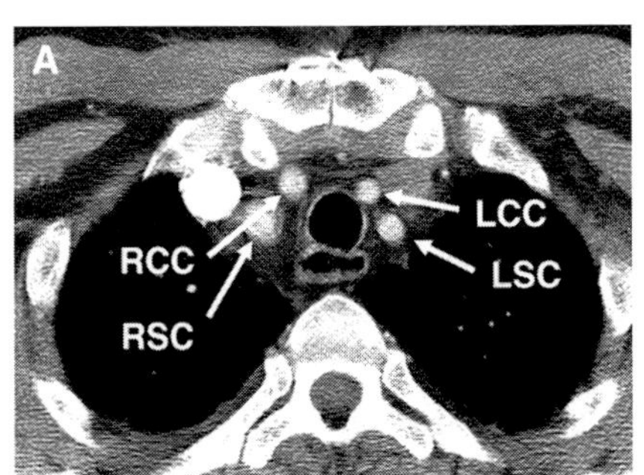

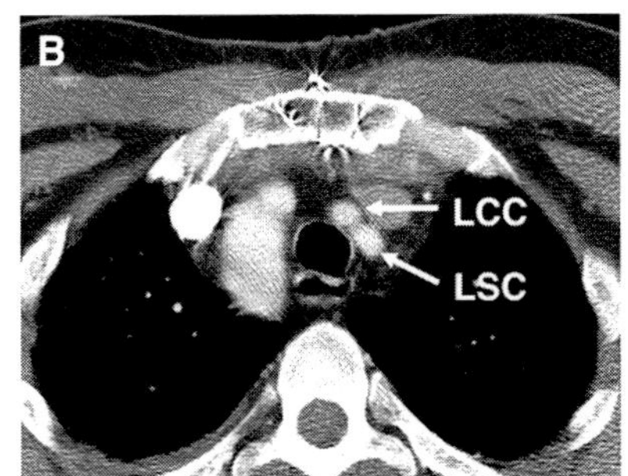

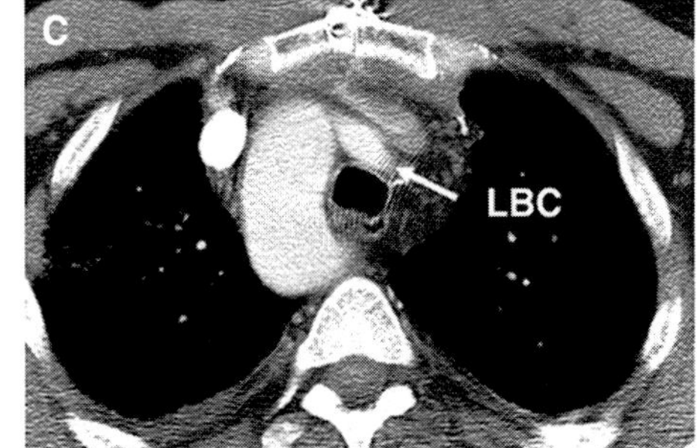

Figure 3 Type 1 right aortic arch. The left common carotid artery (LCC) and left subclavian artery (LSC) arise from a left brachiocephalic artery (LBC). The right common carotid artery (RCC) and right subclavian artery (RSC) arise separately from the right aortic arch.

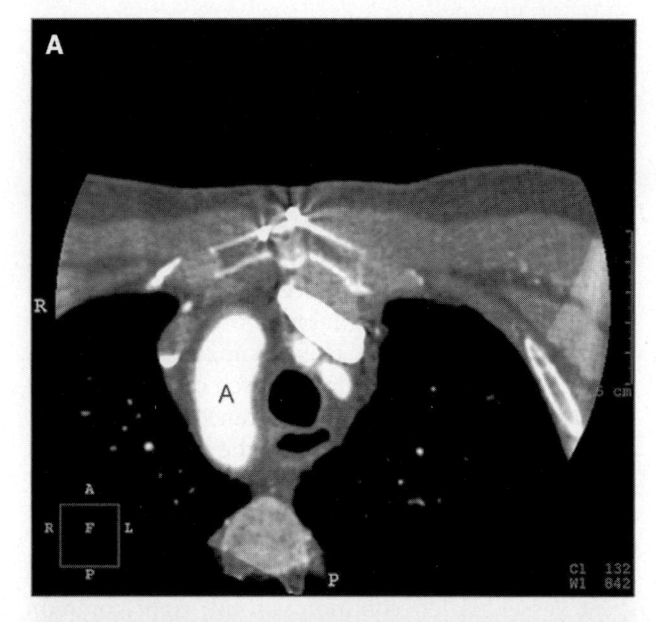

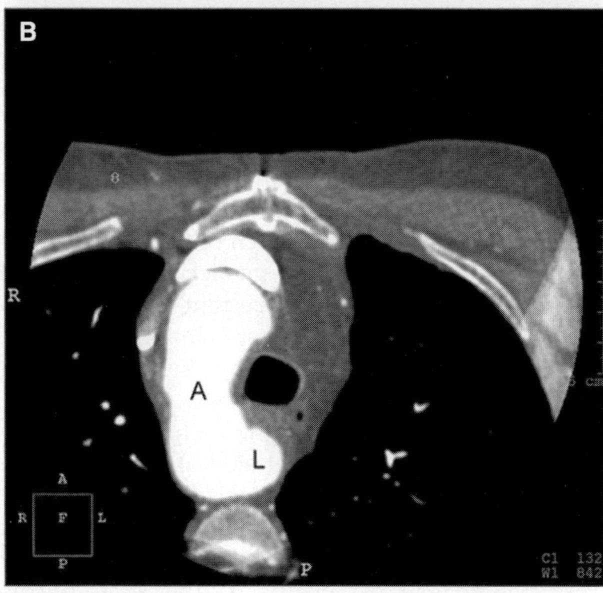

Figure 4 Type 2 right aortic arch. (A and B) The transverse arch (A) is to the right of the trachea. The left subclavian artery (L) arises from the descending aorta.

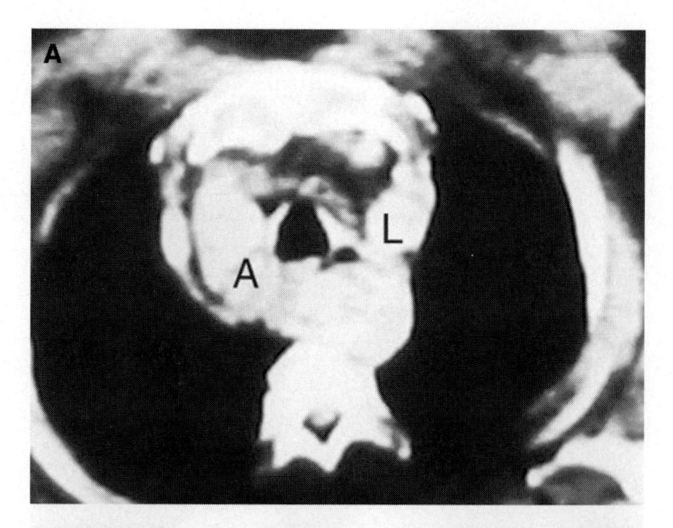

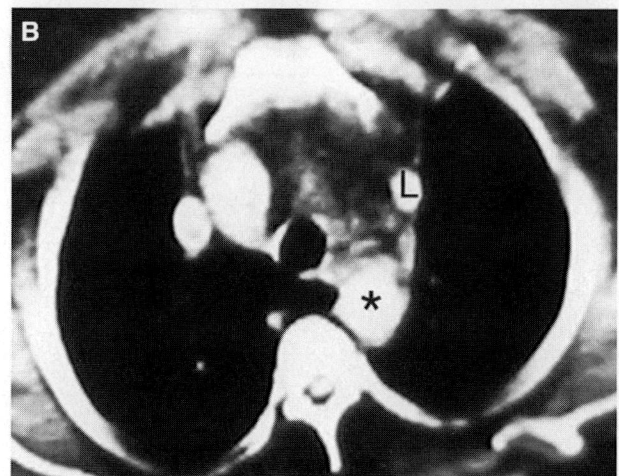

Figure 5 Retroaortic right aortic arch. (A) Scan at the level of the arch and (B) scan below the arch. The transverse arch (A) is to the right of the trachea, but crosses behind the trachea and esophagus to descend on the left (*). The left subclavian artery (L) arises from the descending aorta.

more likely to complain of dysphagia than those in whom the aorta descends on the right.

Left Aortic Arch with Aberrant Right Subclavian Artery

Aberrant origin of the right subclavian artery occurs when the embryological right arch becomes atretic between the origins of the right common carotid artery and the right subclavian artery, and is said to occur in between 1/200 and 1/250 persons. The incidence is increased in Tetralogy of Fallot and coarctation of the aorta. The situation is a mirror image of the Type 2 right aortic arch, with the right subclavian artery arising from the proximal descending aorta. The right ductus almost always disappears and this anomaly is, therefore, rarely associated with a vascular ring. The origin of the aberrant vessel may be quite dilated, in which case it is referred to as the diverticulum of Kommerell. Occasionally the diverticulum of Kommerell enlarges to the point where it compresses on the esophagus (Fig. 6A). Traditionally these have been blamed for dysphagia (dysphagia lusoria), but not all clinicians and investigators accept a causal association. An aberrant right subclavian artery may present as a right supraclavicular mass on the frontal chest radiograph and may be more prone to aneurysm formation than the normally arising right subclavian artery (Fig. 6B).

Coarctation and Pseudocoarctation of the Aorta

Coarctation of the aorta is a rare lesion in adults and is not likely to be discovered incidentally during chest CT for other indications. MRI is the preferred method for evaluation of coarctation because of the lack of

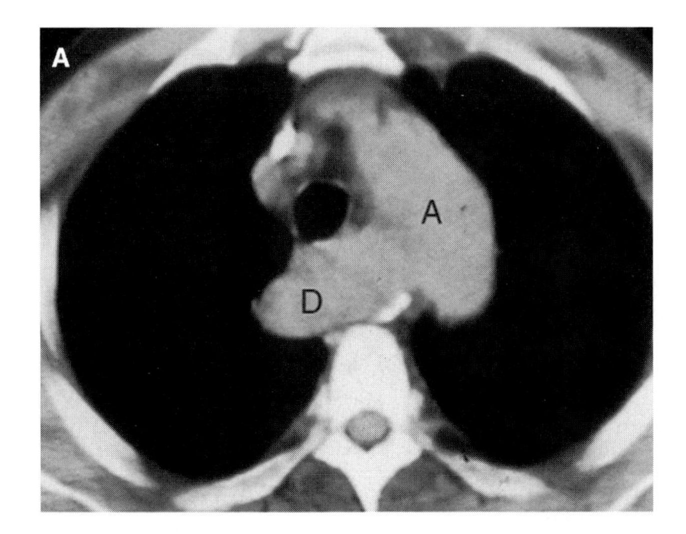

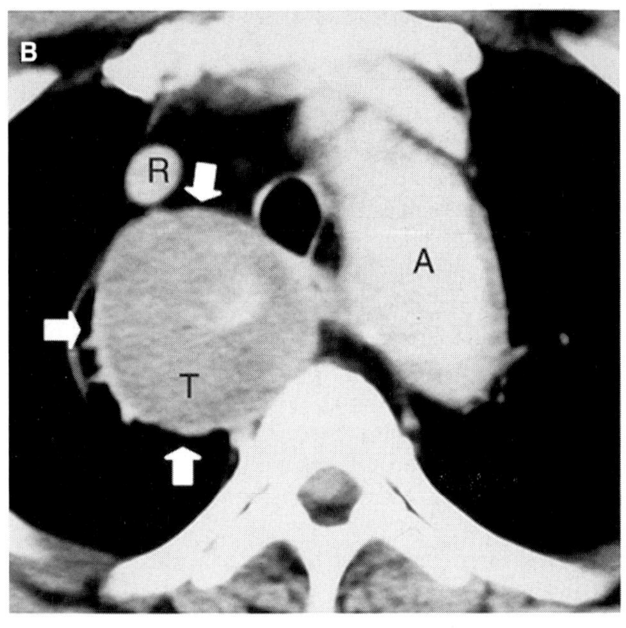

Figure 6 (**A**) Aberrant right subclavian artery. Unenhanced CT shows a large diverticulum of Kommerell (D) arising from the proximal descending aorta. (**B**) Enhanced CT in a different patient shows a large aneurysm (*arrows*) of an aberrant right subclavian artery. Much of the aneurysm is filled with thrombus (T). *Abbreviations*: A, aortic arch; R, right brachiocephalic vein.

radiation and ability to measure pressure gradient, but CT yields excellent anatomic information. The coarctation is almost always just distal to the origin of the left subclavian artery although lower thoracic and abdominal coarctations occur. The area of narrowing may be quite discrete and easily missed on axial images, but should be apparent on reconstructed sagittal images (Fig. 7). Dilatation of the descending aorta and left subclavian artery may be the only clues to the presence of coarctation on the axial images. Dilatation of the ascending aorta is not uncommon and may result from systemic hypertension, a stenotic bicuspid aortic valve, or connective tissue weakness similar to that found in Marfan's disease and other causes of Anuloaortic ectasia.

Pseudocoarctation of the aorta is caused by kinking or folding of the proximal portion of the descending aorta and frequently results in a mass on the frontal chest radiograph. The diagnosis can be suspected from the lateral chest radiograph where the actual kink is sometimes visible. Because CT is the primary modality for evaluation of mediastinal masses, one is more likely to encounter a patient with pseudocoarctation than with coarctation. Pseudocoarctation is thought by some to be a form fruste of coarctation, in part because it also has a high association with bicuspid aortic valve and an increased incidence in Turner's and Noonan's syndromes. By definition there is absent or a trivial pressure gradient across the pseudocoarctation and surgical repair is rarely necessary. On axial CT images one sees a dilated proximal descending aorta that usually extends higher than normal. The left subclavian artery may arise from either above or below the kink. Sagittal and coronal reconstructions nicely demonstrate the folded aorta and great vessel origins (Fig. 8).

Cervical Aortic Arch

Cervical arch is a rare anomaly, most commonly seen on the right side with the arch extending into the high right paratracheal region, displacing the trachea. It is usually asymptomatic in adults although children may present with either a vascular ring or tracheal compression. Clinically it may present as a pulsating neck mass. The diagnosis is straightforward on axial or reconstructed images as the cervical portion of the aorta can be readily demonstrated to be continuous with the ascending aorta and separate from the great vessels (Fig. 9).

ACUTE AORTIC DISEASES

This group of diseases comprises three conditions that typically present with acute chest pain: aortic dissection, aortic IMH, and penetrating atherosclerotic ulcer (PAU) of the aorta. The widespread availability and use of cross-sectional techniques, including TEE, helical CT, and MR angiography, have allowed greater recognition of these disorders. This section focuses on the pathologic and imaging findings in these acute aortic diseases, with an emphasis on the characteristic CT features of each entity (4).

Aortic Dissection

Aortic dissection is the most common and lethal of the acute aortic disorders, with a reported incidence of 0.2–0.8% (5). Risk factors for the development of aortic dissection include hypertension, cystic medial necrosis due to connective tissue disease (i.e., Marfans

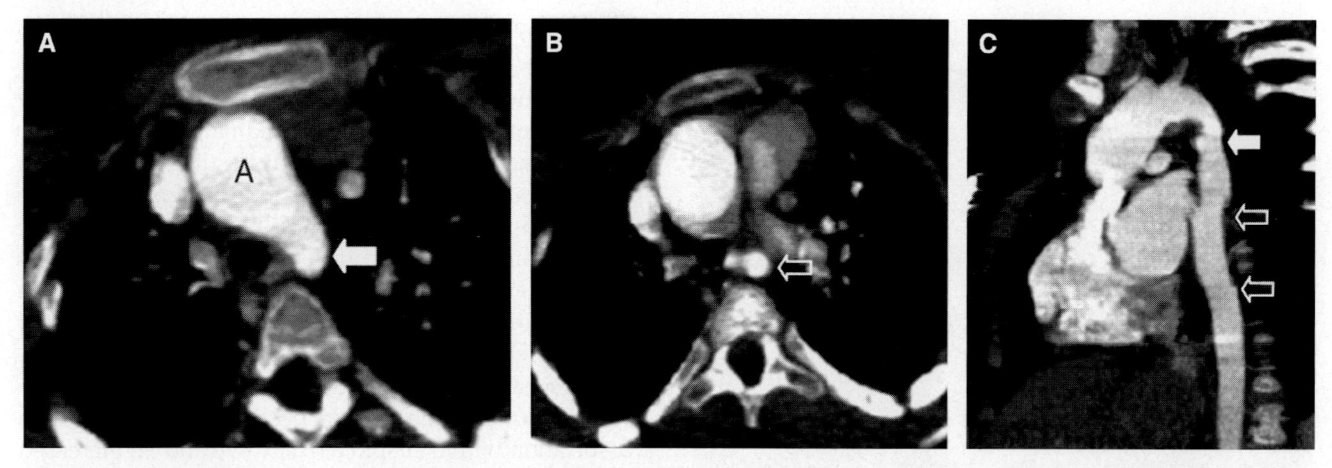

Figure 7 Coarctation of the aorta. (**A** and **B**) Scans through the aortic arch show a dilated ascending aortic arch (**A**), which tapers rapidly as it nears the descending aorta (*solid arrow*). The descending aorta (*open arrow*) (**B**) is diminutive. (**C**) Parasagittal MIP through the aorta shows the focal narrowing in the proximal descending aorta (*solid arrow*). Misregistration artifacts from poor cardiac gating are present in the descending aorta (*open arrows*).

and Ehlers–Danlos syndromes), congenital lesions such as bicuspid aortic valve and aortic coarctation, pregnancy, trauma, and arteritis. Patients who develop IMH may, in a minority of cases, develop communications with the aortic lumen thereby progressing to true dissection. Thoracic aortic aneurysms (TAAs) are more prone to dissection, as aortic wall tension is directly related to luminal diameter (Laplace's law). There is a male predominance for the diagnosis in most reported series. Symptoms on presentation include chest pain radiating to the back, syncope, and shortness of breath. Acute aortic dissection is defined as dissection detected within 2 weeks of the onset of symptoms, while chronic dissection is older than 2 weeks (6). Since the clinical presentation may mimic myocardial infarction, pulmonary embolism, and other conditions, the diagnosis may be delayed.

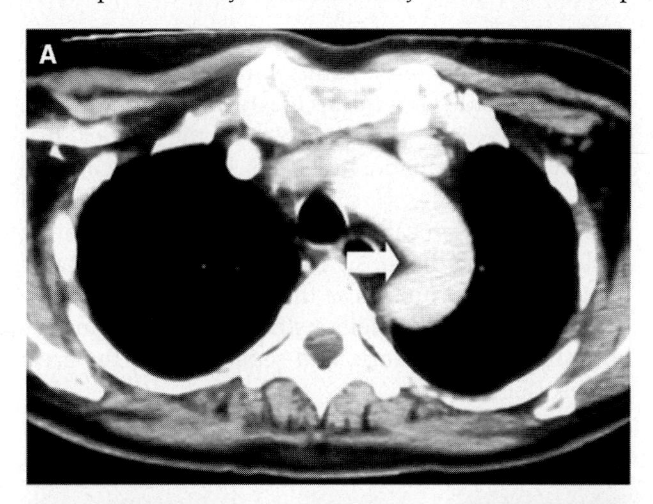

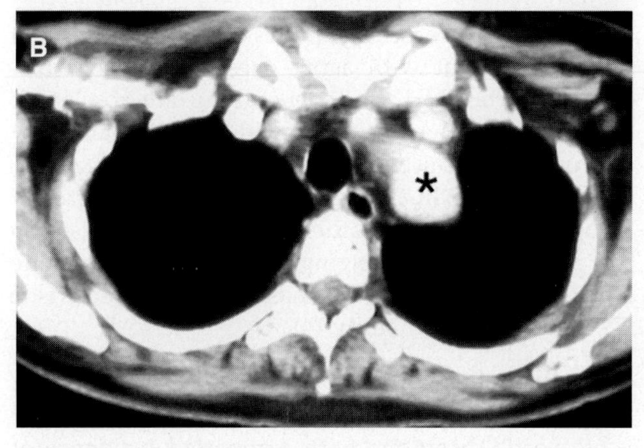

Figure 8 Pseudocoarctation of the aorta. (**A**) Scan through the arch shows unfolding or kinking of the arch just proximal to the descending aorta (*arrow*). (**B**) Scan above the arch shows protrusion of the top of the arch (*) behind the brachiocephalic vessels.

The main pathologic feature of aortic dissection is an intimal tear within a weakened vessel wall that allows aortic blood to form a false channel that runs parallel to the true aortic lumen within the outer two-thirds of the aortic media (Fig. 10). There are two classification systems for aortic dissection that are based on the origin of the intimal tear and the extent of aortic involvement: the Debakey classification and the Stanford classification. In the Debakey system, a Type I dissection arises from a tear in the ascending aorta at the sinotubular junction and involves both ascending and descending aorta, while a Type II dissection affects only the ascending aorta. When the intimal tear arises just distal to the ligamentum arteriosum and extends distally to involve the descending aorta, it is classified as a Type III dissection. Debakey Type III dissections can be further subclassified as Type IIIa when the dissection is limited to the descending aorta and IIIb when there is extension into the abdominal aorta and iliac arteries (7). The Stanford classification divides aortic dissection into two categories: Type A dissections involve the ascending aorta with or without extension distally into the arch or descending aorta,

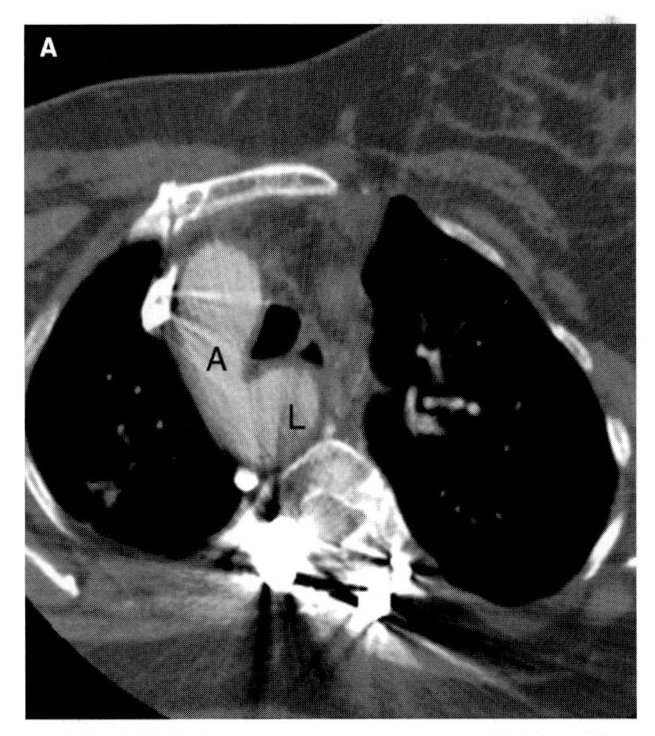

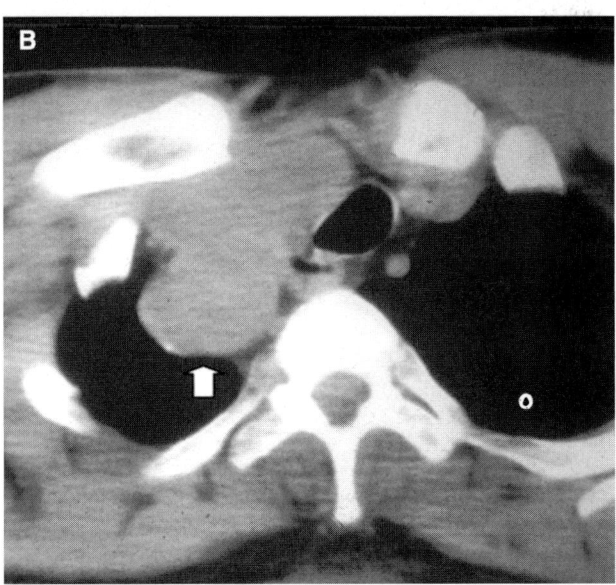

Figure 9 Cervical aortic arch. (**A** and **B**) The aortic arch (A) is on the right of the trachea. The left subclavian artery (L) arises from the descending aorta as occurs with a typical Type 2 right arch. The top of the arch extends into the lower neck (*arrow*).

and Type B dissections are limited to the descending aorta. Approximately two-thirds of aorta dissections are Type A and one-third are Type B. The Stanford classification system has become the more widely utilized system, as there has been significant data published on the therapeutic and prognostic implications of Type A versus Type B aortic dissection.

The chest radiograph is of limited value in the evaluation of suspected acute aortic dissection as there are no reliable or sensitive plain film findings. In chronic dissection, weakening of the aortic wall eventually results in dilatation, but acutely there are almost never any findings unless the aorta has ruptured, in which case a pleural effusion will be present.

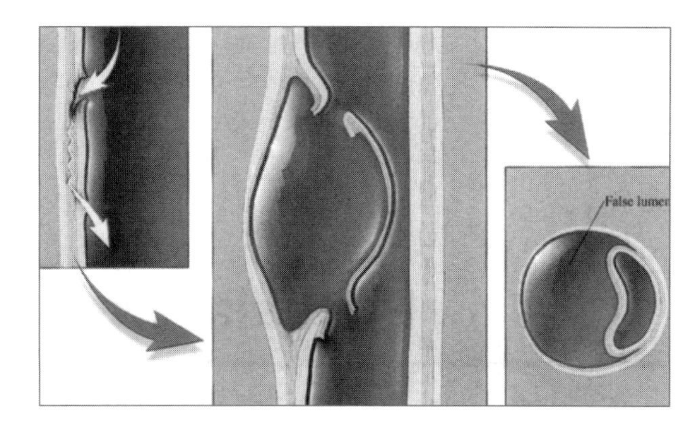

Figure 10 Diagram illustrating the pathogenesis of aortic dissection. Initial tear in the aortic intima (*left image*) results in dissection of blood into the aortic media (*middle image*), and eventual formation of a false lumen (*right image*). *Source*: From Ref. 71.

Emergent cross-sectional imaging will almost invariably be necessary when acute aortic dissection is suspected. In institutions where TEE is available on an emergent basis, this exam, although invasive and quite operator dependent, can be performed at the bedside and provides rapid assessment of the aorta, including the presence or absence of an intimal flap, the status of the aortic valve, the presence of pericardial fluid, and the functional status of the myocardium. Limitations include availability; the inability to assess the status of the great vessels; and occasional difficulty in visualizing the entirety of the ascending aorta, arch, and descending aorta. Prior to the advent of helical CT in the early 1990s, MR appeared to be the modality of choice, with a reported sensitivity and specificity of 98% (8). In addition to its high accuracy for diagnosis, additional advantages of traditional (spin-echo and gradient-echo) MR include lack of need for iodinated contrast and the simultaneous evaluation of the aorta and great vessels, heart, and pericardial space in multiple planes. More recently the development of contrast-(i.e., gadolinium)-enhanced MR angiography has provided exquisite detail of the aorta and arch vessels with significantly reduced acquisition times, allowing complete aortic evaluation in a single-breath-hold acquisition. Recent studies have confirmed the excellent accuracy of MR for imaging aortic dissection but the more widespread availability of MDCT and the greater ease of monitoring unstable patients in the CT suite have made this technique the most widely utilized imaging procedure for evaluation of suspected acute aortic disease, including dissection. MR is of particular value in monitoring the success of nonoperative management of dissection and in the postoperative follow-up of surgically managed patients.

Conventional contrast angiography, while often utilized in the past for detecting the presence and extent of disease in aortic dissection, has been largely supplanted by the cross-sectional modalities described above. Angiography has been shown to be less sensitive than spiral CT, MR, and TEE for the diagnosis of dissection and is usually reserved for cases where percutaneous techniques at managing aortic dissection, such as percutaneous fenestration of the aorta and stent graft obliteration of the lumen, are indicated.

MDCT has become the primary imaging modality in the diagnosis of suspected acute aortic dissection due to its widespread availability and high image acquisition speed; proximity to the emergency room at most institutions; uniform high quality axial and multiplanar reconstructed images; and ability to simultaneously assess the entire aorta and arch vessels, pericardial space, and the remainder of the thorax. In a 1996 study by Sommer and colleagues, helical CT had a 100% sensitivity and specificity in the detection of aortic dissection (9). A recent meta-analysis of English-language reports published from 1980 to 2005 on the diagnosis of thoracic aortic dissection by helical CT, MRI, and TEE showed that all three imaging techniques were equally reliable for confirming or excluding the diagnosis of dissection (10).

The technique used for the evaluation of acute aortic dissection is shown in Table 1. Initial unenhanced scans are performed to detect medially displaced intimal calcifications or to visualize an intimal flap in patients with severe anemia (11), with either finding indicating the presence of a false lumen. In addition, the presence of an aortic IMH that may mimic aortic dissection clinically is depicted on unenhanced scans as a crescentic region of intramural high attenuation that can be mistaken for a thickened aortic wall if only contrast-enhanced scans are obtained. In patients with significant renal insufficiency, either of these findings on unenhanced CT may be sufficient for appropriate diagnosis and triage without the risk of inducing contrast-mediated renal failure.

The contrast-enhanced CT scans obtained in patients with suspected dissection should begin above the aortic arch to include the proximal arch vessels and extend to the level of the common iliac arteries inferiorly. Since a large number of axial images are obtained with the use of thin collimation and overlapping reconstruction from MDCT, the study should be interpreted on a workstation where cine viewing is possible and multiplanar reformatted images, particularly oblique sagittal reconstructions, can be created.

The CT diagnosis of aortic dissection is made by detection of an intimal flap separating the true from false lumen (Fig. 11). In Type A dissections, the false lumen is typically seen along the right anterolateral wall of the ascending aorta and spirals as it extends distally to lie along the left posterolateral wall of the descending aorta. While it is often helpful in Type A dissections to determine the presence of involvement of the arch vessels, this does not usually alter the surgical approach to the patient. CT findings associated with dissection include pericardial or pleural effusion and aortic dilatation.

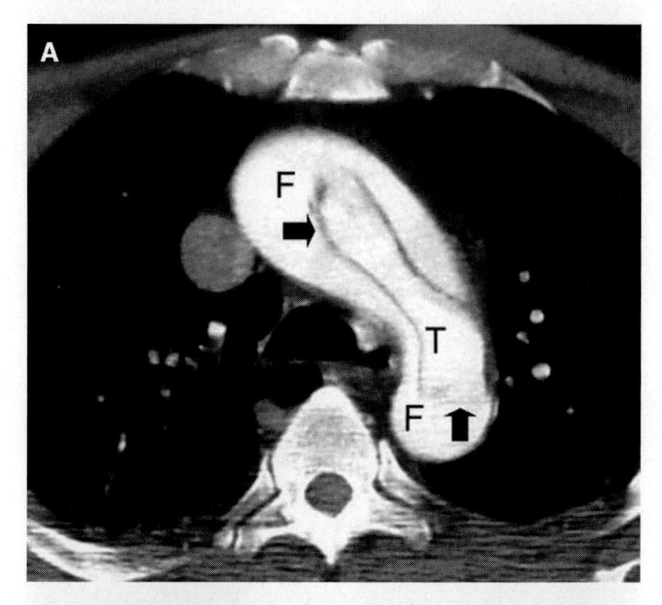

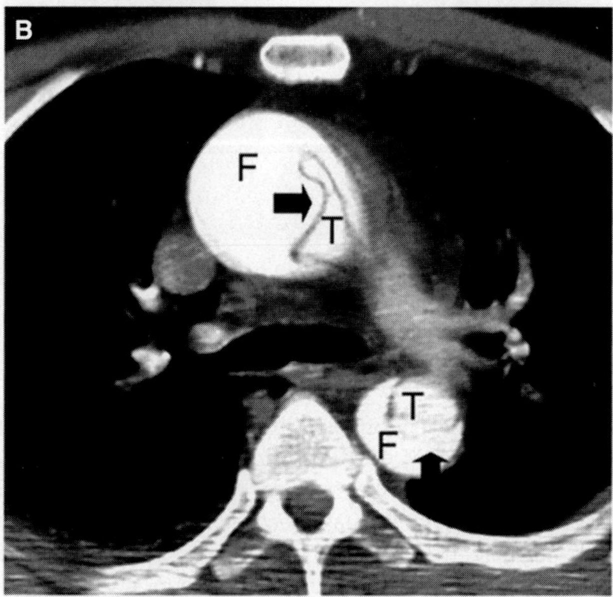

Figure 11 Stanford type A (DeBakey type 1) aortic dissection. (**A** and **B**) CT scans through and just below the arch shows an extensive intimal flap (*arrows*) and dilated ascending aorta. The true lumen (T) is considerably smaller than the false lumen (F).

While the primary goal of imaging is to establish the presence of a dissection, the complications of aortic dissection are also readily depicted on spiral CT. These include aortic branch vessel occlusion, aneurysm formation, hemopericardium, and rupture with mediastinal or pleural hemorrhage. Myocardial infarction resulting from proximal extension of a dissection and aortic regurgitation are best evaluated by TEE.

Computer-generated two-dimensional (multiplanar reformations or MPR) and three-dimensional (multiplanar volumetric reformations or MPVR) reconstructions are not necessary to make the diagnosis of dissection, but may be useful in delineating the extent of involvement of the aorta and branch vessels (Fig. 12) (12). Volumetric reconstructions (MPVRs) performed with maximum intensity projection (MIP) and shaded surface display rendering techniques have a limited ability to depict intimal flaps and, therefore, are the least valuable of the reconstruction algorithms in evaluating aortic dissection.

There are several pitfalls in the interpretation of CT aortography for the diagnosis of dissection. These include factors that can produce the false appearance of an intimal flap and insufficient vascular enhancement to allow detection of an intimal flap (13). The most common cause of a pseudodissection is a curvilinear streak artifact in the ascending aorta related to the pulsatile movement of the aortic wall between end diastole and end systole (Fig. 13) (14). These artifacts are typically seen along the left anterior and right posterior aspects of the ascending aorta and are minimized by use of a 180° linear interpolation reconstruction algorithm (15) and by retrospective cardiac gating, which limits image reconstruction to the late diastolic phase of the cardiac cycle thereby reducing systolic motion. Other common causes of streak artifacts in the aorta include dense contrast in the left brachiocephalic vein (from a left arm contrast injection) or superior vena cava, mediastinal clips or indwelling tubes or catheters. In addition, any high-attenuation structure that contacts the enhancing aortic lumen can simulate an enhancing false lumen and produce the appearance of an intimal flap. These include an enhanced left brachiocephalic, superior intercostal or left inferior pulmonary vein, and curvilinear atelectasis of the left lower lobe.

The natural history of medically managed acute Type A dissection is associated with a 3 month mortality rate of 90% (6), rendering surgical repair the treatment of choice in acute Type A dissection in operative

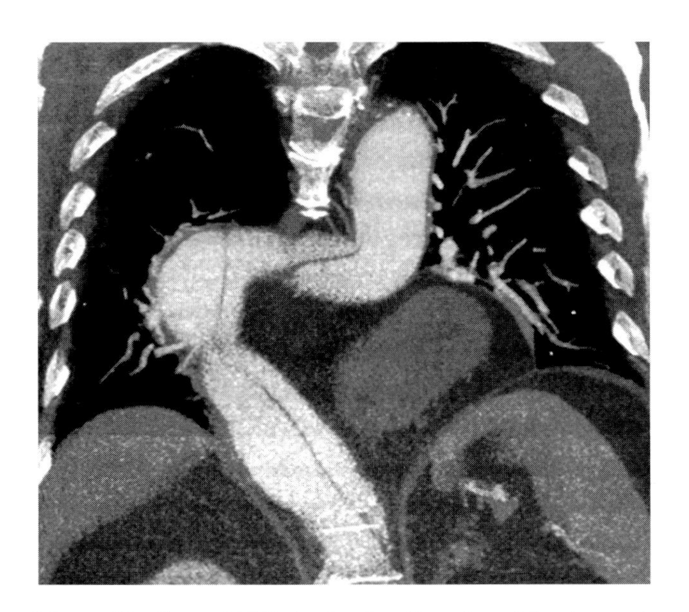

Figure 12 Coronal MIP of extensive dissection of the descending aorta extending into the abdomen.

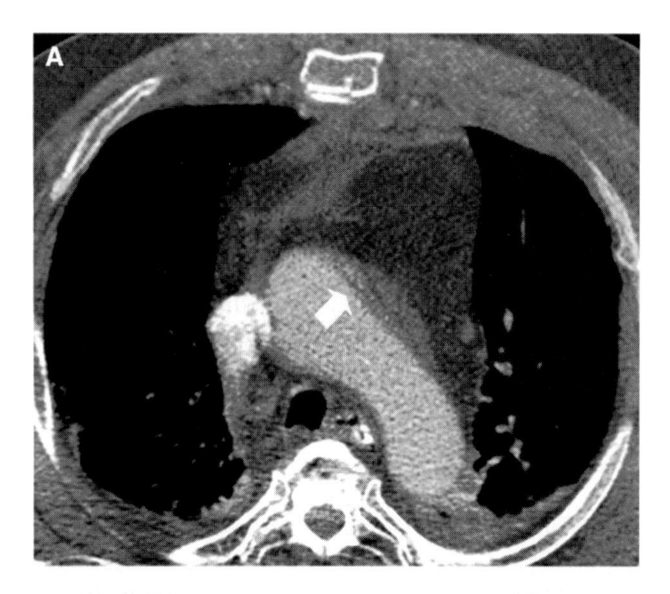

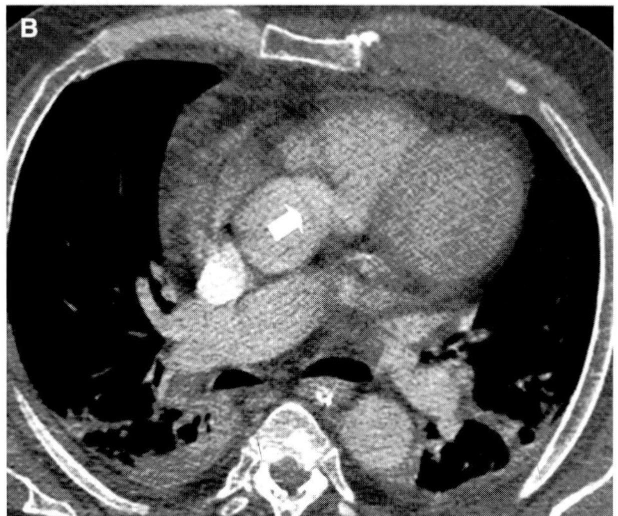

Figure 13 Ascending aortic pulsation artifact. Pulsation artifacts (*arrows*) in the (**A**), transverse arch and (**B**) the ascending aorta mimic intimal flaps.

candidates. Alternatively, the survival rate for medically managed Type B dissection is 73% at 1 year: This in combination with a high rate of paraplegia and death (up to 65%) in surgically managed Type B dissections warrants medical therapy in this group unless there is the development of aneurysm, rupture, or proximal extension into the arch and ascending aorta. Although the traditional approach to Type A dissection is immediate surgery and Type B medical management, recent data suggest that some Type A dissections, particularly where the diagnosis is delayed several days after onset of symptoms or patients are considered poor surgical candidates, may be managed with semi-elective surgery or even aggressive medical therapy alone with good outcomes. Patients with Type B dissections complicated by ischemic injury to the kidneys, spinal cord, bowel, or legs; rapid enlargement; rupture; intractable pain; or proximal extension require surgical repair.

Intramural Hematoma

IMH of the aorta is an acute clinical entity that represents a hemorrhage confined to the aortic media in which there is no intimal tear (Fig. 14). It is thought to arise from rupture of the vasa vasorum within the aortic media and as in aortic dissection tends to affect hypertensive patients, although it can result from trauma or develop as a complication of a PAU. Since only first recognized as a distinct radiographic entity in 1985 (16), it is likely that a significant percentage of cases of IMH have been traditionally misclassified as "atypical" aortic dissections. In support of this concept is the finding that at one institution a retrospective review of 214 patients originally classified as aortic dissection showed 17 (8%) that met the imaging criteria for IMH (17).

Patients with IMH tend to be older at age of presentation than those with aortic dissection,

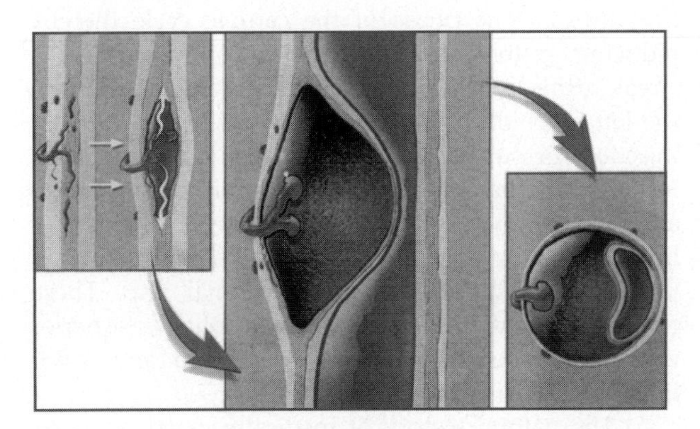

Figure 14 Diagram illustrating the pathogenesis of intramural aortic hematoma. Rupture of the vaso vasorum (*left image*) creates a hematoma within the aortic wall (*middle image*). The aortic intima remains intact (*right image*). *Source*: From Ref. 71.

particularly when compared to Type A dissection associated with Marfan's syndrome. As in classic dissection, pain radiating to the back is the most common presenting complaint. Unlike classic dissection, most patients with IMH (70%) have involvement limited to the descending aorta, and branch vessel occlusion is very uncommon. Based on a similar mode of presentation to classic dissection and severity of this disorder, most experts recommend classifying IMH in a manner analogous to that of aortic dissection (i.e., Type A with ascending aortic involvement and Type B limited to the descending aorta).

TEE can depict IMH but this diagnosis is often difficult to distinguish sonographically from mural thrombus within a dilated aorta. CT has 96% sensitivity for the detection of IMH (18). Unenhanced CT demonstrates a high-attenuation crescent-shaped thickening of the aortic wall that extends in the cephalocaudal direction without significant compromise of the vascular lumen (i.e., there is a concave interface between the hematoma and the aortic lumen) (Fig. 15A). There may be medial displacement of intimal calcifications and the aorta is often dilated or aneurysmal. Following intravenous contrast administration, there is lack of enhancement of the hematoma, no intimal flap is identified, and the hematoma appears hypodense relative to the enhancing aortic lumen (Fig. 15B). It may be difficult to distinguish IMH from atherosclerotic thickening of the aorta or thrombus within an aortic aneurysm. The presence of a high-attenuation smooth crescentic intramural density on precontrast scans that does not enhance and the absence of an intimal flap usually allows for accurate diagnosis. While the distinction from an acutely thrombosed aortic dissection is more difficult, an IMH, unlike a dissection, does not typically spiral around the circumference of the aorta, as it extends longitudinally. MRI, particularly with the use of dynamic cine gradient-echo (GRE) sequences, is particularly accurate for assessing IMH and is used as the primary method of diagnosis in some institutions (19,20). Aortography is insensitive to the detection of IMH, as the thickened aortic wall is difficult to appreciate and distinguish from atherosclerotic disease.

The prognosis for patients with IMH depends on the type or extent of hematoma formation, the age of the patient, and the presence of comorbid conditions. Most centers with experience managing IMH recommend an operative approach to Type A IMH, since there is a high rate of rupture with resultant pericardial tamponade or mediastinal hemorrhage or the development of intimal disruption with dissection in these patients (17,19,21). Most patients with Type B IMH have good short-term outcome with aggressive medical control of hypertension; however, one study

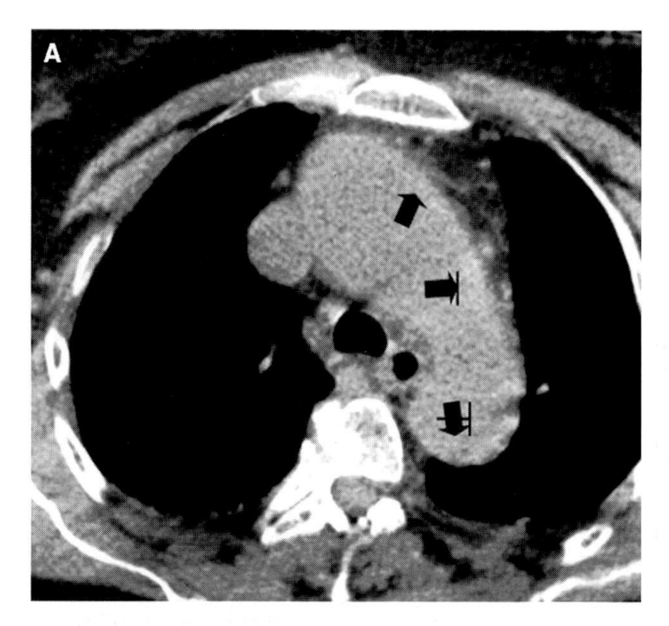

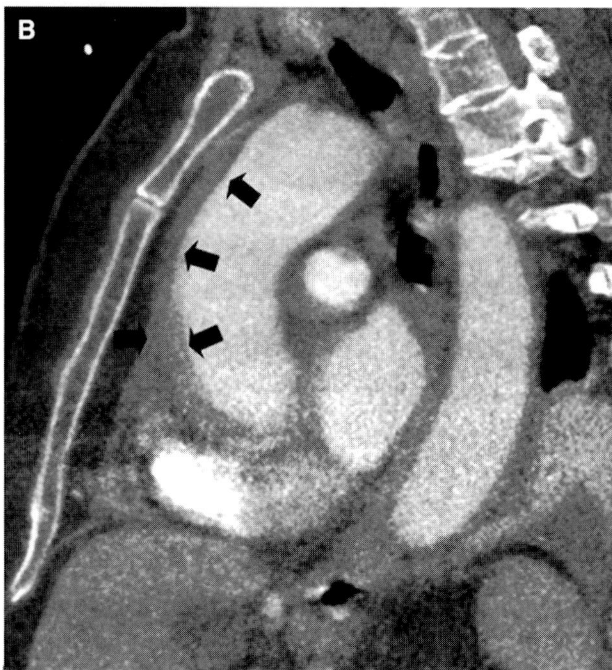

Figure 15 Intramural hematoma. (**A**) Unenhanced axial scan through the transverse arch shows increased attenuation of the outer portion of the aorta (*arrows*) owing to acute intramural hemorrhage. (**B**) Sagittal reconstruction of an enhanced, gated CT shows the hemorrhage as apparent aortic wall thickening (*arrows*).

that evaluated findings on initial CT examinations in patients with type B IMH predictive of progression (i.e., aneurysm formation, ulcer formation, frank dissection, or aortic rupture) found a maximal aortic diameter of 4 cm and a maximum wall thickness of 10 mm or greater to be predictive of progression of disease (22). Another feature of IMH as seen on initial MDCT that may be of prognostic value is the presence of a PAU in association with the hematoma, as one study found a significantly higher incidence of disease progression in those with IMH who had PAUs (23).

In those patients with IMH managed nonoperatively, close clinical and cross-sectional imaging follow-up within the first 30 days of presentation is recommended. Findings on follow-up CT imaging that suggest worsening of IMH include progressive longitudinal aortic involvement, progressive luminal dilatation, penetrating ulcer (Fig 16), enlarging IMH, or the development of typical dissection. Detection of these findings on follow-up CT should prompt consideration of open surgical or endovascular stent graft repair (24).

In the subset of patients with IMH who are managed nonoperatively, the 10-year survival rates excluding non IMH-related deaths are approximately 80–90%, supporting a conservative management approach past the initial presentation period (25).

Penetrating Atherosclerotic Ulcer

PAU is an ulcer that develops within an atherosclerotic portion of the thoracic, or rarely the abdominal,

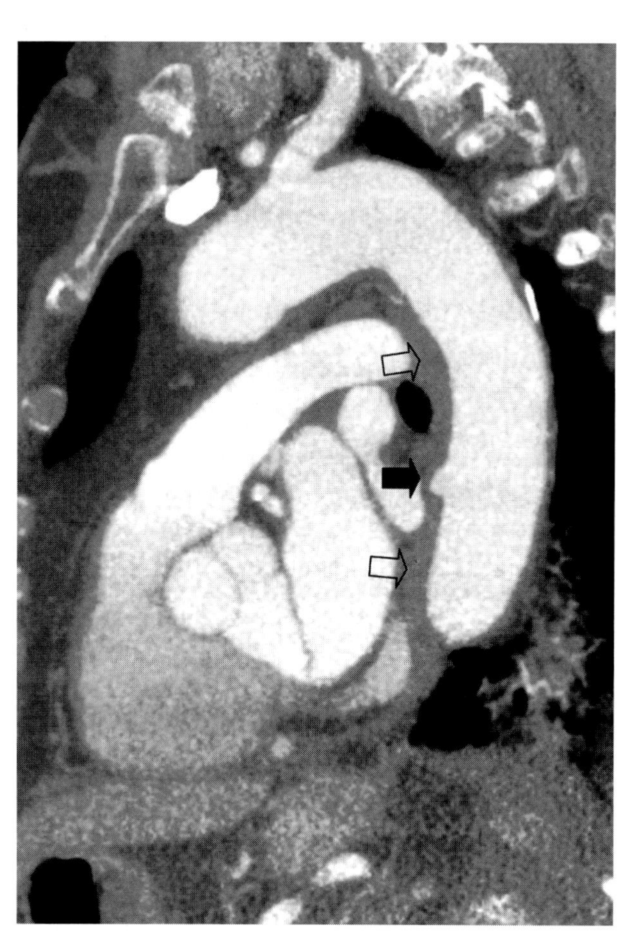

Figure 16 Penetrating ulcer complicating intramural hematoma. The old hematoma is visible as a "thickened" aortic wall (*open arrows*) with a penetrating ulcer (*solid arrow*) protruding into it.

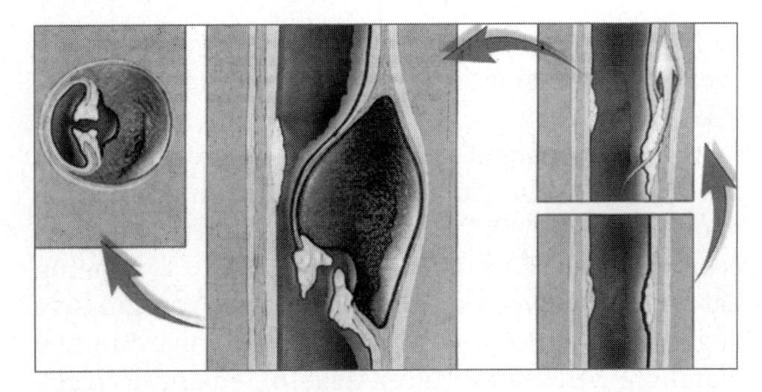

Figure 17 Diagram illustrating the pathogenesis of penetrating atherosclerotic aortic ulcer. Atheromatous plaque in the aortic wall (*left image*) eventually penetrates into the media (*middle image*) resulting in an intramural hematoma. *Source*: From Ref. 71.

aorta. It penetrates through the internal elastic lamina into the aortic media and associated with a localized IMH (Fig. 17) (26). This most often develops in elderly hypertensive patients with severe atherosclerotic disease and most commonly affects the descending thoracic aorta (90%) (17). While ulcerated atherosclerotic plaques limited to the aortic intima may be detected as incidental findings on contrast-enhanced thoracic CT, most patients with PAU present with chest and back pain indistinguishable from Type B aortic dissection. In most cases the ulcerating lesion is limited in extent by the locally advanced atherosclerotic disease in the adjacent portion of the aorta, although extension along the length of the aorta or through the media and adventitia with pseudoaneurysm formation can occur. As with IMH, the diagnosis of PAU in patients presenting with acute aortic syndromes was likely under-recognized in the era prior to cross-sectional imaging with CT: In the above mentioned series from Coady and colleagues at Yale University, 19 (9%) of 214 patients initially diagnosed as aortic dissection were found to have PAU on review of imaging, surgical, and pathologic studies (17).

Contrast-enhanced MDCT with axial and multiplanar reconstructions is the primary method of diagnosis of PAU. The characteristic finding is a localized ulceration penetrating through the aortic intima within the mid to distal third of the descending aorta (Fig. 18) (27,28). There may be inward displacement of intimal calcifications, allowing distinction from an ulcerated atherosclerotic plaque limited to the intima. Focal thickening of the adjacent aortic wall is seen, representing the associated IMH. The cephalocaudal extent of the ulceration is most easily appreciated on coronal or sagittal reconstructions. While MR and TEE can depict the ulceration and associated IMH without the need for intravenous contrast, the lower inherent spatial resolution of these techniques and more widespread access to CT makes contrast-enhanced MDCT the modality of choice for suspected PAU. Aortography can depict PAU projecting from the aortic lumen only if filmed in tangent to the ulcer crater.

Complications of PAU include progression to classic aortic dissection, embolization of material from the ulcer into the distal arterial circulation, extensive IMH formation, and development of a pseudoaneurysm with subsequent rupture. Branch vessel occlusion does not occur in uncomplicated PAU. Most patients with descending PAUs, particularly those with significant contraindications to surgery, can be managed conservatively in the acute setting (29). Nevertheless, several series have shown a tendency for PAUs to progress to aneurysm formation with an incidence of rupture exceeding 40%. This rate of rupture is significantly higher than that seen in classic aortic dissection or IMH (28,30), and has led some to advocate an aggressive surgical approach for patients with PAU. Nonetheless, it is clear that nonoperated patients should be followed closely with repeated cross-sectional imaging studies obtained within days of initial presentation to detect complications that might warrant surgical intervention. Patients who require surgical repair typically undergo replacement of the diseased aortic segment with an interposition graft (31), a procedure that is more extensive than repair of an intimal flap in aortic dissection and is associated with a higher incidence of paraplegia due to spinal cord ischemia (32). More recently, endovascular stent-graft repair has been performed as an alternative to open surgical repair (see section "Postoperative Aorta").

TRAUMATIC AORTIC INJURY

TAI to the aorta accounts for approximately 15% of all deaths due to motor vehicle accidents. While 90% of patients with TAI die before reaching a medical facility, those who survive to reach the hospital have 30–40% mortality within the first 24 h (33). It is in these patients that a rapid and accurate diagnosis of TAI is critical to survival.

The mechanism responsible for TAI in cases of blunt trauma is felt to be a shear injury to the aorta from rapid deceleration. The injury is usually the result of a high-speed motor vehicle accident but can also develop from a vertical fall or other deceleration injury. Those portions of the aorta that are relatively fixed in position are most prone to injury from shearing effects: in survivors of TAI these include the aortic isthmus (90%); aortic root (5–10%); and rarely the descending aorta at the diaphragmatic hiatus or at the site of a hyperextension injury in the thoracic spine. The resultant aortic injury can range from a focal intimal tear or IMH to complete laceration or transection of the aortic wall. Injuries

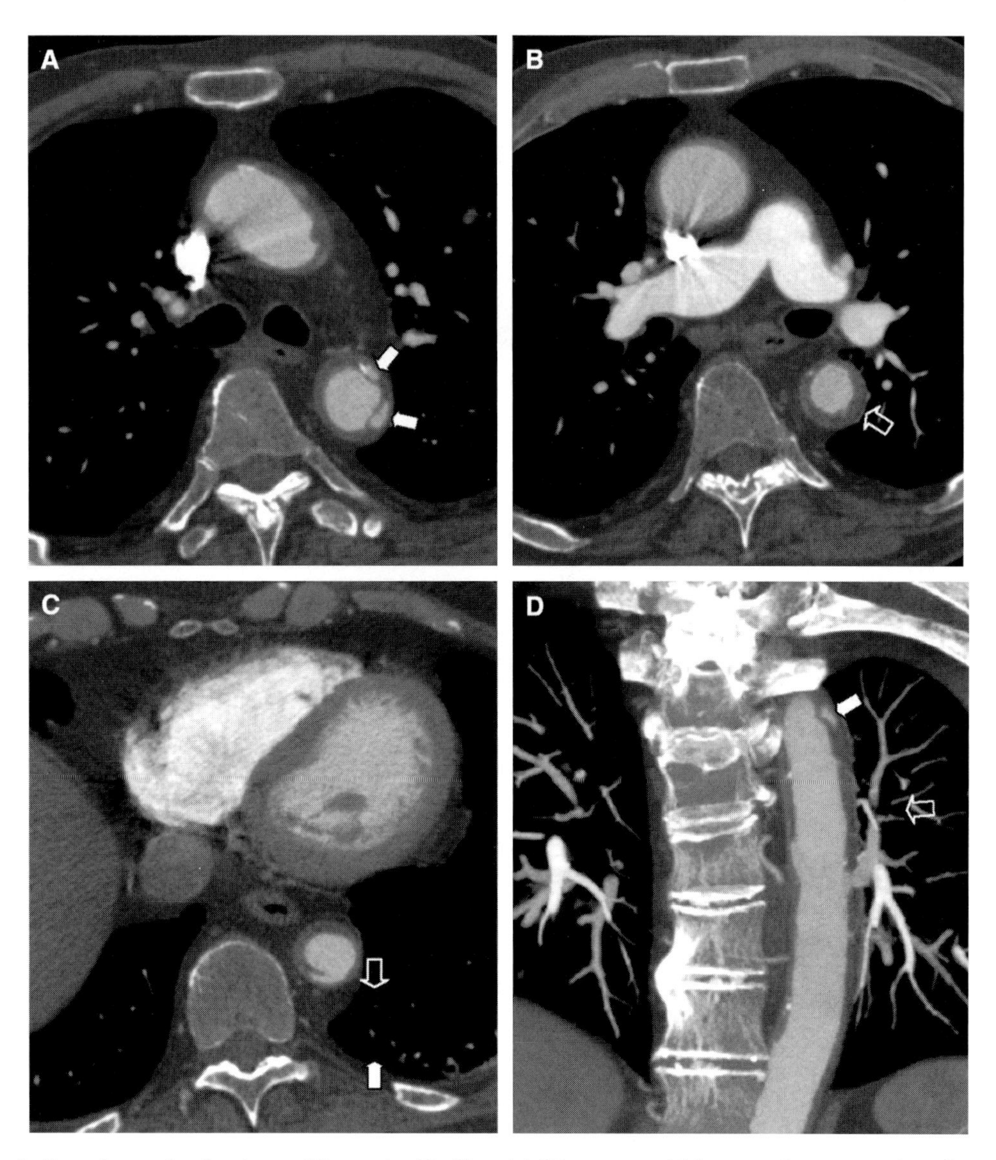

Figure 18 Penetrating atherosclerotic ulcers of the aorta. (**A–C**), axial CT scans, and (**D**), coronal reconstruction, demonstrates multiple penetrating ulcers (*solid arrows*) and extensive atherosclerosis mixed with intramural hematoma (*open arrows*) are present in the descending aorta.

to the ascending aorta are almost invariably fatal, as they result in pericardial tamponade and aortic valve disruption. While injuries to the aortic isthmus can likewise be fatal, containment of a mural aortic injury by the adventitia or periadventitial tissues can prevent exsanguination and allow a patient to survive long enough to develop a pseudoaneurysm.

The initial imaging evaluation of suspected aortic injury remains the portable chest radiograph, usually obtained with the trauma patient in the supine position. Radiographic abnormalities suggesting an aortic injury include widening of the mediastinum, obscuration of the aortic knob, thickening of the right paratracheal stripe, a left apical cap, and rightward deviation of the trachea or indwelling nasogastric tube, all findings of a mediastinal hematoma, which results from bleeding from small vessels. A normal portable chest radiograph, particularly an erect film, has a high-negative predictive value for excluding aortic injury (approximately 98%) (34).

It is well recognized that only a small minority of patients that undergo evaluation for TAI will be found to have such an injury, in large part because the clinical evaluation of the trauma patient is difficult and the chest radiograph is a sensitive but nonspecific indicator of TAI. The initial role of CT in the evaluation of TAI was limited due to relatively slow scan speeds and limited resolution in the uncooperative trauma patient. Both the increased availability of MDCT scanners in trauma centers, with their inherent rapid acquisition time and high contrast and spatial resolution, along with increased utilization of helical CT for the evaluation of head, spine, abdominopelvic, and musculoskeletal injuries have led to renewed interest in the use of helical CT in this setting. The early efforts to determine the role of CT in the evaluation of TAI focused on patients with a low to moderate suspicion for TAI and equivocal chest radiographs who were selected for angiography based on the detection of mediastinal hematoma. This was mostly done in an attempt to reduce the percentage of negative catheter aortograms performed (35,36). More recently, several large series comparing helical CT to conventional angiography for the diagnosis of TAI have shown that helical CT is an accurate and cost-effective technique that provides direct evaluation of the aorta while obviating the need for conventional aortography in most clinical settings (37–39). It is a safe and highly accurate examination with a negative predictive value for aortic injury approaching 100%.

The technique of CT aortography is similar to that described for the evaluation of other aortic diseases (Table 1). In the blunt trauma patient, the evaluation of the thoracic aorta and chest is often only part of a more extensive evaluation of the abdomen, pelvis, head, and spine. Since nearly one-third of patients with aortic injury have an abdominal visceral injury or pelvic fracture, most experts recommend performing an abdominal and pelvic CT as a direct extension of the thoracic examination (40).

The helical CT diagnosis of TAI includes both direct and indirect findings. The detection of a periaortic hematoma, particularly around the aortic isthmus, is an indirect and nonspecific sign of aortic injury but at some centers will lead to an aortogram even in the presence of a normal aorta on CT. An anterior or posterior mediastinal hematoma usually indicates an injury to the sternum or thoracic spine, respectively. In the absence of a periaortic hematoma or aortic abnormality on a good quality helical CT, one can confidently exclude TAI. Hemopericardium or hemothorax are additional indirect signs of TAI but are most often due to other injuries. Direct findings of TAI (Fig. 19) include linear intraluminal filling defects that reflect either intimal or mural flaps from aortic laceration or transection, pseudoaneurysm formation, abrupt caliber change, and active contrast extravasation.

The distinction between minimal aortic injuries and nontraumatic aortic entities such as a ductus diverticulum, prominent origin of a bronchial artery, and atherosclerosis can be difficult and these abnormalities may result in a false positive CT aortogram (40). The subtle aortic abnormality produced by a small intimal flap, mural hematoma, or small pseudoaneurysm may be seen on only two or three contiguous images. Aortography is recommended to delineate such subtle injuries and can usually distinguish between a normal variant (e.g., ductus diverticulum) or atherosclerotic plaque and a true aortic injury. In selected cases, however, transesophageal or intravascular ultrasound may be necessary to better define the aortic abnormality.

AORTIC ANEURYSM

An aortic aneurysm is defined as an abnormal permanent dilatation of the aorta. Since the aorta normally dilates with advancing age, the "normal" diameter is age dependent, but always less than 4 cm in diameter in the midascending aorta and less than 3 cm in the descending aorta (41). A more recent study that assessed thoracic aortic diameters throughout life as measured on helical CT found a diameter (mean ± standard deviation) of the ascending aorta of 3.09 ± 0.41 cm and of the distal descending aorta at the diaphragm of 2.43 ± 0.35 cm (42). These authors recommended a definition of TAA of mean + two standard deviations, which defines an ascending aneurysm as >3.91 cm and descending aneurysm as >3.13, a virtually identical result to that suggested by the work of Aronberg. Approximately 75% of TAAs affect the descending aorta, where atherosclerotic disease is most common. In addition, the aortic diameter tapers as it extends distally, with the descending aorta never larger than the ascending aorta. The prevalence of aneurysm increases with age, with an overall incidence of approximately 450 per 100,000 people and a male:female ratio of approximately 3:1 (43). Concomitant abdominal aortic aneurysm is seen in up to 28% of patients, so the entire thoracoabdominal aorta should be imaged when evaluating TAAs (43).

The etiologies of TAA include atherosclerosis, connective tissue diseases such as Marfan's and Ehlers–Danlos syndromes, trauma, aortitis (including syphilis, mycotic aneurysms, and noninfectious inflammatory diseases), and aortic dissection. A genetic predisposition to TAA is supported by studies that show a familial aggregation of cases (44).

TAA are generally divided into true aneurysms and pseudoaneurysms (i.e., false aneurysms) based on their gross and pathological appearance. True aortic aneurysms are usually fusiform in shape and are composed of all three anatomic layers (intima, media, and adventitia). These most commonly arise in the descending thoracic aorta as the result of atherosclerotic disease. Pseudoaneurysms have an absent intimal layer and are contained by the adventitia or periadventitial tissues. They are usually saccular in shape, have a narrow neck where they arise from the aorta, and develop as the result of blunt or penetrating trauma, a PAU, or infection. Pseudoaneurysms may affect any portion of the thoracic aorta, although traumatic pseudoaneurysms are most often found at

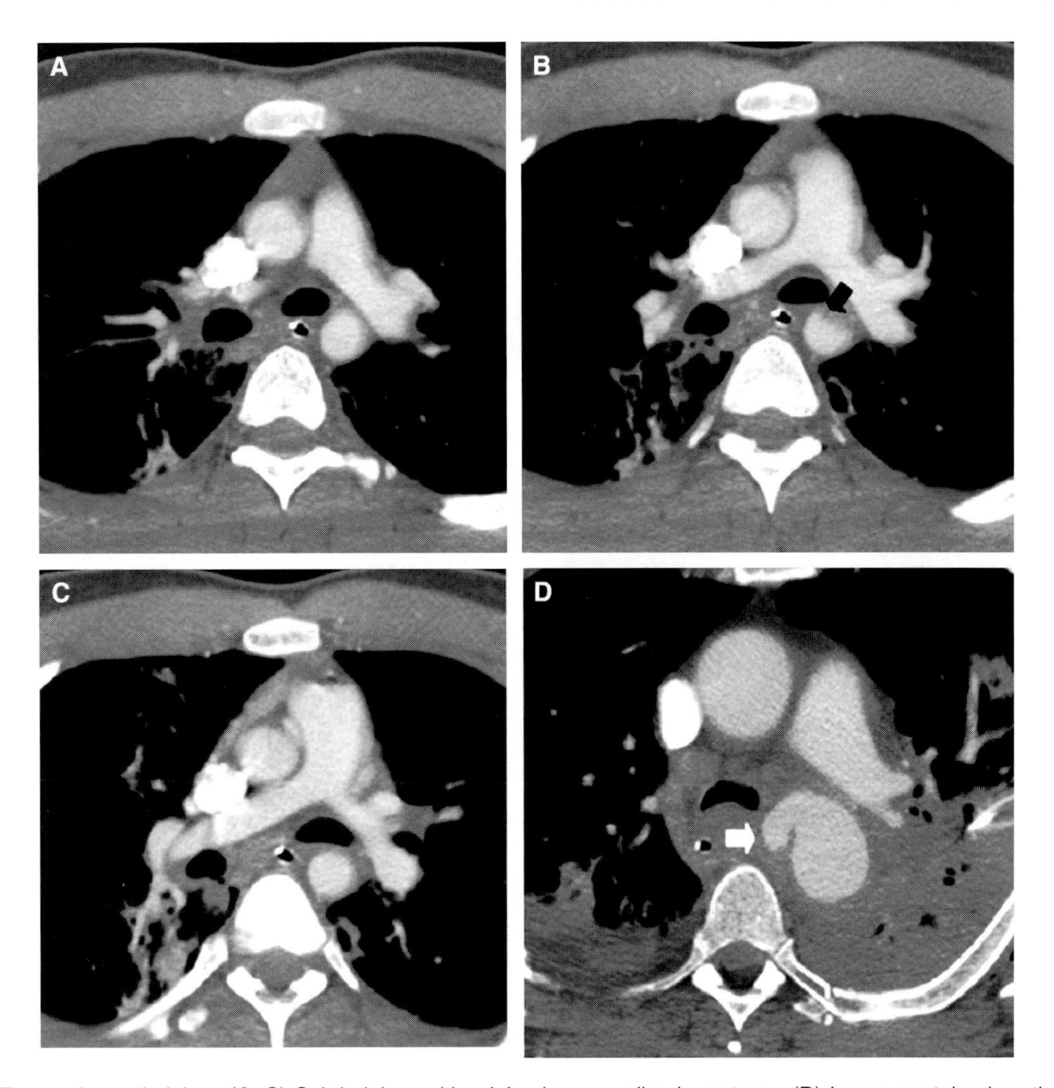

Figure 19 Traumatic aortic injury. (**A–C**) Subtle injury with minimal surrounding hematoma. (**D**) Large, contained aortic tear (*arrow*) with moderate mediastinal hematoma. The tear (*arrow*) is limited in cranial-caudal extent and would likely be missed on thicker slices.

the aortic isthmus, and those resulting as a complication of PAU are usually seen in the descending aorta.

Plain film findings of aortic aneurysm include a mediastinal mass with peripheral calcification that is contiguous with the aorta, widening of the aortic knob or prominence of the ascending or descending aorta, and mediastinal widening. Aortography can considerably underestimate the size of the aneurysm due to mural thrombus and is rarely obtained in the evaluation of TAA.

MDCT aortography and MR have virtually replaced conventional aortography for the detection and characterization of thoracoabdominal aortic aneurysms. Spiral CT allows accurate diagnosis of aortic aneurysm and readily distinguishes this from other mediastinal masses. It demonstrates all features of TAAs, including an accurate assessment of the shape, length, and diameter of the aneurysm; the presence of mural thrombus and calcification; and the relationship of the aneurysm to adjacent intrathoracic structures (45). Spiral CT is no longer limited by an inability to evaluate the coronary arteries in patients with ascending aortic aneurysms or delineate the intercostal supply to the spinal cord at T8-L1 in those with descending TAAs.

While it may be difficult to distinguish mural thrombus in an aortic aneurysm from an IMH or thrombosed aortic dissection, there are several CT findings that aid in this distinction. In a thrombosed aneurysm, the residual aortic lumen is generally smooth and the thrombus circumferential (Fig. 20), while IMH and thrombosed dissection produces a more irregular interface with the aortic lumen. When present, atherosclerotic intimal calcifications are seen at the peripheral edge of thrombus, whereas they are displaced medially by IMH and thrombosed dissection. Despite these characteristic features, the distinction between a thrombosed aneurysm and IMH or

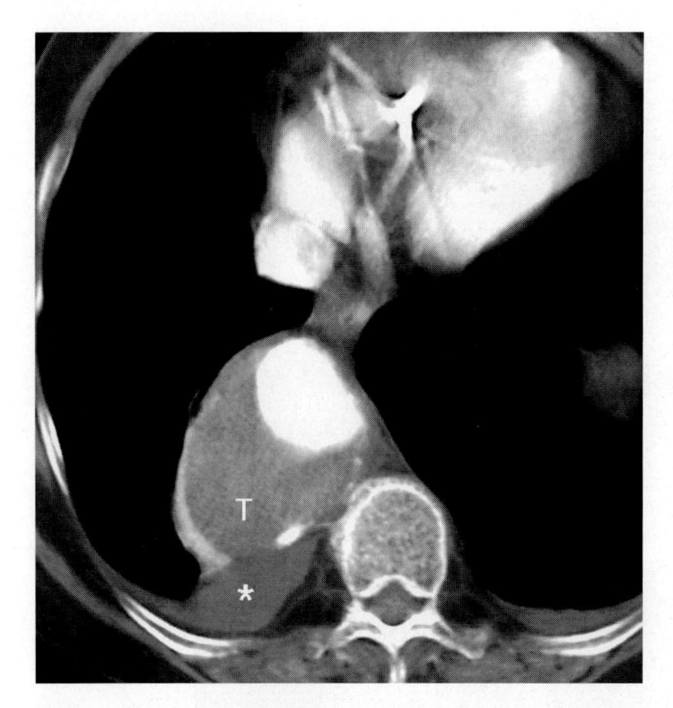

Figure 20 Large descending thoracic aortic aneurysm contains mostly thrombus (T). Pleural fluid posteriorly (*) is from bleeding from the aneurysm.

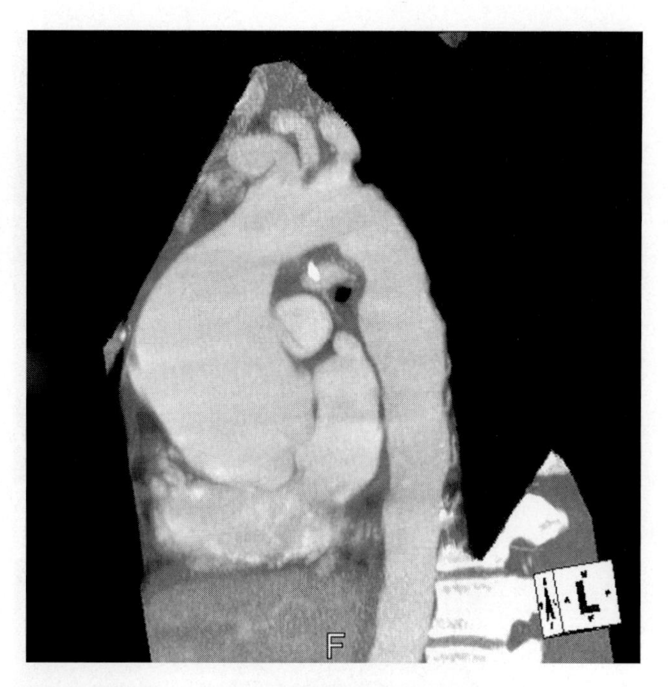

Figure 21 Anuloaortic ectasia.

thrombosed dissection may be difficult in selected cases, particularly when the thrombus within an aneurysm is calcified (46,47).

There is no direct relationship between the etiology of a TAA and its radiologic appearance, except in the case of anuloaortic ectasia. Patients with connective tissue abnormalities of the ascending aorta have anuloaortic ectasia, which is characterized by dilated sinuses of Valsalva with effacement of the sinotubular junction (where the sinuses of Valsalva and ascending aorta meet). Classically it presents with classic pear-shaped aneurysmal aorta with a smooth taper to a normal aortic arch (Fig. 21). This appearance is best appreciated on coronal reformations through the ascending aorta. The most common cause of anuloaortic ectasia is Marfan's syndrome, but about a third of cases are idiopathic (48). Other causes include homocystinuria, Ehlers–Danlos syndrome, and osteogenesis imperfecta. It is critical to identify anuloaortic ectasia as the cause of an ascending aortic aneurysm as the surgery is different from that of other types of aneurysm (see below).

Atherosclerotic aneurysms appear as continuous fusiform dilatations of the descending aorta with smooth mural thrombus that can be either crescentic or concentric. Mycotic aneurysms arising from bacterial infection of a diseased aortic wall are most often saccular with focal dilatation and eccentric thrombus and mural calcification (49). They have a propensity to affect the ascending aorta likely due to its proximity to the regions affected by endocarditis, which is often an associated condition (50). Traumatic pseudoaneurysms following blunt trauma most often develop near the aortic isthmus and are usually saccular with a narrow neck (Fig. 22). Mural calcification is common in chronic cases. Aneurysms arising as a complication of PAUs are most often seen as saccular aneurysms of the descending aorta. Aortitis due to noninfectious diseases, particularly connective tissue diseases such as rheumatoid arthritis; Reiter's syndrome; and ankylosing spondylitis usually produces fusiform aneurysms of the ascending aorta (Fig. 23).

As in other aortic diseases, the axial reconstructions provide the primary means of helical CT interpretation; however, there are advantages of specific types of reformations unique to the evaluation of aortic aneurysms that differ from those performed for aortic dissection and its variants. MPRs of volumetric data provide a more accurate measurement of the diameter of a TAA than axial scans, particularly in the descending aorta where the dilated lumen may course oblique to the scan plane. MPRs also allow display of intraluminal contents, particularly mural thrombus and atherosclerotic changes (12). In patients with aneurysms complicated by dissection, curved planar reformats (CPRs) best depict the relationship of the intimal flap to the great vessel ostia. Shaded surface display, a three-dimensional volume-rendering technique, is useful in displaying complex relationships of aneurysms to adjacent mediastinal vessels but does not provide visualization of aneurysm contents.

MR using standard spin-echo techniques can provide information regarding TAAs analogous to

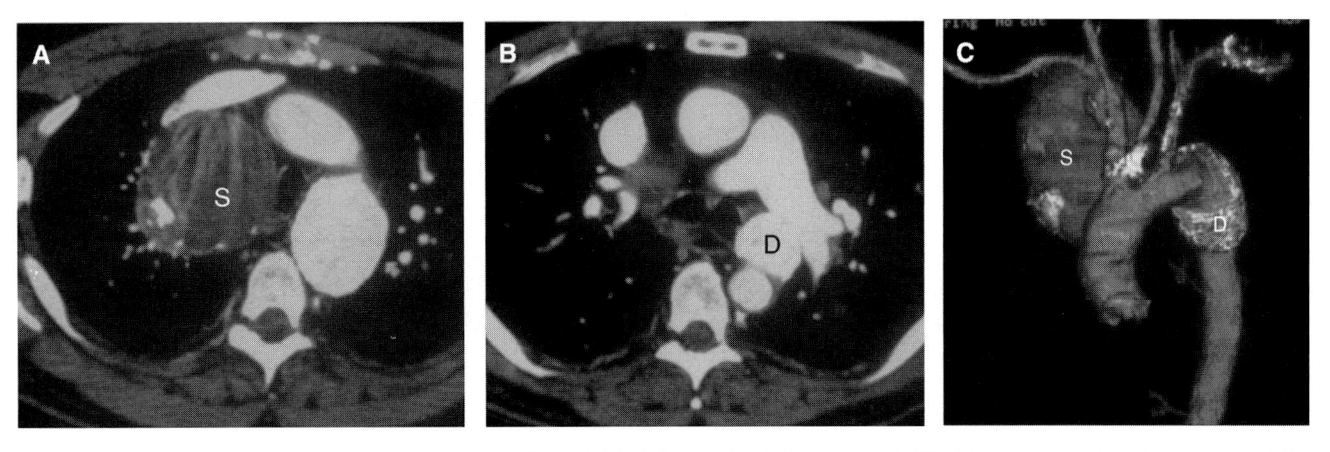

Figure 22 Chronic traumatic pseudoaneurysms. (**A** and **B**) Enhanced axial scans and (**C**) 3D reconstruction demonstrate false aneurysms of the right subclavian artery (S) and proximal descending aorta (D). The subclavian aneurysm is mostly thrombus-filled.

MDCT, although without the use of ionizing radiation or intravenous contrast. MR depicts mural thrombus as intermediate signal material on Tl-weighted images but cannot detect calcification within the wall of an aneurysm. Oblique sagittal MR scans of the aorta allow simultaneous display of the entire length of the thoracic and upper abdominal aorta, which is beneficial in patients with thoracoabdominal aneurysms (51). MR is particularly useful in the follow-up of patients with known TAAs and in those with contraindications to intravenous contrast administration. Unlike CT, MR images must be acquired in the desired plane and cannot be reconstructed into other planes postacquisition.

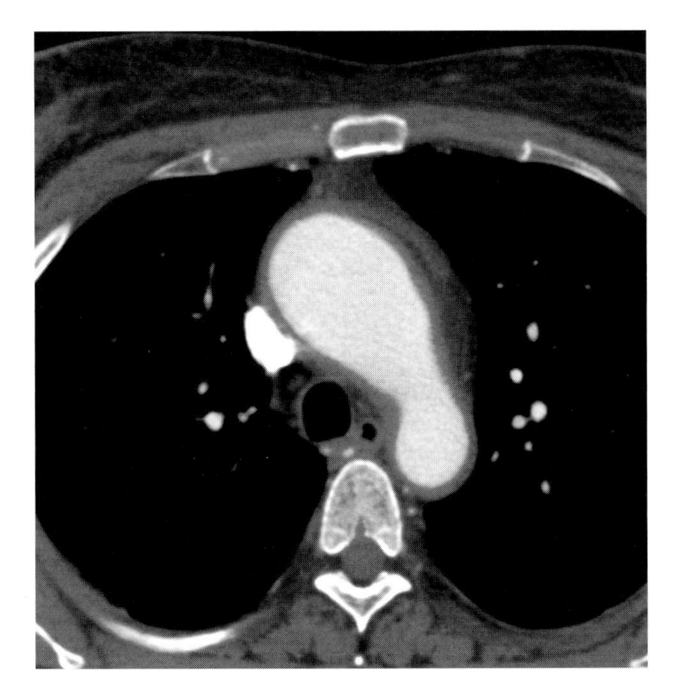

Figure 23 Ascending aneurysm from Takayasu's arteritis. The aortic wall is uniformly thickened and the ascending aorta dilated.

Complications of TAA, including progressive dilatation, dissection, and hemorrhage, are easily assessed by CT. In particular, helical CT is the modality of choice in the setting of suspected acute aortic rupture, as it can detect active contrast extravasation or high-attenuation hematoma within the pleural or pericardial space or mediastinum (52). A crescent of high-attenuation material within the mural thrombus of a TAA represents acute or impending contained aneurysm rupture (53). A contained rupture of the posterior aortic wall in close apposition to the spine may show a draped aorta sign, thought to be indicative of a deficient aortic wall (54). Aortobronchial fistula results from communication between the aorta and bronchial tree and most often arises as a complication of an atherosclerotic TAA or as a postsurgical complication of aneurysm repair. The fistulous communication in an aortobronchial fistula is between the descending aorta and left bronchopulmonary tree in nearly 90% of cases (55). Patients usually present with massive hemoptysis. Helical CT does not often demonstrate the fistula itself but shows an aortic aneurysm adjacent to consolidated lung (56). Management consists of surgical repair of the aortic and bronchial defects, with approximately three-fourths of patients successfully repaired. Similarly, aortoesophageal fistula is a catastrophic and often fatal complication of TAA, resulting from communication between the descending aorta and esophagus. Patients presented with massive upper gastrointestinal hemorrhage with endoscopy often fail to delineate the source of bleeding. CT may demonstrate the aneurysm and its intimate relationship to the esophagus; mediastinal hematoma or rarely contrast extravasation into the esophagus may be seen. Immediate surgical repair is mandatory (57).

The natural history of TAA is directly related to its size. While TAAs can present due to mass effect on adjacent mediastinal structures, the most serious complication is aortic rupture, which occurs in up to 70% of affected patients (58). While aortic rupture usually results in exsanguination into the mediastinum, lung, or pleural space, sometimes a communication will develop with the tracheobronchial tree or esophagus producing hemoptysis or hematemesis, respectively. The risk of rupture increases with increasing size of the aneurysm, and TAAs have been observed to dilate at a mean rate of 0.12 cm/yr (59). Based on these data, elective surgical repair has been recommended for ascending aortic aneurysm diameters of 5–5.5 cm and descending aortic aneurysms of 5.5–6.5 cm (59). Surgical treatment generally consists of the placement of a Dacron graft within the diseased aortic segment: Ascending aortic aneurysms that involve the aortic anulus and valve, most often seen in patients with anuloaortic ectasia, require a composite graft (i.e., combined aortic valve with prosthetic ascending aortic graft) with reimplantation of the coronary arteries.

AORTITIS

There are a number of autoimmune disorders that can produce aortitis. These noninfectious inflammatory processes include many of the connective tissue diseases such as rheumatoid arthritis, ankylosing spondylitis, Reiter's syndrome, giant cell arteritis, Behcet's disease, and relapsing polychondritis. These diseases weaken the aortic wall and predispose to aneurysm formation with a predilection for involvement of the ascending aorta. The most common noninfectious cause of aortitis is Takayasu's arteritis, usually seen in young Asian women. This is a vasculitis of unknown etiology that primarily affects the thoracic aortic arch with variable involvement of the abdominal aorta and pulmonary arteries. This disease produces inflammation of the media and adventitia that most commonly results in arterial stenosis and occlusion, hence the use of the descriptor "pulseless" disease. Aneurysmal dilatation of the aorta is a less common manifestation of the disease (60).

Patients with thoracic aneurysms resulting from the aortitis associated with connective tissue disease usually have fusiform dilatation of the ascending aorta (Fig. 23) with variable involvement of the aortic valve annulus. Fine curvilinear calcification may be seen in the wall of the aneurysm. The CT features of Takayasu's arteritis of the aorta have been described (61). Unenhanced CT demonstrates high attenuation of the thickened aortic wall and mural calcifications in the majority of affected patients. Mural enhancement during the arterial phase following contrast administration was seen in 75% of patients with active disease and was 100% specific (Fig. 24). Aortic arch and branch vessel stenoses are present in the majority of patients. Aneurysm formation is uncommon, may be fusiform or saccular in shape, and is often difficult to distinguish from dilatation proximal to a hemodynamically significant stenosis.

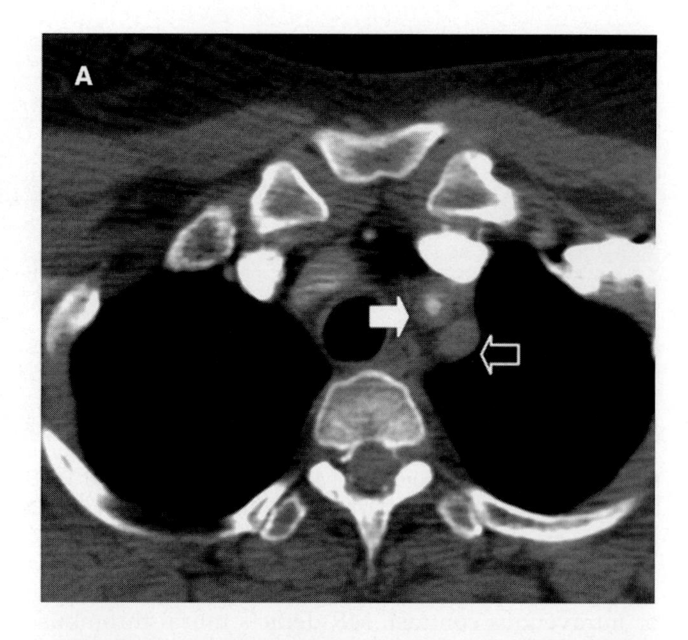

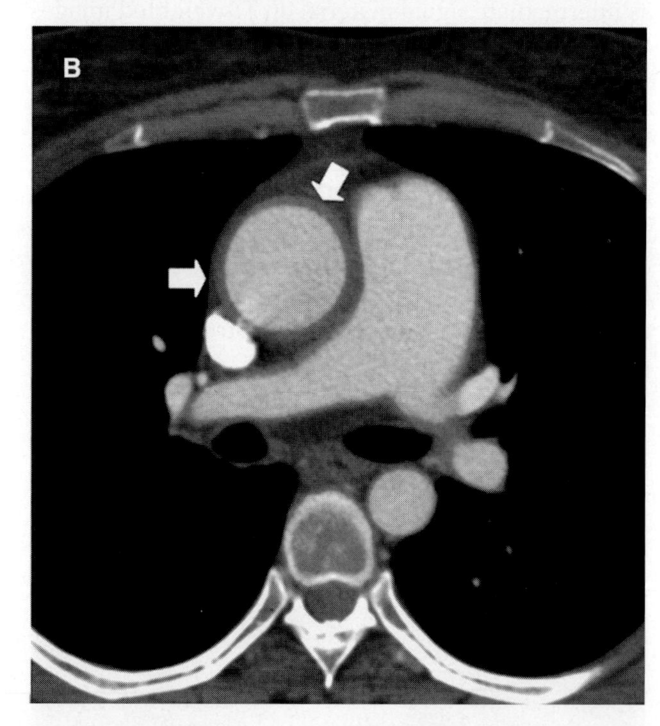

Figure 24 Takayasu's arteritis. (**A**) The left carotid artery (*solid arrow*) is severely narrowed and the left subclavian artery (*open arrow*) is occluded. (**B**) The ascending aorta is minimally dilated with a slightly thickened, enhancing wall (*arrows*).

POSTOPERATIVE AORTA

An effective imaging evaluation of the postoperative aorta cannot be accomplished without an understanding

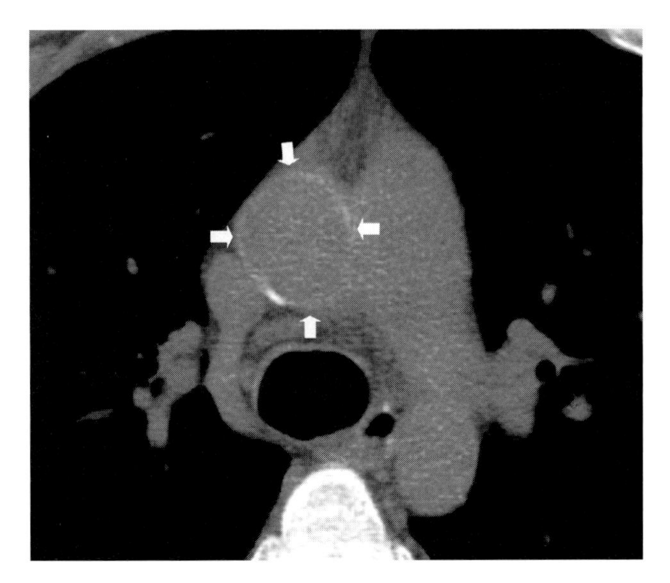

Figure 25 Unenhanced CT of the aorta in a patient with an aortic interposition graft. The graft (*arrows*) is slightly higher in attenuation than blood in the aorta.

of the surgical techniques utilized in aortic repair and the resultant alterations in aortic anatomy. A familiarity with those procedures most commonly employed at the specific institution and their imaging manifestations should allow for rapid distinction between a normal postoperative appearance and the development of a postoperative complication that requires intervention.

Two standard techniques are currently employed for the repair of aortic aneurysm and dissection (62): (1) interposition graft and (2) inclusion graft. In interposition graft the diseased segment is excised and the graft is sewn end to end; tributary vessels are reimplanted. Inclusion graft is performed via an aortotomy with insertion of the graft within the diseased aortic lumen, leaving a potential space between the graft and the native aortic wall. This potential space may thrombose or may contain clot and persistent blood flow in combination. A Cabrol procedure, whereby the perigraft space is decompressed into the right atrial appendage, is thought to prevent progression of pseudoaneurysm formation (63). For patients with involvement of the aortic root, a composite graft that includes a prosthetic aortic valve may be utilized.

Noncontrast-enhanced CT of aortic grafts shows the graft as a ring of high attenuation (Fig. 25). While this ring will form the outer boundaries of the aorta when the graft is interposed, inclusion grafts will appear as a ring within a larger circle representing the native aortic wall. Many patients with inclusion grafts demonstrate a peripheral thrombosed space between the graft and the native aortic wall. Occasionally there will be flow in the perigraft space, a finding readily demonstrated on contrast-enhanced spiral CT. The

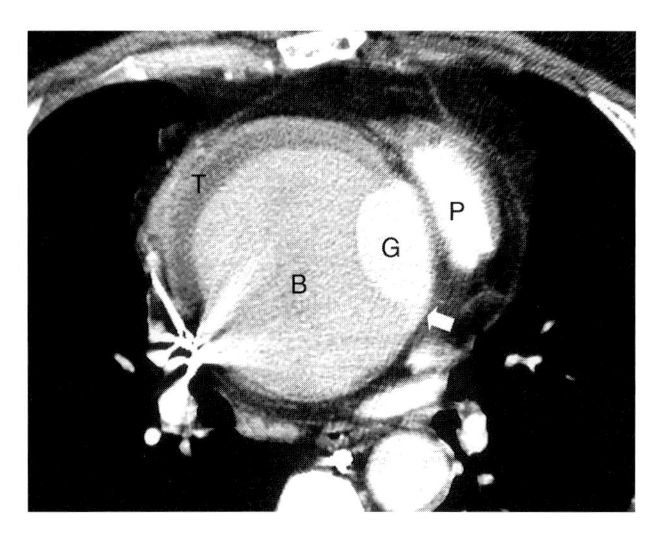

Figure 26 Leaking ascending aortic composite graft. There is substantial blood (B) outside the lumen of the ascending graft (G). The hemorrhage has been contained by the native aorta, which was wrapped around the graft at surgery. Thrombus (T) lines the anterior portion of the pseudoaneurysm. The leak is at the left coronary anastomosis (*arrow*). The main pulmonary artery (P) is compressed.

vast majority of patients with repairs of acute Type A dissections will demonstrate a persistent intimal flap distal to the graft site on spiral CT (64). One of the complications of aortic inclusion graft is aneurysmal dilatation of the aorta, which is readily depicted on spiral CT or MR. Patients who have had composite graft repair of the ascending aorta for connective tissue abnormalities occasionally develop false aneurysms as a result of leakage of blood from a suture line, frequently one involving the reimplanted coronary artery (Fig. 26).

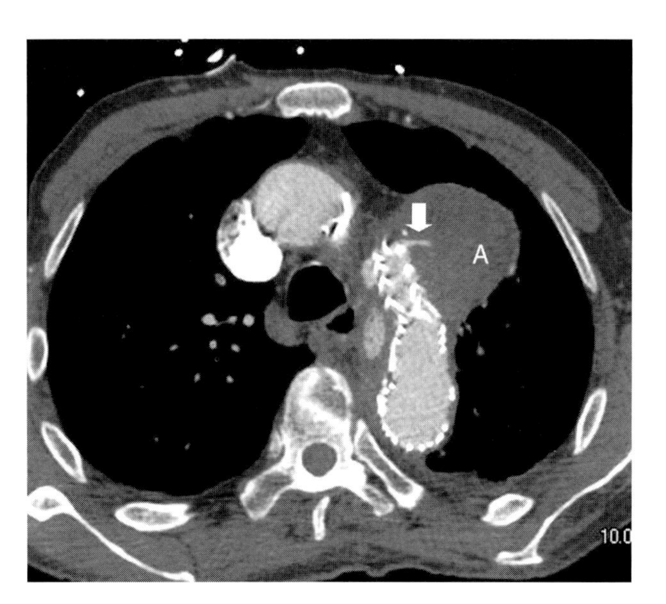

Figure 27 Type 1 endograft leak. A small jet of contrast (*arrow*) enters the pseudoaneurysm (A) from the proximal portion of the aortic endograft. *Source*: Courtesy of Laura Heynemann.

Endoluminal repair of aortic aneurysms, penetrating ulcers, fistulas, mycotic aneurysms, traumatic tears, and dissections can be achieved in some patients using endovascular stent grafts. Thoracic stent grafts consist of a metallic skeleton covered by synthetic material. The stents may have metallic barbs or be uncovered proximally or distally. At most institutions these are placed in collaboration with interventional radiology and cardiovascular surgery. Stent graft placement for management of TAAs is predominantly used in patients who are poor operative candidates. Spiral CT is the imaging modality of choice for both pre- and postprocedure evaluation of stent graft repairs of TAAs (65,66).

CT is used prior to stent graft placement to determine if the patient's anatomy is suitable for placement and to determine the size stent graft to be used. Generally, stent grafts are 10% to 15% greater in diameter than the diameter of the aortic on either side of the graft and should be at least 15 mm longer than the length of the aneurysm on either end. Stent grafts used to repair dissections are generally shorter and cover only the tear site. Ideally, stent grafts in the proximal descending aorta should be located more than 15 mm from the left subclavian artery. If covering of the subclavian origin is required to repair the aneurysm, surgical bypass of the subclavian or a fenestrated graft may be required. Following successful aortic aneurysm repair with an endograft, the excluded portion of the aneurysm usually decreases in size. In dissection repairs the false lumen may disappear or thrombose.

Routine follow-up of stent grafts is usually performed at discharge, and variable intervals afterward using contrast-enhanced CT. The metal frame of the graft is easily recognizable (66). Early complications of stent graft placement include misplacement of the graft and arterial trauma. Late complications are generally well demonstrated by CT (Fig. 27) (68) and include leaks, migration, mechanical failure, infection, and rupture of the aorta. Leaks may occur at either end of the graft when there is incomplete sealing of the graft with the aortic wall, from failure of the covering membrane of the graft, erosion of the aortic wall by the graft frame, or from separation of stents when multiple stents are used. They present on CT as enlargement of the preexisting aneurysm or as extra aneurysmal hematoma (67). Treatment of leaks is usually achieved by insertion of a longer stent graft.

SUMMARY

Multidetector row, helical CT is now the imaging modality of choice for the evaluation of thoracic aortic disease. Diagnostic quality has improved as a result of the isotropic voxel capabilities of current 40 and 64 detector scanners with two- and three-dimensional reconstructions and the use of retrospective ECG gating, which is particularly useful in evaluation of the ascending aorta. MDCT is readily available and rapidly performed in almost all patients, providing excellent anatomic detail of acute aortic pathology and in the follow-up of nonoperatively managed and surgically repaired aorta.

REFERENCES

1 Edwards JE. Anomalies of the derivatives of the aortic arch system. Med Clin North Am 1948; 32:925.
2 Kersting-Sommerhoff BA, Sechtem UP, Fisher MR, Higgins CB. MR imaging of congenital anomalies of the aortic arch. Am J Roentgenol 1987; 149:9–13.
3 Katz M, Konen E, Rozenman J, Szeinberg A, Itzchak Y. Spiral CT and 3D reconstruction of vascular rings and associated tracheobronchial anomalies. J Comput Assist Tomogr 1995; 19:564–8.
4 Manghat NE, Morgan-Hughes GJ, Roobottom CA. Multidetector row computed tomography: imaging the acute aortic syndrome. Clin Radiol 2005; 60:1256–67.
5 Levinson DC, Edmeades DT, Griffith GC. Dissecting aneurysm of the aorta: its clinical electrocardiographic and laboratory features: a report of fifty-eight autopsied cases. Circulation 1950; 1:360–87.
6 Prete R, Von Segesser LK. Aortic dissection. Lancet 1997; 349:1461–4.
7 DeBakey ME, McCollum CH, Crawford ES, et al. Dissection and dissecting aneurysms of the aorta: twenty-year follow-up of 527 patients treated surgically. Surgery 1982; 92:1118–34.
8 Nienaber CA, von Kodolitsch Y, Nicholas V. The diagnosis of thoracic aortic dissection by noninvasive imaging procedures. N Engl J Med 1993; 328:1–9.
9 Sommer T, Fehske W, Holzknecht N, et al. Aortic dissection: a comparative study of diagnosis with spiral CT, multiplanar transesophageal echocardiography, and MR imaging. Radiology 1996; 199:347–52.
10 Shiga T, Wajima Z, Apfel C, Inoue T, Ohe Y. Diagnostic accuracy of transesophageal echocardiography, helical computed tomography, and magnetic resonance imaging for suspected thoracic aortic dissection. Arch Intern Med 2006; 166:1350–6.
11 Demos TC, Posniak HV, Churchill RJ. Detection of the intimal flap of aortic dissection on unenhanced CT images. Am J Radiol 1986; 146:601–3.
12 Rubin GD. Helical CT angiography of the thoracic aorta. J Thorac Imag 1997; 12:128–49.
13 Batra P, Bigoni B, Maning J, et al. Pitfalls in the diagnosis of thoracic aortic dissection at CT angiography. Radiographics 2000; 20:309–20.
14 Posniak HV, Olson MC, Demos TC. Aortic motion artifact simulating dissection on CT scans. Am J Radiol 1993; 161:557–8.
15 Loubeyre P, Angelie E, Grozel F, Albidi H, Minh VAT. Spiral CT artifact that simulates aortic dissection:

image reconstruction with use of 180° and 360° linear interpolation algorithms. Radiology 1997; 205: 153–7.

16 Yamada T, Takamiya M, Naito H, et al. Diagnosis of aortic dissection without intimal rupture by x-ray computed tomography. Nippon Acta Radiol 1985; 45:699–710.

17 Coady MA, Rizzo JA, Elefteriades JA. Pathologic variants of thoracic aortic dissections: penetrating atherosclerotic ulcers and intramural hematomas. Cardiol Clin 1999; 17:637–57.

18 Patrick TO, Roman WD. Acute aortic dissection and its variants: toward a common diagnostic and therapeutic approach. Circulation 1993; 88:1–10.

19 Murray JG, Manisali M, Flamm SD, et al. Intramural hematoma of the thoracic aorta: MR image findings and their prognostic implications. Radiology 1997; 204: 349–55.

20 Bluemke DA. Definitive diagnosis of intramural hematoma of the aorta with MR imaging. Radiology 1997; 204:319–21.

21 Moriyama Y, Yotsumoto G, Kuriwaki K, et al. Intramural hematoma of the thoracic aorta. Eur J Cadiothorac Surg 1998; 13:230–9.

22 Sueyoshi E, Imada T, Sakamoto I, Matsuoka Y, Hayashi K. Analysis of predictive factors for progression of type B aortic intramural hematoma with computed tomography. J Vasc Surg 2002; 35:1179–83.

23 Ganaha F, Miller DC, Sugimoto K, et al. Prognosis of aortic intramural hematoma with and without penetrating atherosclerotic ulcer. A clinical and radiological analysis. Circulation 2002; 106:342–8.

24 Tittle SL, Lynch RJ, Cole PE, et al. Midterm follow-up of penetrating ulcer and intramural hematoma of the aorta. J Thorac Cardiovasc Surg 2002; 123:1051–9.

25 Moizumi Y, Komatsu T, Motoyoshi N, Tabayashi K. Clinical features and long-term outcome of type A and type B intramural hematoma of the aorta. J Thorac Cardiovasc Surg 2004; 127:412–7.

26 Stanson AW, Kazmier FJ, Hollier LH, et al. Penetrating atherosclerotic ulcers of the thoracic aorta: natural history and clinicopathologic correlations. Ann Vasc Surg 1986; 1:15–23.

27 Hayashi H, Matsuoka Y, Sakamoto I, et al. Penetrating atherosclerotic ulcer of the aorta: imaging features and disease concept. Radiographics 2000; 20:995–1005.

28 Kazerooni EA, Bree RI, Williams DM. Penetrating atherosclerotic ulcers of the descending thoracic aorta: evaluation with CT and distinction from aortic dissection. Radiology 1992; 183:759–65.

29 Cho KR, Stanson AW, Potter DD, Cherry KJ, Schaff HV, Sundt TM III. Penetrating atherosclerotic ulcer of the descending thoracic aorta and arch. J Thorac Cardiovasc Surg 2004; 127(5):1393–401.

30 Harris JA, Bis KG, Glover JL, Bendick PJ, Shetty A, Brown OW. Penetrating atherosclerotic ulcers of the aorta. J Vasc Surg 1994; 19:90–8.

31 Cooke JP, Kazmier FJ, Orszulak TA. Penetrating athero-sclerotic ulcers of the aorta: pathologic manifestations, diagnosis, and management. Mayo Clin Proc 1988; 63:718–25.

32 Levy JR, Heiken JP, Gutierrez FR. Imaging of penetrating atherosclerotic ulcers of the aorta. Am J Radiol 1999; 173:151–4.

33 Parmley LF, Mattingly TW, Manion WC, Jahnke EJ. Nonpenetrating traumatic injury of the aorta. Circulation 1958; 17:1086–101.

34 Mirvis SE, Bidwell JK, Buddemeyer EU, et al. Value of chest radiography in excluding traumatic aortic rupture. Radiology 1987; 163:487–93.

35 Morgan PW, Goodman LR, Aprahamian C, Foley WD, Lipchik EO. Evaluation of traumatic aortic injury: does dynamic contrast-enhanced CT play a role? Radiology 1992; 182:661–6.

36 Raptopoulos V, Sheiman RG, Phillips DA, Davidoff A, Silva WE. Traumatic aortic tear: screening with chest CT. Radiology 1992; 182:667–73.

37 Gavant ML, Menke PG, Fabian T, Flick PA, Graney MJ, Gold RE. Blunt traumatic aortic rupture: detection with helical CT of the chest. Radiology 1995; 197:125–33.

38 Gavant ML, Flick PA, Menke PG, Gold RE. CT aortography of thoracic aortic rupture. Am J Radiol 1996; 166:955–61.

39 Dyer DS, Moore EE, Mestek MF, et al. Can chest CT be used to exclude aortic injury? Radiology 1999; 213:195–202.

40 Gavant ML. Helical CT grading of traumatic aortic injuries. Radiol Clin North Am 1999; 37:553–74.

41 Aronberg DJ, Glazer HS, Madsen K, Sagel SS. Normal thoracic aorta diameters by computed tomography. J Comput Assist Tomogr 1984; 8:247–50.

42 Hager A, Kaemmerer H, Rapp-Bernhardt U, et al. Diameters of the thoracic aorta throughout life as measured by helical computed tomography. J Thorac Cardiovasc Surg 2002; 123:1060–6.

43 Bickerstaff LK, Pairolero PC, Hollier LH, et al. Thoracic aortic aneurysms: a population-based study. Surgery 1982; 92:1103–8.

44 Coady MA, Davies RR, Roberts M, et al. Familial patterns of thoracic aortic aneurysms. Arch Surg 1999; 134:361–7.

45 Quint LE, Francis IR, Williams DM, et al. Evaluation of thoracic aortic disease with the use of helical CT and multiplanar reconstructions: comparison with surgical findings. Radiology 1996; 201:37–41.

46 Heiberg E, Wolverson MK, Sundaram M, Shields JB. CT characteristics of atherosclerotic aneurysm versus aortic dissection. J Comput Assist Tomogr 1985; 9:78–83.

47 Torres WE, Maurer DE, Steinberg HV, Robbins S, Bernadino ME. CT of aortic aneurysms: the distinction between mural and thrombus calcification. Am J Roentgenol 1988; 150:1317–9.

48 Lemon DK and White CW. Anuloaortic ectasia: angiographic, hemodynamic and clinical comparison with with aortic valve insufficiency. Am J Cardiol 1978; 41:482–6.

49 Gonda RL, Gutierrez OH, Azodo MV. Mycotic aneurysms of the aorta: radiologic features. Radiology 1988; 168:343–6.

50 Posniak HV, Olson MC, Demos TC, Benjoya RA, Marsan RE. CT of thoracic aortic aneurysms. Radiographics 1990; 10:839–55.

51 Dinsmore RE, Liberthson RR, Wismer GL, et al. Magnetic resonance imaging of thoracic aortic

aneurysms: comparison with other imaging methods. Am J Roentgenol 1986; 146:309–14.
52 Kucich VA, Vogelzang RL, Hartz RS, LoCicero J, Dalton D. Ruptured thoracic aneurysm: unusual manifestation and early diagnosis using CT. Radiology 1986; 160:87–9.
53 Mehard WB, Heiken JP, Sicard GA. High-attenuating crescent in abdominal aortic aneurysm wall at CT: a sign of acute or impending rupture. Radiology 1994; 192:359–62.
54 Halliday KE, Alkutoubi A. Draped aorta: CT sign of contained leak of aortic aneurysms. Radiology 1996; 199:41–3.
55 Macintosh EL, Parrott JCW, Unruh HW. Fistulas between the aorta and tracheo-bronchial tree. Ann Thorac Surg 1991; 51:515–9.
56 Coblentz CL, Sallee DS, Chiles C. Aortobronchopulonary fistula complicating aortic aneurysm: diagnosis in four cases. Am J Roentgenol 1988; 150:535–8.
57 Amin S, Luketich J, Wald A. Aortoesophageal fistula: case report and review of the literature. Digest Dis Science 1998; 43:1665–71.
58 Kouchoukos NT, Dougenis D. Medical progress: surgery of the thoracic aorta. N Engl J Med 1997; 336:1876–88.
59 Coady MA, Rizzo JA, Hammond GL, et al. What is the appropriate size criterion for resection of thoracic aneurysms? J Thorac Cardiovasc Surg 1997; 113: 476–91.
60 Sharma S, Sharma S, Taneja K, Gupta AK, Rajani M. Morphologic mural changes in the aorta revealed by CT in patients with nonspecific aortoarteritis (Takayasu's arteritis). Am J Roentgenol 1996; 167:1321–5.
61 Park JH, Chung JW, Im JG, et al. Takayasu arteritis: evaluation of mural changes in the aorta and pulmonary artery with CT angiography. Radiology 1995; 196: 89–93.
62 Naidich DP, Webb WR, Muller NL, Krinsky GA, Zerhouni EA, Siegelman SS. Aorta, arch vessels, and great veins. In: Computed Tomography and Magnetic Resonance Imaging of the Thorax. 3rd ed. Philadelphia: Lippincott-Raven, 1999:570–6.
63 Cabrol C, Pavie A, Mesnildrey P, et al. Long-term results with total replacement of the ascending aorta and reimplantation of the coronary arteries. J Thorac Cardiovasc Surg 1986; 91:17–25.
64 Mathieu D, Keta K, Loisance D. Post-operative CT follow-up of aortic dissection. J Comput Assist Tomogr 1986; 10:216–8.
65 Mitchell RS, Dake MD, Semba CP, et al. Endovascular stent-graft repair of thoracic aortic aneurysms. J Thorac Cardiovasc Surg 1996; 111:1054–60.
66 Kato N, Dake MD, Miller DC, et al. Traumatic thoracic aortic aneurysm: treatment with endovascular stent-grafts. Radiology 1997; 205:657–62.
67 Fillinger MF. Postoperative imaging after endovascular AAA repair. Semin Vase Surg 1999; 12:327–38.
68 Armerding MD, Rubin GD, Beaulieu CF, et al. Aortic aneurysmal disease: assessment of stent-graft treatment-CT versus conventional angiogaphy. Radiology 2000; 215:138–46.
69 Garzon G, Fernandez-Velilla F, Milagros M, Acitores I, Ybanez F, Riera L. Endovascular stent-graft treatment of thoracic aortic disease. Radiographics 2005; 25:S229–244.
70 Therasse E, Soulez G, Giroux M, et al. Stent-graft placement for the treatment of thoracic aortic diseases. Radiographics 2005; 25;157–73.
71 Macura KJ, Corl FM, Fishman EK, Bluemke DA. Pathogenesis in acute aortic syndromes: aortic dissection, intermural hematoma, and penetrating atherosclerotic ulcer. AJR 2003; 181:309–316.

9

Noninvasive Assessment of the Solitary Pulmonary Nodule

Bradley S. Sabloff
Department of Diagnostic Imaging, M. D. Anderson Cancer Center, University of Texas, Houston, Texas, U.S.A.

Page H. McAdams
Department of Radiology, Duke University Medical Center, Durham, North Carolina, U.S.A.

Jeremy J. Erasmus
Department of Diagnostic Imaging, M. D. Anderson Cancer Center, University of Texas, Houston, Texas, U.S.A.

INTRODUCTION

A solitary pulmonary nodule (SPN) is defined as "a round opacity, at least moderately well-marginated and no greater than 3 cm in maximum diameter" (*1*). The adjective *small* is occasionally used to characterize a nodule with a maximum diameter of less than 1 cm (*1*). The strict application of this definition is often inappropriate, as poorly marginated or irregular opacities, which are a common initial manifestation of lung cancer, are excluded. In order to encompass these abnormalities, this definition is either not strictly adhered to, or the term SPN is replaced by the more loosely defined term solitary pulmonary opacity. Solitary pulmonary opacities are common, and the increasing use of CT to image the lungs, together with improvements in CT image acquisition and quality, as well as the use of picture archiving and communication systems for image interpretation, has resulted in a high incidence of detection. In fact, in one screening study, the majority of patients who were screened had at least one nodule (*2*). However, most incidentally discovered nodules are benign and, despite an extensive differential diagnosis (Table *1*), are usually the sequelae of pulmonary infection. Nevertheless, lung cancer constitutes an important proportion of solitary pulmonary opacities. According to the American Cancer Society 1 in 13 men and 1 in 17 women will be affected by lung cancer in their lifetimes, and it is estimated that 20–30% of these patients will present with a solitary pulmonary opacity (*3–5*). Because many of the patients with lung cancer who present with a solitary pulmonary opacity are potentially curable if appropriately diagnosed and treated, one of the main goals of imaging is to accurately differentiate these from benign opacities. However, prospective differentiation of benign and malignant opacities before surgical resection can be difficult and can result in inappropriate resection of benign opacities (Fig. *1*). Recently, noninvasive image-based assessment and management of these opacities has evolved in large part due to data extrapolated from ongoing screening studies and from thin-slice helical CT scans studies examining the morphologic features of nodules. This chapter reviews evaluation strategies and recent advances in imaging that can improve the accuracy of differentiating benign and malignant solitary pulmonary opacities.

CLINICAL ASSESSMENT

Management of a nodule depends on the likelihood of malignancy. Clinical risk factors that are associated with an increased risk of developing lung cancer include age, presenting symptoms, smoking (increasing with degree and duration of exposure), and exposure to asbestos, uranium, or radon. There is a positive correlation between advancing age and a higher risk of lung cancer, and patients with hemoptysis are also at increased risk for malignancy (*6*). The patient's past medical history is important as there is an increased risk of lung cancer associated with a history of a prior neoplasm and in patients with pulmonary fibrosis (*6,7*). Family history is also important to determine the likelihood of cancer. In this regard, there is strong evidence for a susceptibility gene to lung cancer, and the risk of developing lung cancer increases in patients who have a first-degree relative with lung cancer (*8*). The overall assessment of an individual's risk for malignancy, based on their clinical risk factors, is important because observation is usually undertaken if the probability of malignancy is low. For instance, in a patient presenting with a new focal abnormal pulmonary opacity and clinical findings of pneumonia,

Table 1 Differential Diagnosis of a Solitary Pulmonary Opacity

Type of cause	Disease
Neoplastic-malignant	Primary lung malignancies (non-small-cell, small cell, carcinoid, lymphoma)
	Solitary metastasis
Neoplastic-benign	Hamartoma
	Arteriovenous malformation
Infectious	Granuloma
	Bacterial (round pneumonia)
	Abscess
	Septic embolus
Noninfectious	Amyloidoma
	Subpleural lymph nodule
	Rheumatoid nodule
	Wegener's granulomatosis
	Focal scarring
	Infarct
Congenital	Sequestration
	Bronchogenic cyst
	Bronchial atresia with mucoid impaction

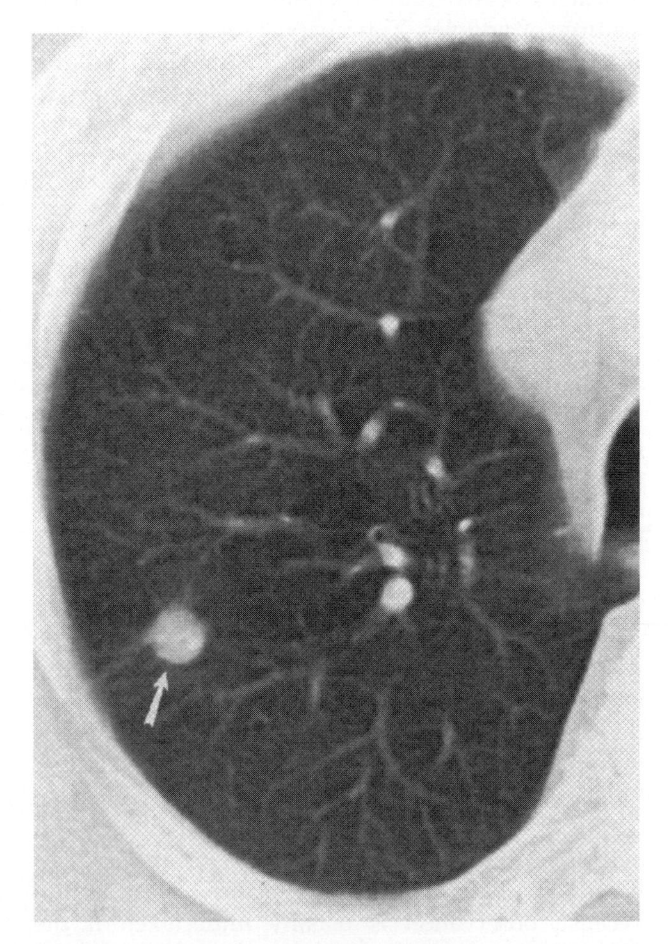

Figure 1 Pulmonary nodule detected on chest radiograph (not shown) in a 61-year-old asymptomatic man with history of cigarette smoking. CT shows a small, well-circumscribed, noncalcified nodule in right upper lobe (*arrow*). Because of the high probability of malignancy, the nodule was resected and revealed a noncaseating granuloma.

radiographic reassessment after a short interval may be all that is necessary to exclude malignancy and confirm a diagnosis of round pneumonia (Fig. 2). In contradistinction, if a new nodule is detected in a young adult with a peripheral sarcoma, the probability that this is a solitary metastasis is high, and resection is commonly performed.

RADIOLOGICAL EVALUATION

Although an increasing number of solitary pulmonary opacities are diagnosed by CT, either incidentally or as part of a lung cancer screening study, many are still initially detected on chest radiographs. If the nodule is diffusely calcified (Fig. 3), or comparison with older

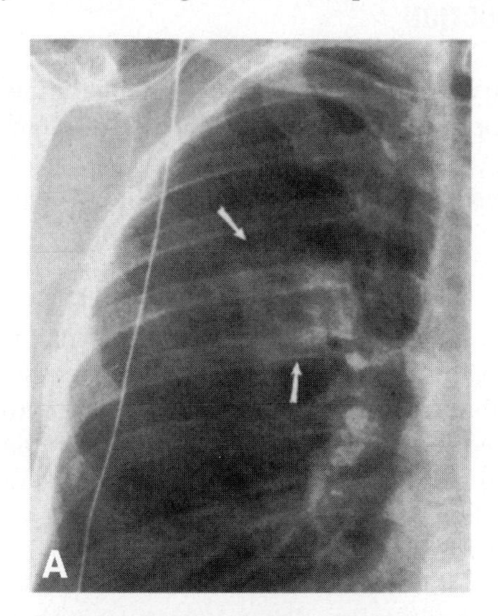

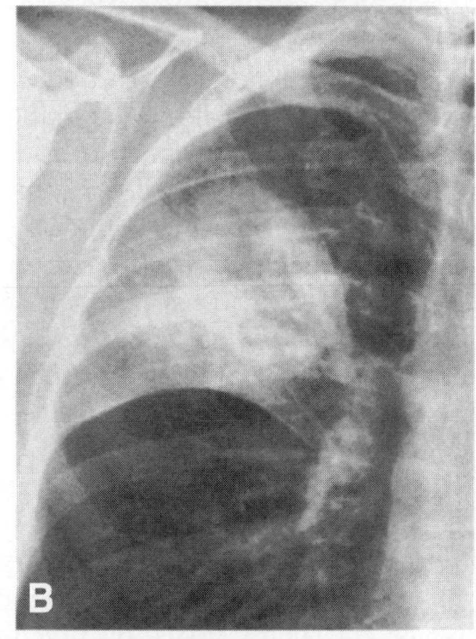

Figure 2 Round pneumonia in a woman who presented with fever and cough. (**A**) Chest radiograph shows poorly marginated opacity in the right upper lobe (*arrows*). (**B**) Follow-up radiograph performed 48 h later shows diffuse consolidation in the right upper lobe. Although more common in children, round pneumonia is occasionally seen in adults.

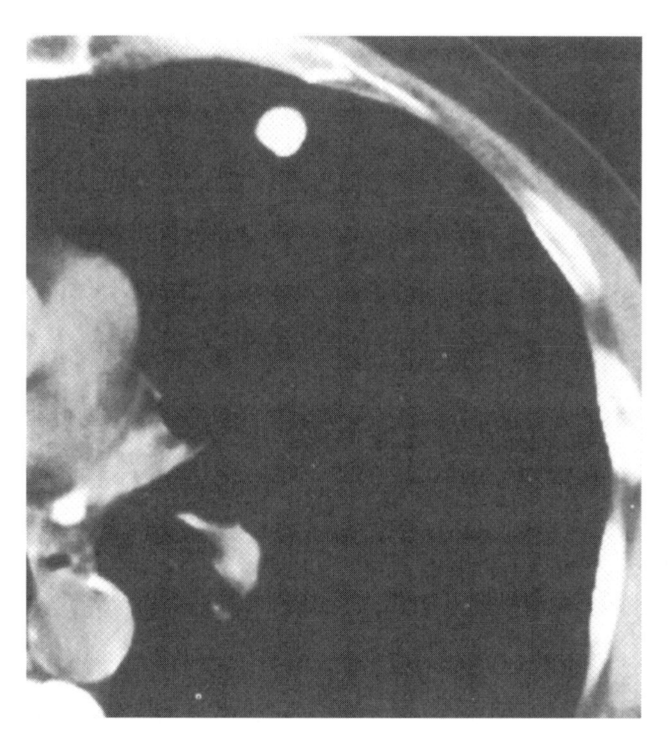

Figure 3 Histoplasmoma. CT shows diffusely calcified nodule in the left upper lobe. Note small calcified lymph node within mediastinum. Diffuse calcification is indicative of a benign etiology and, in the absence of a primary osteosarcoma, no further evaluation is required.

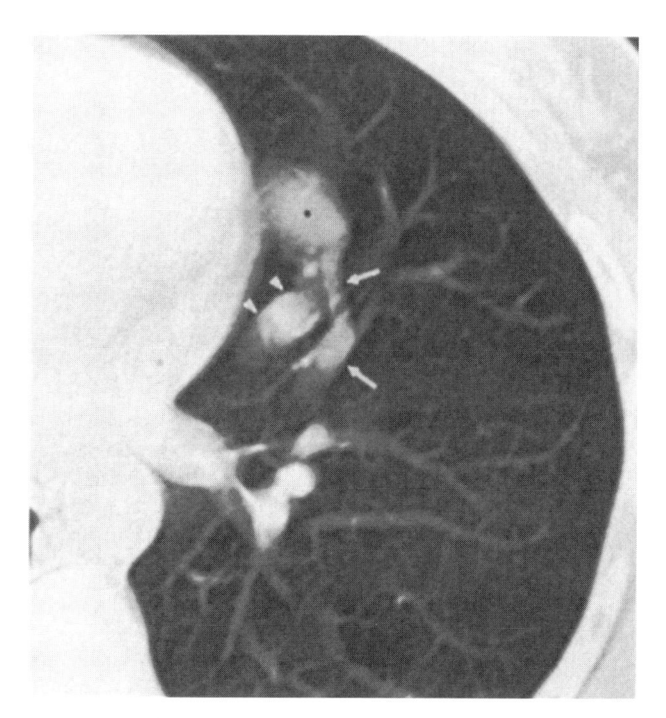

Figure 4 Arteriovenous malformation (AVM) in a woman with hereditary hemorrhagic telangiectasia. Chest radiograph (not shown) shows a small solitary nodule in lingula. CT reveals an enlarged feeding artery (*arrows*) and an enlarged draining vein (*arrowheads*) as well as the nidus of the vascular malformation (*). Morphologic characteristics are diagnostic for arteriovenous malformation. CT also revealed a few smaller AVMs in both lungs (not shown).

radiographs shows stability in size for more than 2 years, the nodule is presumed to be benign, and no further evaluation is recommended. However, many nodules require further radiological evaluation because, one, it can be difficult to determine whether a small nodular opacity is located in the lung on chest radiographs or is calcified or stable in size and, two, preexisting radiographs are often not available for review (*9*). In most cases CT is performed to further evaluate these radiographic abnormalities. The CT is accurate in determining where the abnormality is located and, if in the lung, optimally evaluates morphological characteristics of the nodule (Fig. *4*). The CT is also useful in determining if the nodule is truly solitary and for assessing growth on serial studies. Occasionally, interpretive difficulty occurs with CT as it may not be possible to determine whether a small opacity is a nodule, a vessel, or due to partial volume averaging of adjacent intrathoracic structures. However, the common use of thin section CT, together with cine review of images at a picture archiving and communications systems (PACS) workstation, has improved the ability to correctly determine whether a pulmonary opacity is a nodule (*10*). In those instances where differentiation is not possible or difficult, accurate assessment can often be achieved by either increasing or decreasing the slice collimation. For instance, if a 5-mm slice collimation has been used, obtaining images through the region of abnormality using a slice collimation of 1–2.5 mm is useful in eliminating partial volume averaging. If a 1.25-mm slice collimation has been used, as is common in protocols utilized to evaluate the pulmonary arteries for emboli, the difficulty of differentiating a vessel from a small nodule is often overcome by reconstructing the original data at thicker collimation, or by using maximum intensity projection (MIP) images (Fig. *5*). MIP images are generated from an axial slab of volumetric data obtained when helical CT is performed. By displaying the continuity of vessels, this technique has been shown to improve nodule detection and discrimination from vessels (*11*).

Nodule Morphology

Although there is considerable overlap in the morphology and appearance of benign and malignant solitary pulmonary opacities, several morphologic features are useful in assessing a nodule's malignant or benign potential. These features include the size, margins, contour, internal morphology (attenuation, wall thickness in cavitary nodules, air bronchograms), presence of satellite nodules, and growth rate.

In terms of size, the likelihood of malignancy increases the larger the opacity is. However, small nodule size does not exclude malignancy. In this

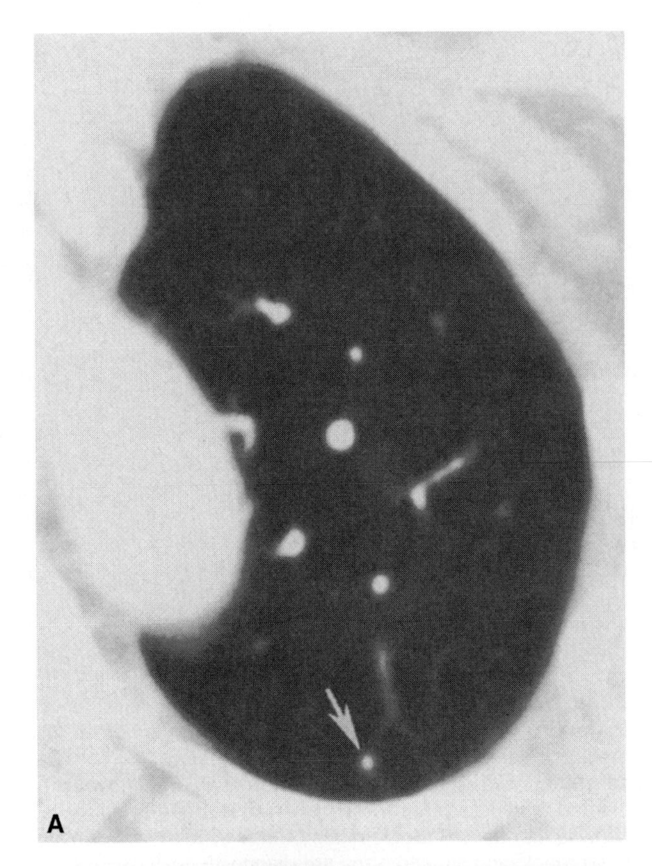

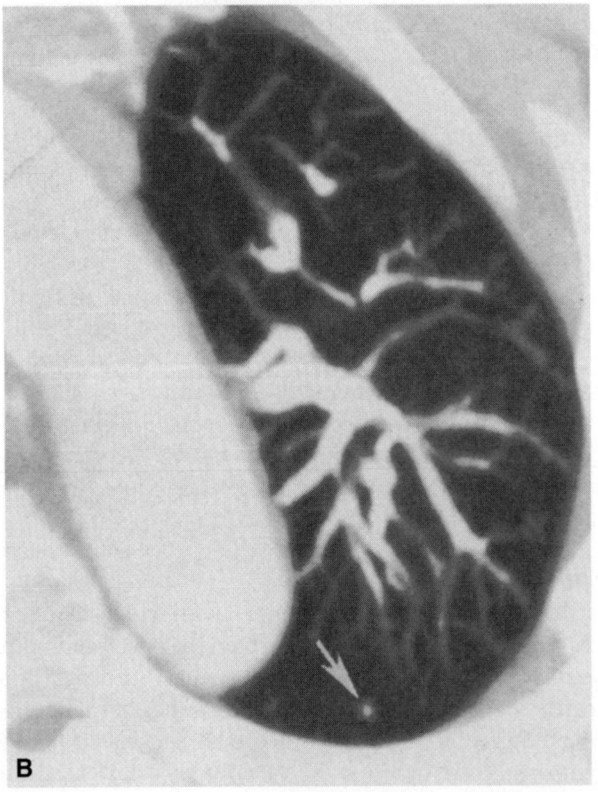

Figure 5 Small nodule visualization using maximal intensity projection (MIP) image. (**A**) CT shows small nodular opacity in left lung (*arrow*). Confident differentiation from pulmonary vessels is difficult. (**B**) Axial MIP image allows nodule (*arrow*) to be more easily differentiated from tubular vessels.

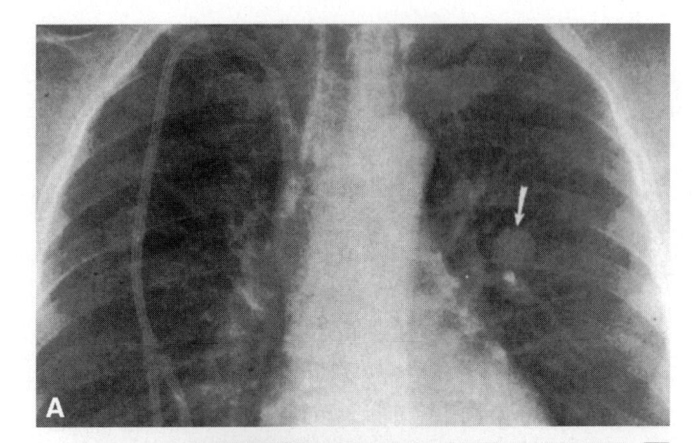

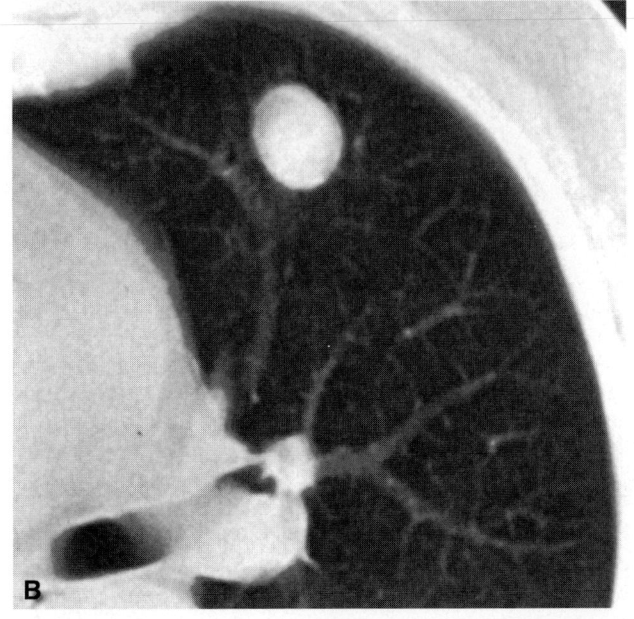

Figure 6 Mucormycosis manifesting as solitary pulmonary nodule in a patient with multiple myeloma. (**A**) Chest radiograph shows well-circumscribed pulmonary nodule (*arrow*). (**B**) CT confirms left upper lobe pulmonary nodule. Note well-defined margins and smooth contour, findings suggestive of a benign etiology.

regard, widespread use and improvements in CT technology, coupled with a recent interest in CT screening for lung cancer, have resulted in the frequent and incidental detection small nodules (1–5 mm (*12–14*). While the majority of these nodules are benign, studies of resected small nodules have shown that a considerable number are either primary or secondary pulmonary malignancies (*15,16*).

Typically, benign nodules have well-defined margins and a smooth contour while malignant nodules have poorly defined or spiculated margins and a lobular or irregular contour (Figs. *6–8*) (*6,17,18*). The lobular contour is attributed to uneven growth rates, while the irregular or spiculated margins are usually due to growth of malignant cells along the interstitium of the lung parenchyma (*19*). However, there is considerable overlap between benign and malignant nodules regarding margins and contour.

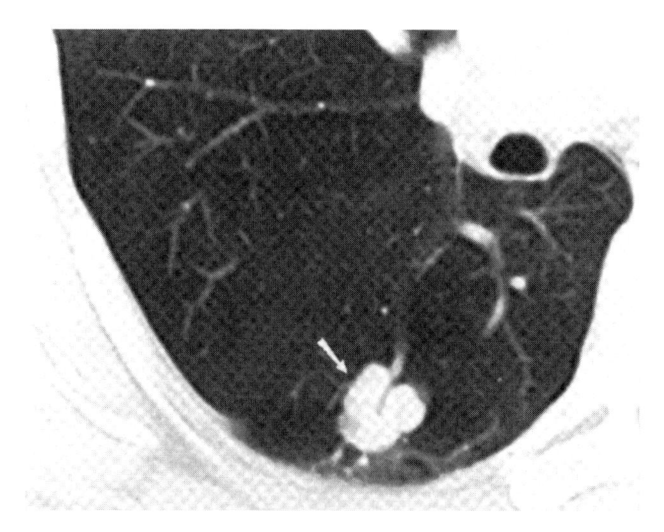

Figure 7 Solitary metastasis from renal cell malignancy. CT shows nodule (*arrow*) with lobular contour in right lower lobe. Lobular contour is due to uneven growth, a finding often associated with malignancy.

For instance, although a spiculated margin with distortion of adjacent vessels (often described as a sunburst or corona radiata appearance) is highly suggestive of malignancy, benign nodules can occasionally have this appearance. Additionally, a smooth nodule margin does not exclude malignancy. Up to 20% of primary lung malignancies have smooth contours and well-defined margins, and most metastatic nodules typically manifest as smooth margins (*6,18*).

Internal morphology of a nodule, with the exception of fat [attenuation of −40 to −120 Hounsfield units (HU)] and calcification, is unreliable in distinguishing a

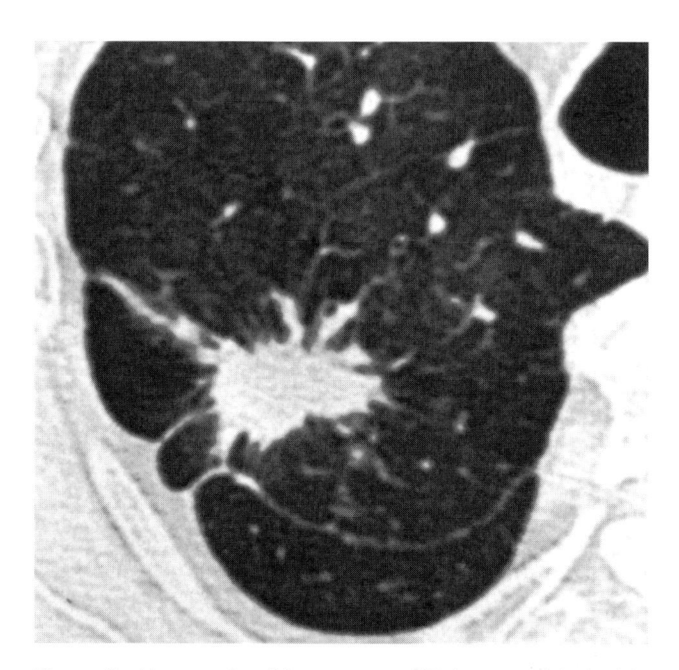

Figure 8 Non-small-cell lung cancer. CT shows nodule in right upper lobe with irregular contour and spiculated margin. Appearance is highly suggestive for malignancy.

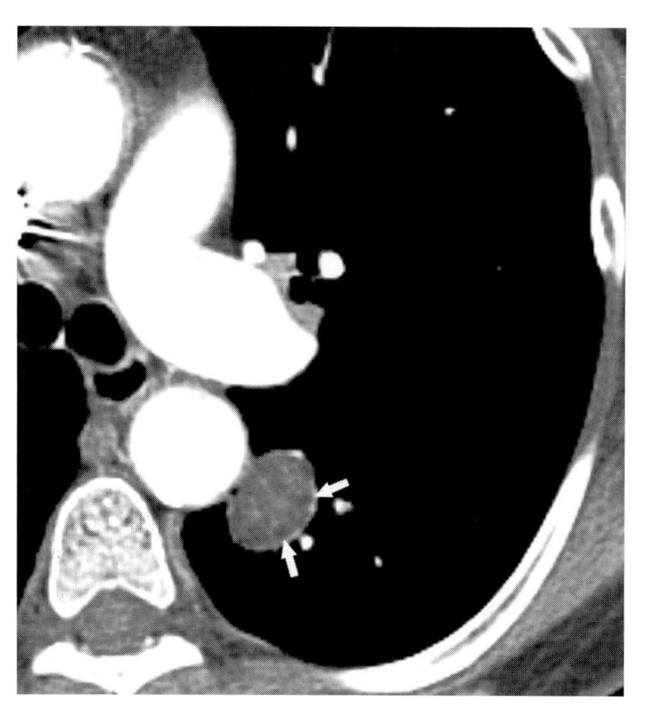

Figure 9 Hamartoma. CT shows well-circumscribed left lung nodule. Low attenuation within nodule (attenuation, 106 HU) (*arrows*) is consistent with fat and diagnostic of hamartoma.

malignant from a benign nodule. Fat within a nodule is a characteristic finding of a hamartoma and is detected by CT in up to 50% of these neoplasms (Figs. *9* and *10*) (*20*). However, the overall clinical impact of this finding in nodule evaluation is small, as hamartomas constitute a

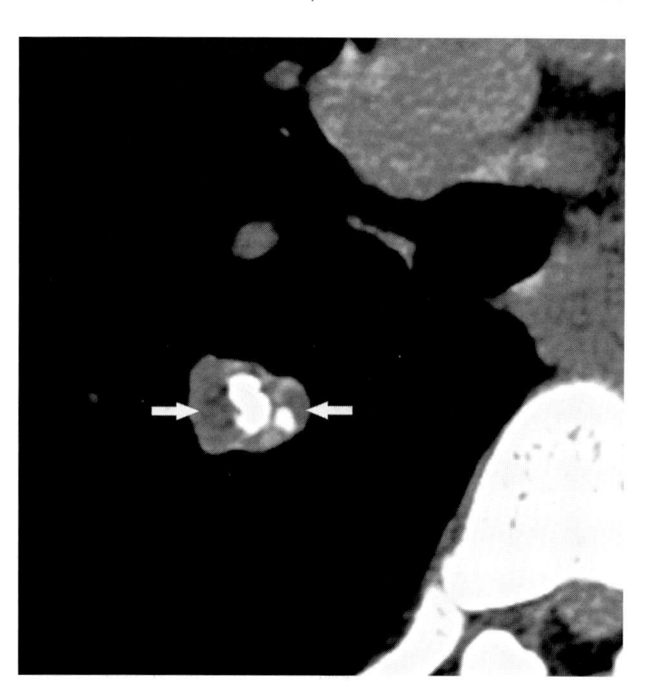

Figure 10 Hamartoma. CT shows well-circumscribed nodule in right upper lobe. Focal punctate calcifications are suggestive of hamartoma. Similar calcifications can, however, be seen in carcinoid tumors. Small focal areas of fat within the nodule are diagnostic of hamartoma (*arrow*).

very small percentage of solitary pulmonary opacities. Additionally, while this finding typically negates further evaluation, lung metastases in patients with liposarcomas or renal cell cancers rarely manifest as fat-containing nodules (*21*). Calcification of a solitary pulmonary opacity can be useful in determining benignity of a nodule and may be detected on chest radiographs. However, chest radiography is not optimal for the detection of calcification and, unless the nodule is obviously calcified, CT is usually performed as it is a considerably more sensitive imaging modality for detecting calcification in a nodule (*9,17,22,23*). Calcification is usually detected visually when thin collimation slices (1–3 mm) are performed through the nodule (Fig. *11*). However, partial volume averaging can make calcification within a small nodule visually inapparent when thicker collimated slices are obtained. In most of these cases reimaging with thin collimation slices should be performed to detect calcification. Measurement of CT attenuation values (CT densitometry) have been used to infer the presence of calcium within a nodule (*17,22,24,25*). The use of this technique is, however, inappropriate if the nodule is spiculated or if the opacity is greater than 3 cm in diameter. A CT attenuation value of 200 HU is usually used to distinguish between calcified and noncalcified nodules. If the density of the nodule is in the benign range (>200 HU), serial radiological observation is performed at 3, 6, 12, 18, and 24 months to confirm the absence of growth. The sensitivity and specificity of this technique for benign disease is not optimal, and the popularity of CT densitometry for discriminating benign from malignant nodules has declined since its inception in the early 1980s (*26,27*). In addition, although it has been proposed that measurement of CT attenuation values obtained at different kilovolt peaks may be useful in detecting visually inapparent amounts of calcium in a nodule, a multi-institutional trial has shown that dual-energy CT is unreliable for distinguishing benign from malignant nodules (*28–30*).

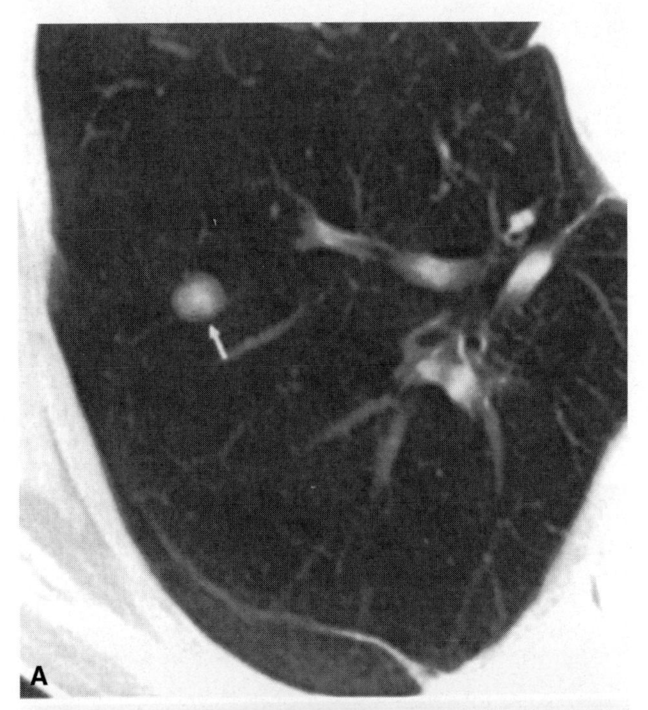

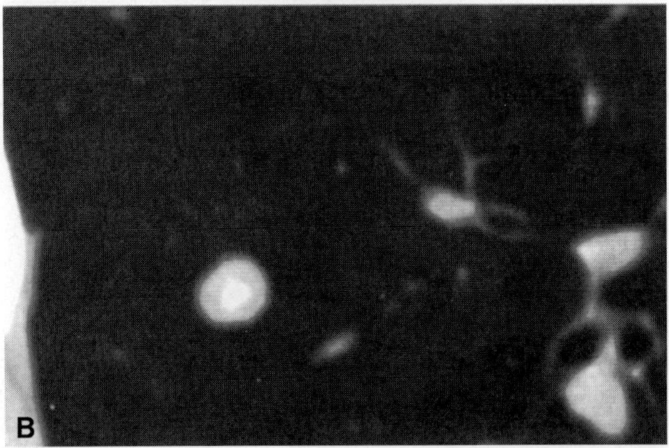

Figure 11 Postinfectious granuloma. (**A**) Standard CT (7-mm collimation, lung window) shows nodule (*arrow*) with possible small, central punctate calcification. (**B**) Thin-section CT (1.5-mm collimation) better demonstrates the central punctate calcification in nodule and is diagnostic of a benign etiology.

Although the majority of benign nodules are not calcified, the presence of calcification can be useful in evaluation as specific patterns of calcification indicate benignity (*6,31*). Benign patterns of calcification include diffusely solid, centrally punctate, laminated, or "popcornlike." However, occasionally, lung metastases in patients with chondrosarcomas or osteosarcomas can manifest as benign patterns of calcification (Figs. *12* and *13*) (*32,33*). Additionally, punctate calcification within a nodule with spiculated margins should be viewed suspiciously as spiculation has a 90% predictive value for malignancy (*33*). Calcification can be detected in up to 13% of all lung cancers on CT, although the incidence in patients with lung cancer manifesting as nodules less than 3 cm is only 2% (Fig. *14*) (*31,34,35*). Typically, this calcification is stippled, eccentric, or amorphous and suggests a high probability of malignancy, although a similar pattern can occasionally be seen in benign nodules (*35*).

The widespread use of thin collimation CT images has increased the detection of soft tissue nodules with low attenuation. Soft tissue nodular opacities are classified into three categories of attenuation: (*i*) nonsolid or ground-glass (where the underlying lung parenchyma and vessels can be seen through the lesion) (Fig. *15*), (*ii*) partially solid (Fig. *16*), or (*iii*) solid. Importantly, it has been shown that incidence of malignancy varies according to the degree of soft tissue attenuation. Partially solid nodular opacities have the highest incidence of malignancy, with an incidence of malignancy of 40–50% in lesions less than 1.5 cm, while

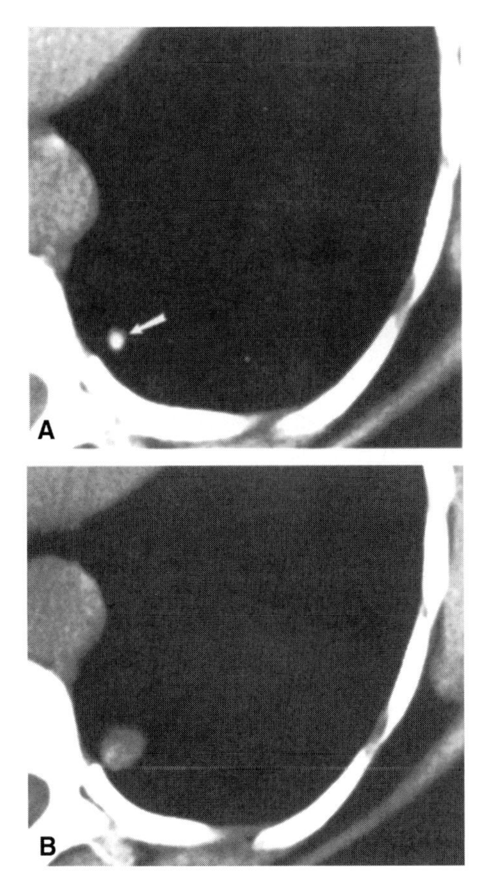

Figure 12 Metastatic osteosarcoma. (**A**) CT shows small, high attenuation nodule in lower lobe (*arrow*). The appearance is suggestive of a benign etiology. (**B**) CT obtained 3 months later reveals interval growth of nodule. Resection revealed metastatic osteosarcoma.

nonsolid nodular opacities have an incidence of malignancy of 34%. While nodular opacities with solid attenuation are the most common opacity detected, they have the lowest incidence of malignancy, as many infections, particularly mycoses and tuberculosis, manifest as solid nodules. However, despite the lower incidence of malignancy in solid nodules, most primary lung cancers and metastases manifest as solid nodules (*33*).

Cavitation occurs in both benign and malignant nodules and in both primary and metastatic tumors. Up to 15% of primary lung malignancies will cavitate and typically occur most frequently in squamous cell cancer subtypes. Malignant cavitary nodules typically have thick, irregular walls, while benign cavitary nodules have smooth, thin walls (Figs. 17–19) (*18*). It has been reported that 97% of cavitary nodules with a wall thickness greater than 16 mm are malignant and 93% with a wall thickness less than 4 mm are benign (*36,37*). Although these measurements can be of some value in nodule evaluation, cavity wall thickness cannot be used to confidently differentiate benign and malignant nodules.

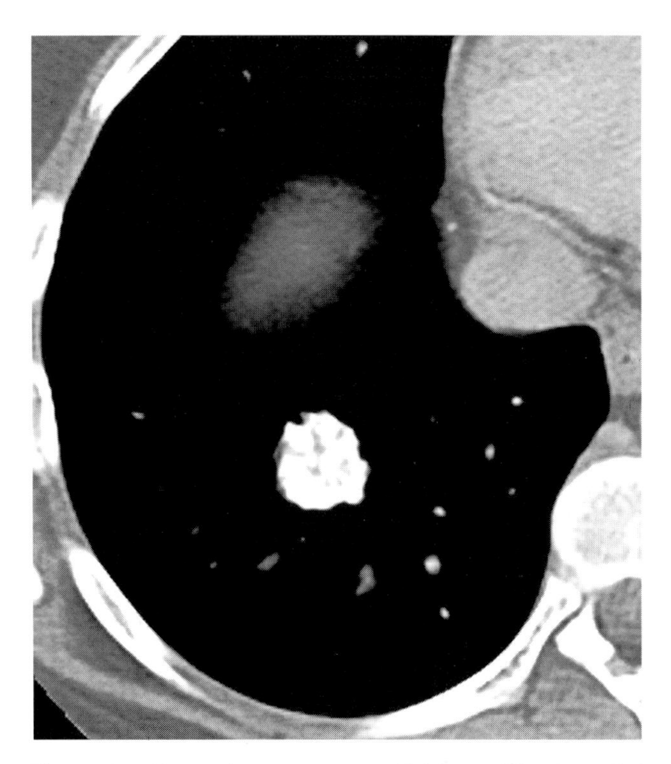

Figure 13 Metastatic osteosarcoma. CT shows diffusely ossified nodule in lower lobe. The appearance is suggestive of a benign calcified nodule secondary to infection.

Additional morphologic imaging features that can be used in assessing the malignant or benign potential of a solitary pulmonary opacity include air

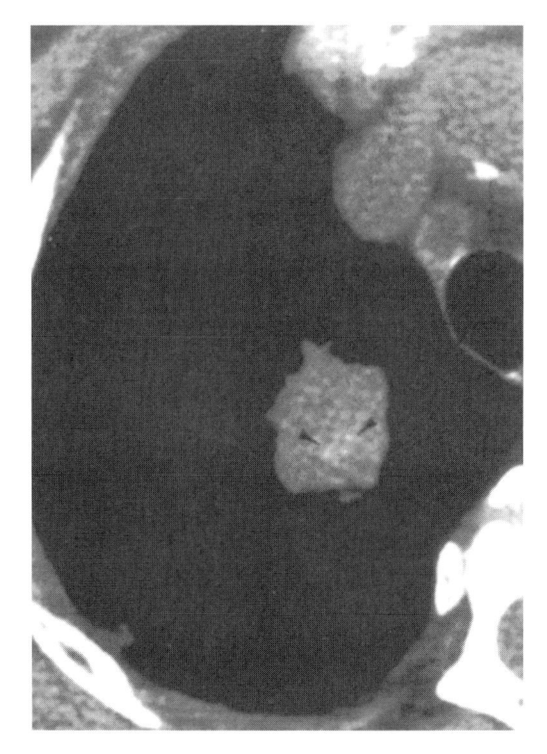

Figure 14 Non-small-cell lung cancer. CT reveals amorphous calcification in nodule, a pattern typical of malignancy (*arrowheads*). Adenocarcinoma was confirmed at resection.

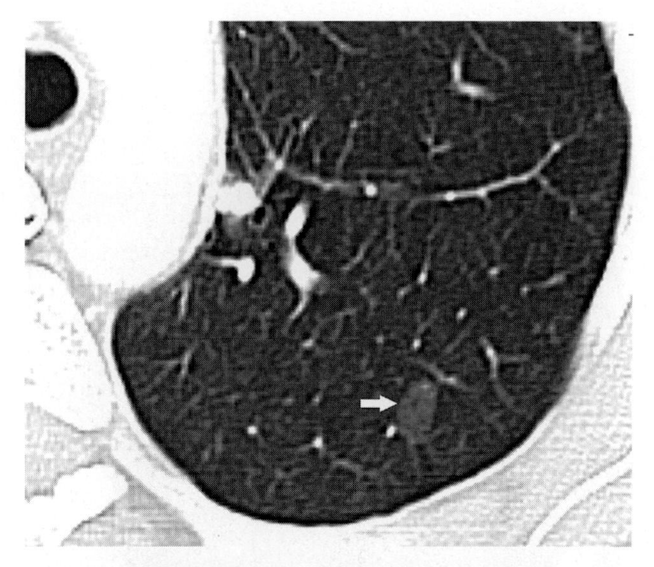

Figure 15 Primary adenocarcinoma of lung. CT shows nodule with ground-glass attenuation (*arrow*). Up to one-third of ground-glass nodular opacities are malignant.

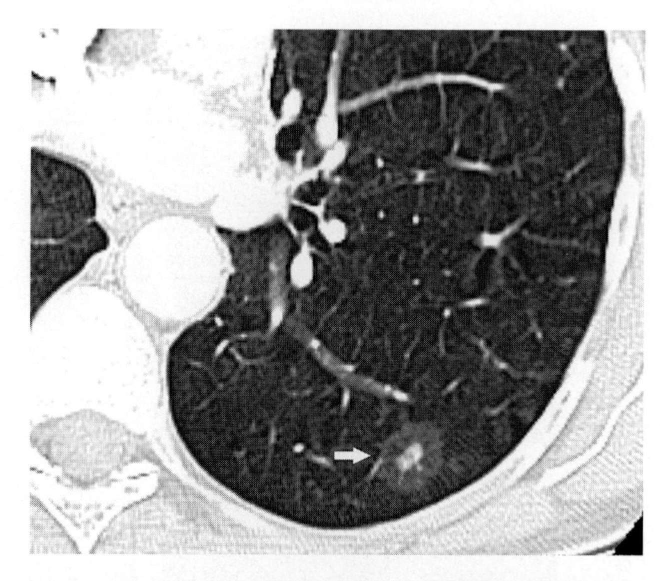

Figure 16 Bronchioloalveolar cancer. CT shows nodule with ground-glass attenuation with small solid component (*arrow*). Partially solid nodular opacities have the highest incidence of malignancy (up to 50%) when compared to nodules with solid or ground-glass attenuation alone.

bronchograms and satellite nodules. In one study, air bronchograms occurred more frequently in malignant nodules (30%) than benign nodules (6%) (Fig. *20*) (*38*). Satellite nodules, small nodules adjacent to a dominant nodule, are more frequently associated with benign lesions; however, 10% of dominant nodules are malignant.

Nodule Growth

Evaluation of growth is performed by reviewing preexisting chest radiographs or chest CTs. The majority of malignant nodules double in volume between 30 and 400 days (*39*). Nodular opacities that double in volume more rapidly than 30 days are usually infectious or inflammatory in origin (Fig. *21*), whereas those that double in volume more slowly than 400 days are usually benign pulmonary neoplasms or sequelae of prior pulmonary infections. It is generally accepted that the absence of visible growth over a 2-year period is reliable in determining benignity of a nodular opacity (*40–42*). However, the use of stability in size for 2 years to infer benignity has recently been questioned by Yankelevitz and Henschke, and they have recommended that this criterion be used with caution (*43*). In a screening study analyzing the growth rates of small lung cancers, Hasegawa et al. found that approximately 20% (12 of 61) of these opacities had a volumetric doubling time greater than 2 years. These nodular opacities were typically well-differentiated adenocarcinomas (*44*). Interestingly, the volumetric doubling times were shorter in smokers than nonsmokers, and solid lesions had a shorter doubling time compared to partly solid lesions, which in turn had a shorter doubling period compared to nonsolid lesions (*44*).

The concern raised about conferring benignity to a lesion based on the absence of growth over 2 years is particularly important when the accuracy of growth assessment in small nodules is considered. To detect growth on a radiograph requires a nodule to change in diameter by 3–5 mm (*43,45*). The small change in diameter (approximately 26%) that occurs when a small nodule doubles in volume makes it difficult to assess interval growth in these nodules. For example, a 4 mm nodule will increase to only 5 mm in diameter after doubling in volume, and consequently will appear stable on the chest radiograph. Although this change in diameter can theoretically be detected by CT, slight differences in the level at which the image is obtained occurs commonly from study to study and makes the confident detection of a small diameter change difficult. Additionally, it has recently been shown that there is significant inter- and intraobserver variability in lesion measurement, particularly in lesions with spiculated margins, thus further clouding the issue of using linear measurement to assess the growth rate and benignity or malignancy of a nodular opacity (*46,47*). However, the use of CT does in most cases allow an accurate assessment of growth, and it has been recently reported that growth can be detected in lung cancers as small as 5 mm when CT imaging is repeated within a 30 day interval (*48*). Furthermore, the measurement of serial volumes, rather than diameters, and computer-calculated doubling of volume of small nodules has been suggested to be an accurate and potentially useful method to assess growth (*49,50*). Presently, however, there is no consensus as to what parameters should be measured, when the first and

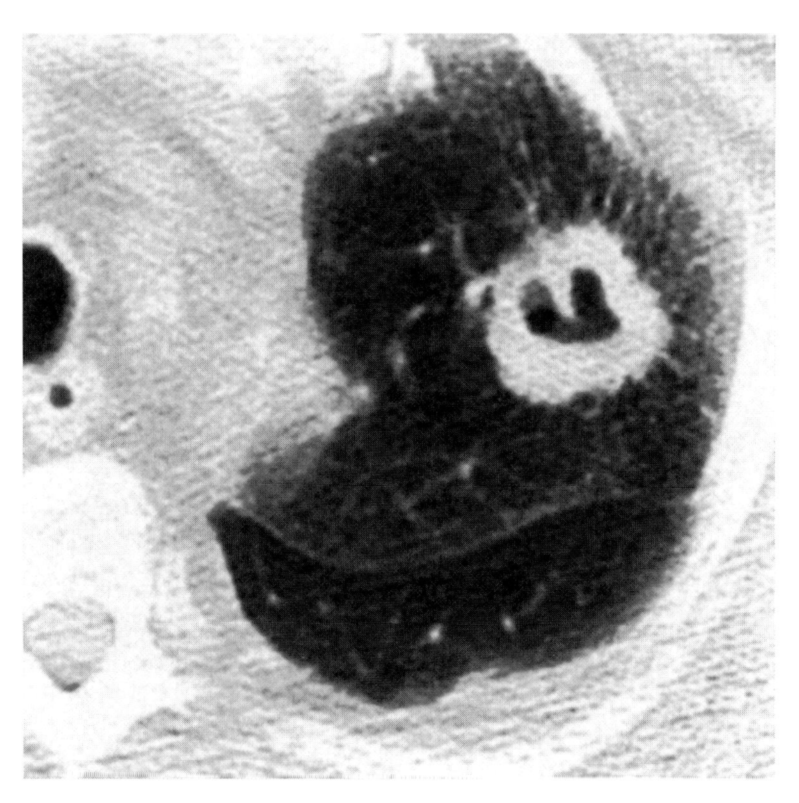

Figure 17 Squamous-cell lung cancer. CT shows thick-walled cavitary nodule in left upper lobe. Thick walls and eccentric cavitation are suggestive, but not diagnostic, of malignancy.

subsequent serial CTs should be performed, or the period of time required to ascertain that a small nodule is benign based on absence of growth.

Nodule Enhancement and Metabolism

Perfusion and metabolism of malignant pulmonary nodules is qualitatively and quantitatively different from that of benign nodules. Contrast-enhanced CT can be used to differentiate between benign and malignant nodules because the intensity of enhancement is directly related to the vascularity of the nodule, which is increased in malignant nodules

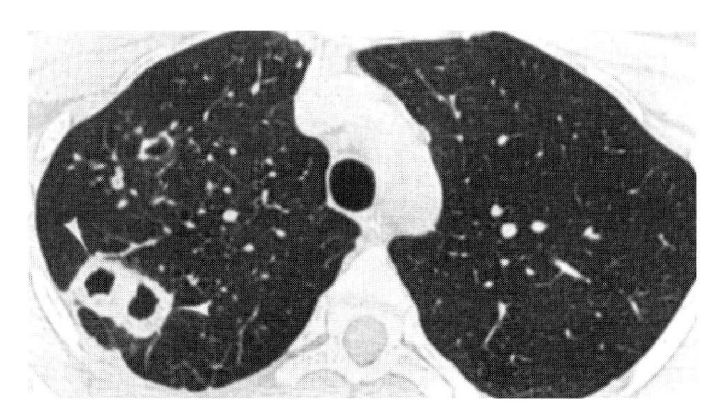

Figure 18 Nontuberculous mycobacterium infection (*Mycobacterium avium intracellulare*). CT shows well-circumscribed, cavitary nodule (*arrowheads*) with thick walls in right upper lobe. Note bronchiectasis and scattered branching tubular opacities, findings often associated with *M. avium intracellulare* infection.

(*51–53*). This technique has been shown in a multi-institutional prospective trial to be useful in determining the likelihood of malignancy of nodules that are indeterminate in etiology after standard radiological evaluation (*53*). 3-mm collimation images of the nodule are obtained before and after the intravenous administration of contrast (2 mL/s; 300 mg iodine/mm; 420 mg iodine/kg). Serial 5 s spiral acquisitions (3-mm collimation scans with 2-mm reconstruction intervals; 120 kVp, 280 mA, pitch of 1 : 1; standard reconstruction algorithm; 15 cm field of view) are performed at 1, 2, 3, and 4 min after the administration of contrast. Enhancement is determined by subtracting the precontrast attenuation of the nodule from the maximal nodule attenuation after contrast administration. Typically, malignant nodules enhance more than 20 HU, while benign nodules enhance less than 15 HU (Fig. *22*) (*53*). When a cut off of 15 HU is used the negative predictive value for malignancy is 96% (*53*). There are, however, several potential limitations to clinical application of this technique. Many nodules do not fulfill the selection criteria used in this study. For instance, nodules smaller than 5 mm in diameter and nodules that were not relatively spherical were excluded. The technique does, however, have clinical utility: a nodule that enhances less than 15 HU is almost certainly benign (sensitivity 98%, specificity 58%, accuracy 77%) and can be managed conservatively

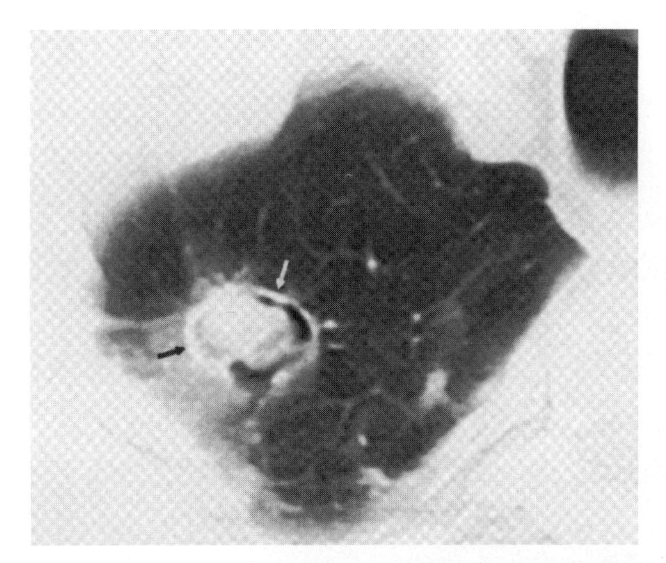

Figure 19 Squamous-cell lung cancer. CT shows thin-walled cavitary nodule in right upper lobe (*arrows*). Soft tissue within nodule is due to necrotic lung. Extensive necrosis can occasionally result in thin walls and erroneously suggest a benign etiology.

with serial radiological assessment. While the use of contrast-enhanced CT can reduce the number of nodules that need to be followed over time, a significant proportion of benign nodules will enhance. Such nodules remain indeterminate in etiology and require additional radiological evaluation.

The use of contrast-enhanced CT to determine nodule enhancement requires important attention to technical details. First, it is important to carefully follow the imaging protocol as outlined above.

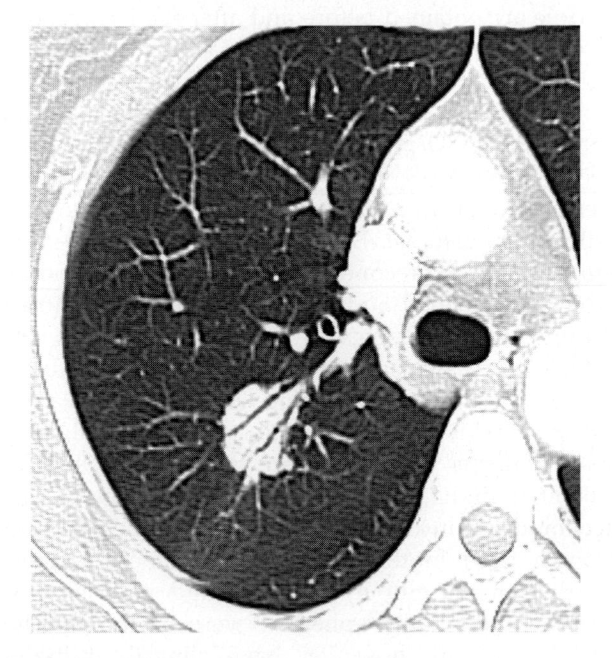

Figure 20 Primary well-differentiated adenocarcinoma of lung. CT shows nodule with air bronchograms. Although more frequent in malignant nodules, air bronchograms also occur in benign nodules.

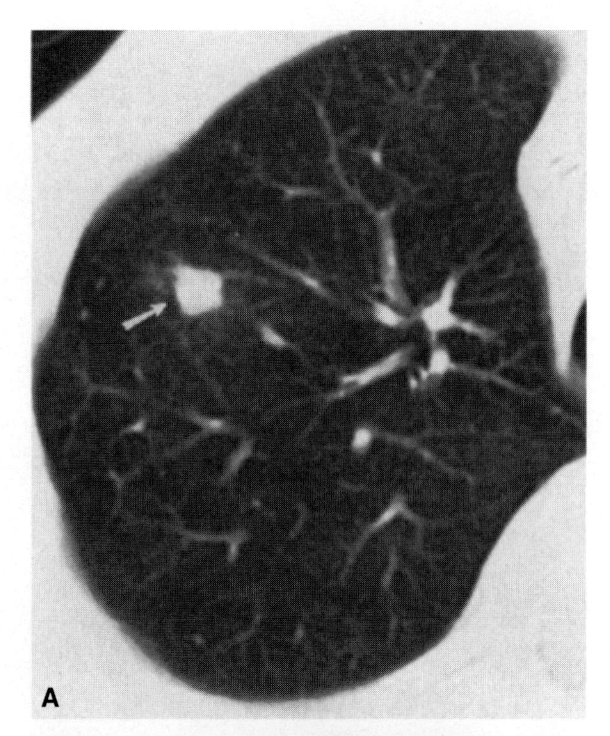

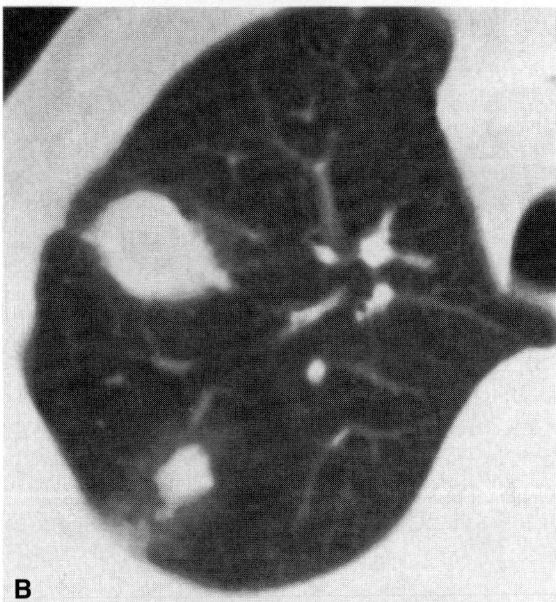

Figure 21 Nocardia infections in heart transplant recipient. (**A**) CT shows small, well-circumscribed, right upper-lobe nodule (*arrow*). (**B**) CT 1 week later shows marked increase in size of right upper lobe nodule and interval development of smaller right upper lobe pulmonary nodules. Transthoracic needle aspiration biopsy confirmed diagnosis of *Nocardia* infection. Rapid growth is indicative of a benign, in this case infectious, etiology.

Second, with regard to obtaining region of interest (ROI) measurements, the circular or oval ROI is centered on the image closest to the nodule equator and should comprise roughly 70% of the diameter of a nodule. All ROI measurements should be made on mediastinal window settings in order to ensure that partial volume averaging is minimized.

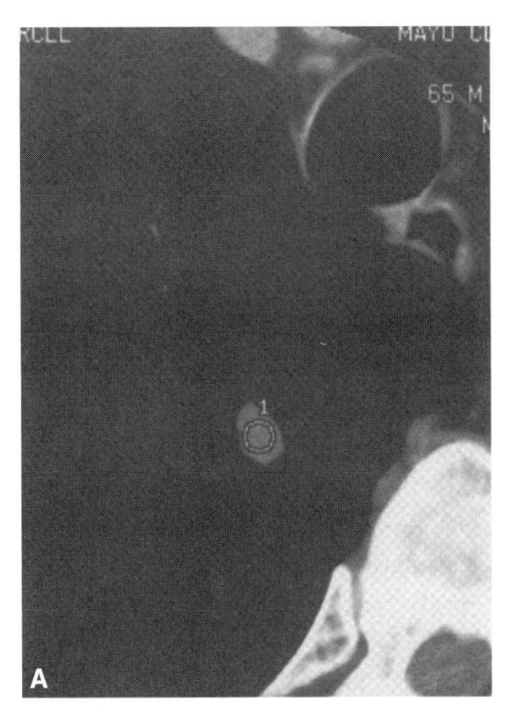

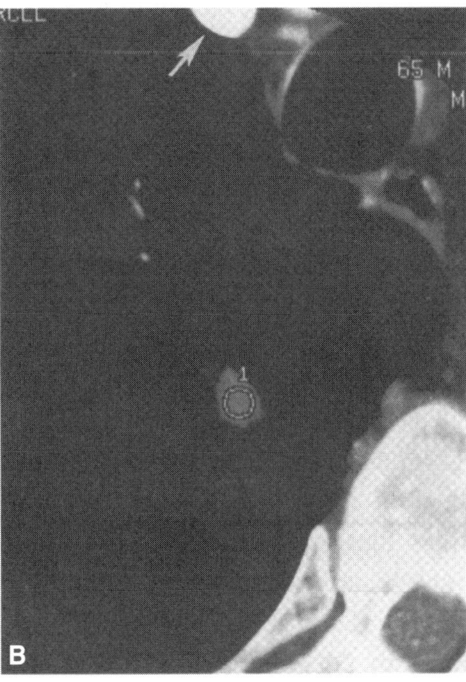

Figure 22 Benign pulmonary nodule. (**A**) Noncontrast CT shows right lung nodule with attenuation value of 28 HU. (**B**) Contrast CT shows no visual enhancement of nodule. Attenuation value measured 33 HU. The findings are consistent with a benign diagnosis. Note contrast in mediastinal vessels (*arrow*). *Source*: Courtesy of Tom Hartman, Mayo Clinic, Rochester, Minnesota.

Careful inspection of the bronchovascular structures adjacent to the nodule will allow one to obtain ROI measurements at similar levels in the *z*-axis of the nodule on serial scans. Third, this technique should only be performed on nodules that are relatively homogeneous in attenuation, without evidence of fat, calcification, cavitation, or necrosis.

Recently, there has been an effort to combine vascular enhancement and morphologic characteristics of a nodule with computer-aided diagnosis (CAD) to assist in differentiating benign from malignant nodules. In a study by Shah et al., a CAD system using quantitative features to describe the nodule's size, shape, attenuation, and enhancement properties was used to assist in the differentiation of benign and malignant nodules. The study showed that CAD using volumetric and contrast-enhanced data from 35 CT data sets of SPNs with a mean diameter of 25 mm (range, 6–54 mm) is useful in assisting in the differentiation of benign and malignant solitary pulmonary opacities (*54*).

Positron emission tomography (PET) can be used as an additional study to evaluate a solitary pulmonary opacity detected radiologically or as an alternative to contrast-enhanced CT to differentiate benign from malignant nodules. Similar to contrast enhancement, metabolism of glucose is typically increased in malignant nodules compared to benign nodules. PET, using the D-glucose analog FDG, can be used to image this increase in glucose metabolism, allowing differentiation of malignant from benign nodules (Fig. 23) (*55–59*). Sensitivity and specificity for detection of malignancy in nodules 10 mm or greater in diameter is about 90% with FDG-PET imaging (*55,58–65*). Because the probability of malignancy is high when a nodule has increased FDG-uptake, these nodules should be either biopsied, resected, or remain under close surveillance. When FDG-uptake by a nodule 10 mm or greater in diameter is low, the likelihood of malignancy is generally low. However, the usefulness of FDG-PET in the evaluation of a solitary pulmonary opacity is not predicated on diagnostic accuracy alone, but rather on clinical risk factors for malignancy, the radiologic appearance of the opacity, and how patient management will be altered. For instance, in a patient with a low pretest likelihood of malignancy (20%) being considered for serial radiologic observation, a negative PET will reduce the likelihood of malignancy to 1% and thereby justify conservative management (*65,66*). However, in a patient with a high pretest likelihood of malignancy (80%) a negative PET will only reduce the likelihood of malignancy to 14% (*65,66*). Accordingly, biopsy or resection rather than a PET would be more appropriate management strategy in this patient.

It is important to emphasize that the published data regarding FDG-PET evaluation of solitary pulmonary opacities indicating high sensitivity, specificity, and accuracy mostly pertains to solid nodules of 1 cm or greater in diameter. However, FDG-uptake in ground glass and partially solid nodules that are malignant is variable and unreliable in differentiating

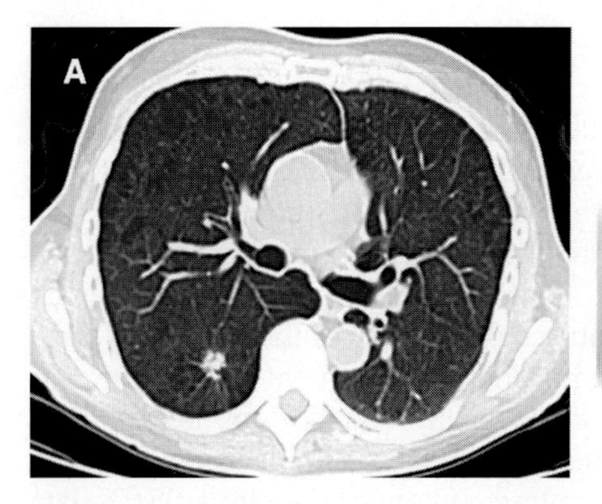

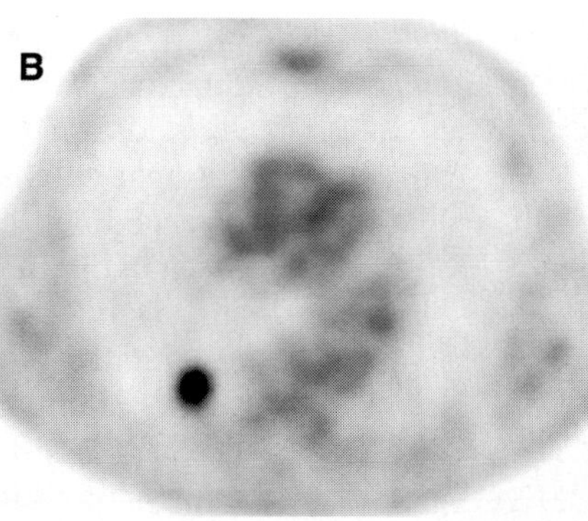

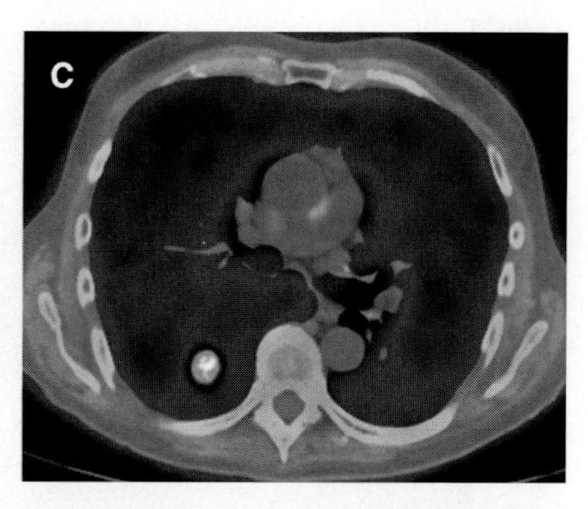

Figure 23 Non–small cell lung cancer manifesting as hypermetabolic nodule on FDG-integrated CT-PET scan. (**A**) Axial CT, (**B**) PET, and (**C**) integrated CT-PET show increased uptake of FDG in spiculated right lung nodule. Note emphysematous lung disease. The findings are suggestive of malignancy, and resection revealed lung cancer. (*See color insert for* **C**.)

benign from malignant nodular opacities (Fig. 24). In a recent study, 9 of 10 well-differentiated adenocarcinomas manifesting as ground-glass nodular opacities were falsely negative on PET, while 4 of 5 benign ground-glass nodular opacities were falsely positive (*67*). The sensitivity (10%) and specificity (20%) for ground-glass opacities in this study were significantly lower than that for solid nodules (90% and 71%, respectively). Limitations in spatial resolution can also result in false-negative studies when lesions smaller than 10 mm in diameter are evaluated (*67,68*). Otherwise, false-negative PET results are uncommon, but tend to occur with carcinoid tumors and bronchioloalveolar cell carcinomas (*69–71*). In an attempt to detect the small percentage of malignant nodules falsely designated benign after FDG-PET imaging, radiologic assessment, biopsy, or resection can be performed according to the recommendations of the Fleischner Society (see below). Although the high specificity of PET imaging for benign lesions can substantially reduce the number of benign nodules resected, benign neoplasms and nodules due to infection and inflammation (tuberculosis, histoplasmosis, rheumatoid arthritis, etc.) can result in false-positive diagnoses (Fig. 25).

The recent introduction of integrated CT-PET scanners has introduced the near-simultaneous acquisition of coregistered, spatially matched functional and morphologic data. The temporal and spatial fusion of these two sets of images can be useful when used as the initial imaging modality in solitary pulmonary opacity characterization (*72*). In a study comparing CT-PET and helical dynamic CT (HDCT) in the evaluation of SPNs, CT-PET was more sensitive (96% vs. 81%) and accurate (93% vs. 85%) than HDCT (*72*). However, it is important to emphasize that in contradistinction to dedicated PET imaging, integrated CT-PET uses CT data instead of transmission data from a germanium-68 source for PET attenuation correction. This has introduced artifacts and quantitative errors that can affect the emission image and, consequently, PET scan interpretation (*73*). For instance, patient breathing introduces a mismatch between the CT attenuation map and the PET emission data as the PET data is obtained during quiet breathing, while the CT data is usually obtained during suspended respiration (*74,75*). Besides localization errors, this misregistration results in incorrect attenuation coefficients applied to the PET data that can affect the standardized uptake value (SUV), the

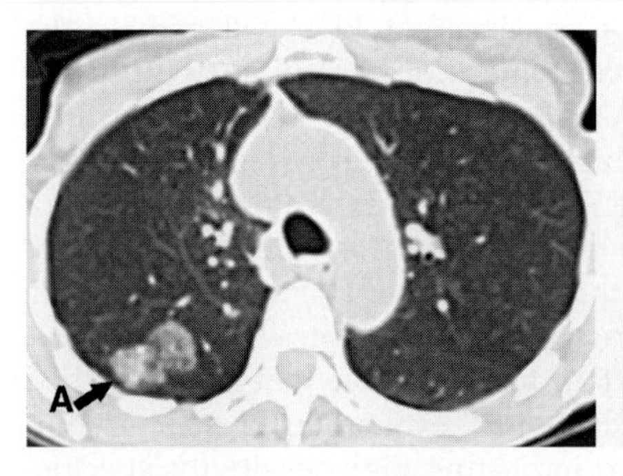

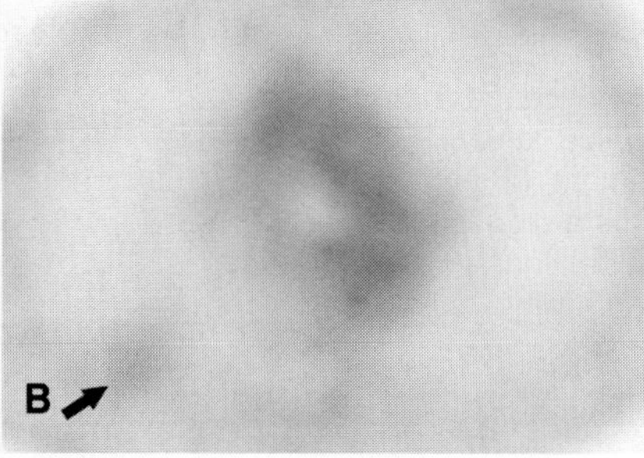

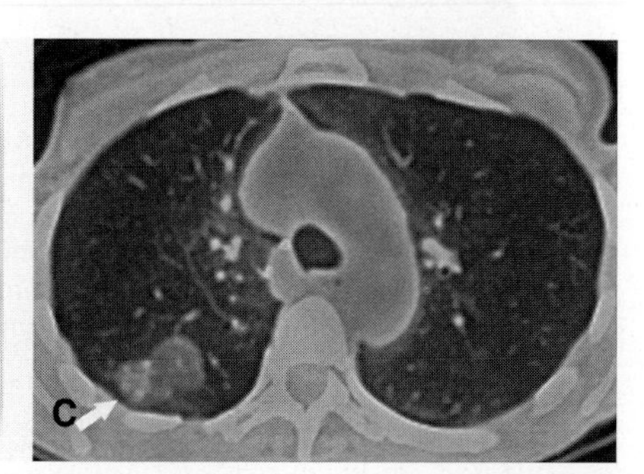

Figure 24 Bronchioloalveolar cell cancer manifesting as hypometabolic nodule on FDG-integrated CT-PET scan. (**A**) Axial CT, (**B**) PET, and (**C**) integrated CT-PET show bilobed, partially solid (ground-glass nodule with small solid soft tissue component) nodule with minimal FDG-uptake when compared to mediastinum (*arrows*). CT appearance raises the possibility of malignancy, while minimal FDG-uptake is suggestive of benignity. Note that FDG-uptake in malignant, partially solid nodules is unreliable in differentiating these nodules from benign nodular opacities. (*See color insert for* **C**.)

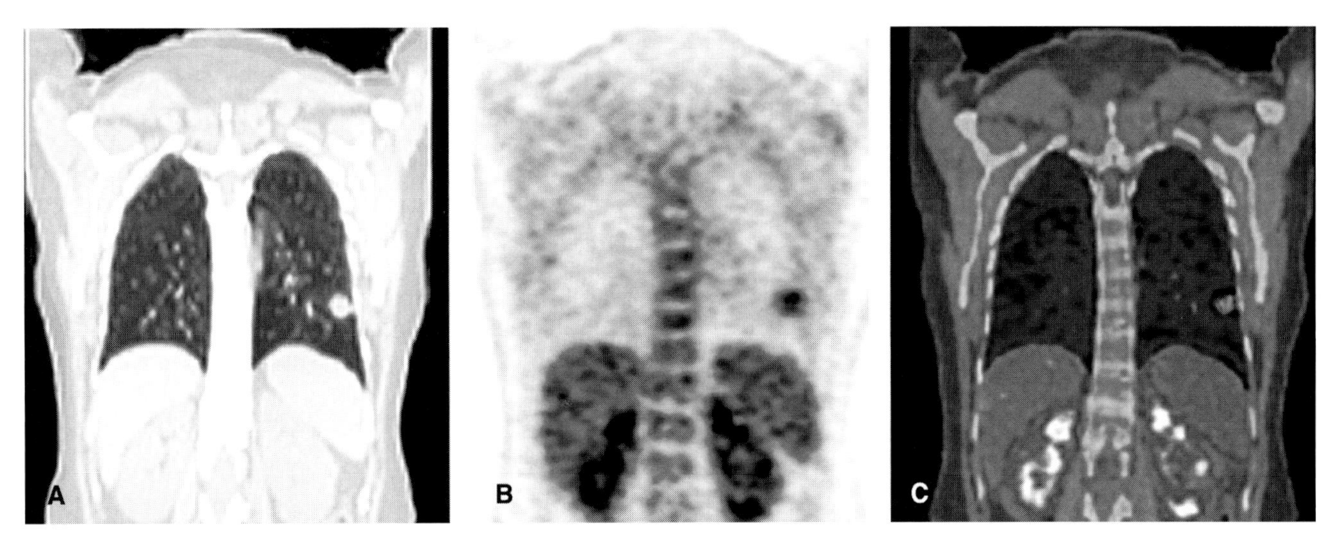

Figure 25 Necrotizing granuloma manifesting as hypermetabolic nodule on FDG-integrated CT-PET scan. (**A**) Coronal CT, (**B**) PET, and (**C**) integrated CT-PET show nodule in left lower lobe with increased FDG-uptake within nodule. Findings are suggestive of malignancy. Transthoracic needle aspiration biopsy was inconclusive for malignancy, and surgical resection revealed necrotizing granuloma. (*See color insert for* **C**.)

most commonly used parameter to quantify the intensity of FDG-uptake (74,76,77). In this regard, the SUV is generally lower than expected and can potentially result in a false-negative study. Strategies to reduce the affect of respiratory mismatch of the CT and PET images include obtaining the CT scan in end expiration, which most closely approximates the PET data acquisition. In this process, however, the anatomic detail of a diagnostic CT is compromised and small nodules may be obscured. A more recent approach advocates the use of respiratory-averaged CT to improve SUV quantification (Fig. *26*) (*78*).

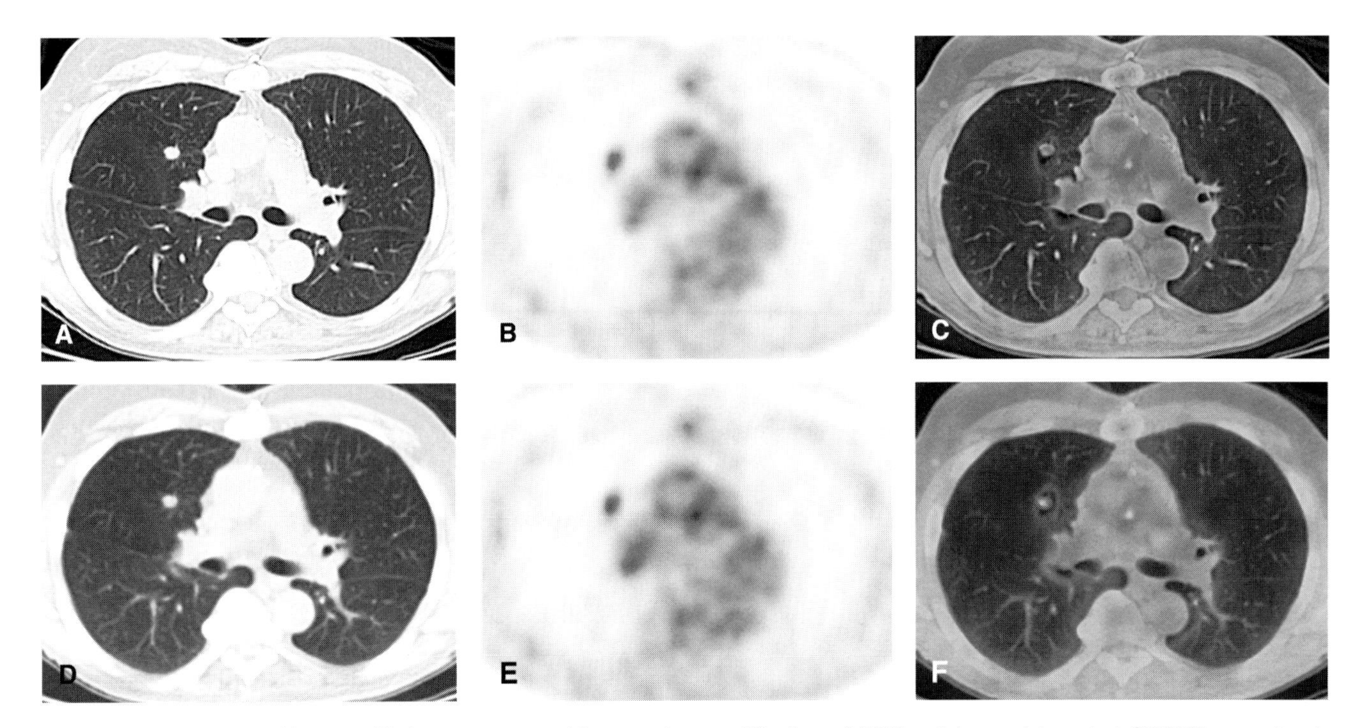

Figure 26 A 73-year-old man with lung cancer and inaccurate quantification of FDG uptake on integrated CT-PET scan due to respiratory motion. (**A**) Axial CT, (**B**) PET, and (**C**) integrated CT-PET show hypermetabolic right upper lobe nodule. 4D CT, acquired over several respiratory cycles was used to correct attenuation correction (AC) of PET for respiration. Axial images of respiratory-averaged CT (**D**), PET (**E**), and integrated CT-PET (**F**) show visual increase in FDG-uptake by nodule. PET-AC using four-dimensional CT shows a 25% increase in lesion standardized uptake value (SUV) (from 2.7 to 3.4). Note respiration-induced attenuation artifact can have implications for lesion characterization. (*See color insert for* **C** *and* **F**.)

Respiratory-averaged CT used for attenuation correction of a PET scan has shown differences of more than 50% in some lesions as compared with the standard method of CT attenuation with CT data in the midexpiratory phase (*78,79*).

DECISION ANALYSIS

Following clinical assessment, nodules will be categorized as (*1*) benign, (*2*) malignant, or (*3*) indeterminate in etiology. Benign nodules, either because of their pattern of calcification or stability over a long period of time, require no further evaluation. Nodules with malignant characteristics such as spiculation need further expeditious evaluation and generally require biopsy or resection. However, many nodules remain indeterminate in etiology after comprehensive noninvasive radiological assessment. At this point, a decision to observe with radiologic reassessment, biopsy, or resect the nodule is made. Commonly used guidelines from the American College of Chest Physicians (*66*) and in *The New England Journal of Medicine* review by Ost and colleagues (*80*) for following these indeterminate pulmonary nodules have included multiple CTs obtained over a 2-year period to determine nodule stability. However, recently the detection of pulmonary nodules has increased with new technological advancements and many of these nodules are small (less than 7 mm) and benign. This, together with the radiation exposure, cost, limited resources, and patient anxiety resulting from serial radiologic evaluation, resulted in the recent publication of recommendations for the management of pulmonary nodules discovered incidentally on routine and screening CT by the Fleischner Society (*8*). The Fleischner recommendations integrate lesion morphology, growth rate, patient age, and smoking history (*8*). In terms of the recommendations, the size of the nodular opacity is important as there is a positive relationship between size and the likelihood of malignancy. In this regard, small nodules (less than 4 mm) have a less than 1% chance of being a primary lung cancer, even in people who smoke, while the risk increases to 10–20% in nodules in the 8 mm range (*8*).

Fleischner Society Recommendations

The following lists the Fleischner Society's recommendations for an incidentally discovered nodule in an adult patient (*8*).

Low-risk populations (little or no history of smoking, and no other risk factors)

1. Nodules equal to or smaller than 4 mm have a very small likelihood of malignancy, and no reassessment is necessary.
2. Nodules greater than 4 mm but less than or equal to 6 mm. Reassessment CT at 12 months, and, if stable, no further evaluation is required. The exception is the nonsolid or partially solid nodule for which reassessment may need to be continued to exclude the risk of an indolent adeno-carcinoma.
3. Nodules greater than 6 mm but less than or equal to 8 mm. Reassessment CT at 6–12 months and, if stable, again at 18–24 months.
4. Nodules greater than 8 mm. Either reassessment CT scans at 3, 9, and 24 months to assess for stability in size or further evaluation with contrast-enhanced CT, CT-PET, or biopsy or resection.

High-risk populations (history of smoking, or other exposure or risk factor)

5. Noduls equal or smaller than 4 mm. Reassessment at 12 months, and, if stable, no further evaluation is required. The exception is the nonsolid or partially solid nodule for which reassessment may need to be continued to exclude the risk of an indolent adenocarcinoma.
6. Nodules greater than 4 mm but less than or equal to 6 mm. Reassessment CT at 6–12 months and, if stable, again at 18–24 months.
7. Nodules greater than 6 mm but less than or equal to 8 mm. Reassessment CT at 3–6 months and, if stable, again at 9–12 months and 24 months.
8. Nodules greater than 8 mm. Either reassessment CT at 3, 9, and 24 months to assess stability, or perform contrast-enhanced CT, CT-PET, or biopsy or resection.

A noncontrast, thin collimation, limited coverage, low-dose CT scan is recommended by the Fleischner Society when the only indication for the study is nodule reassessment (*8*). Importantly, these recommendations do not apply to patients with a history of malignancy, young patients less than 35 years in whom the risk of lung cancer is low, and in those patients with fever in which the nodules may be infectious (*8*).

SUMMARY

Solitary pulmonary opacities, including SPNs, are a common radiological abnormality that are often detected incidentally. Although the majority are benign, lung cancer constitutes an important proportion of SPNs. The goal of management is to correctly differentiate these malignancies from benign nodules so that appropriate treatment can be initiated. The detection of specific patterns of calcification and stability in size for 2 years or more have historically been the only reliable findings useful for determining nodule benignity. More recently, the ability to distinguish benign and malignant SPNs has improved with assessment of nodule perfusion and metabolism using contrast-enhanced CT and FDG-CT-PET imaging. Despite the availability of different modalities and strategies to differentiate benign from malignant nodules, some nodules will remain indeterminate in etiology after extensive radiological evaluation. However, new management recommendations and imaging modalities have improved reassessment imaging protocols and preoperative identification of benign nodules.

ACKNOWLEDGMENT

Many thanks to Lisa Allen for her assistance in preparing this manuscript and Dr. Tinsu Pan for his technical assistance.

REFERENCES

1 Austin JH, Müller NL, Friedman PJ, et al. Glossary of terms for CT of the lungs: recommendations of the Nomenclature Committee of the Fleischner Society. Radiology 1996; 200:327–31.
2 Swensen SJ, Jett JR, Hartman TE, et al. CT screening for lung cancer: five-year prospective experience. Radiology 2005; 235:259–65.
3 American Cancer Society. Cancer Facts and Figures 2006. Atlanta: American Cancer Society, 2006.
4 Viggiano RW, Swensen SJ, Rosenow EC III. Evaluation and management of solitary and multiple pulmonary nodules. Clin Chest Med 1992; 13:83–95.
5 Mountain CF. Revisions in the international system for staging lung cancer. Chest 1997; 111:1710–7.
6 Gurney JW, Lyddon DM, McKay JA. Determining the likelihood of malignancy in solitary pulmonary nodules with Bayesian analysis.Part II. Application. Radiology 1993; 186:415–22.
7 Lee HJ, Im JG, Ahn JM, Yeon KM. Lung cancer in patients with idiopathic pulmonary fibrosis: CT findings. J Comput Assist Tomogr 1996; 20(6):979–82.
8 MacMahon H, Austin JH, Gamsu G, et al. Guidelines for management of small pulmonary nodules detected on CT scans: a statement from the Fleischner Society. Radiology 2005; 237:395–400.
9 Berger WG, Erly WK, Krupinski EA, Standen JR, Stern RG. The solitary pulmonary nodule on chest radiography: can we really tell if the nodule is calcified? AJR Am J Roentgenol 2001; 176:201–4.
10 Seltzer SE, Judy PF, Adams DF, et al. Spiral CT of the chest: comparison of cine and film-based viewing. Radiology 1995; 197:73–8.
11 Coakley FV, Cohen MD, Johnson MS, Gonin R, Hanna MP. Maximum intensity projection images in the detection of simulated pulmonary nodules by spiral CT. Br J Radiol 1998; 71:135–40.
12 Henschke CI, McCauley DI, Yankelevitz DF, et al. Early lung cancer action project: overall design and findings from baseline screening. Lancet 1999; 354:99–105.
13 Kaneko M, Eguchi K, Ohmatsu H, et al. Peripheral lung cancer: screening and detection with low-dose spiral CT versus radiography. Radiology 1996; 201: 798–802.
14 Sone S, Takashima S, Li F, et al. Mass screening for lung cancer with mobile spiral computed tomography scanner. Lancet 1998;351:1242–5.
15 Munden RF, Pugatch RD, Liptay MJ, Sugarbaker DJ, Le LU. Small pulmonary lesions detected at CT: clinical importance. Radiology 1997; 202:105–10.
16 Ginsberg MS,Griff SK, Go BD, Yoo HH, Schwartz LH, Panicek DM. Pulmonary nodules resected at video-assisted thoracoscopic surgery: etiology in 426 patients. Radiology 1999; 213:277–82.
17 Zerhouni EA,Stitik FP, Siegelman SS, et al. CT of the pulmonary nodule: a cooperative study. Radiology 1986; 160:319–27.
18 Zwirewich CV, Vedal S, Miller RR, Müller NL. Solitary pulmonary nodule: high-resolution CT and radiologic pathologic correlation. Radiology 1991; 179:469–76.
19 Heitzman ER, Markarian B, Raasch BN, Carsky EW, Lane EJ, Berlow ME. Pathways of tumor spread through the lung: radiologic correlations with anatomy and pathology. Radiology 1982; 144:3–14.
20 Siegelman SS, Khouri NF, Scott J, et al. Pulmonary hamartoma: CT findings. Radiology 1986; 160:313–7.
21 Muram TM, Aisen A. Fatty metastatic lesions in 2 patients with renal clear-cell carcinoma. J Comput Assist Tomogr 2003; 27:869–70.
22 Siegelman SS, Khouri NF, Leo FP, Fishman EK, Braverman RM, Zerhouni EA. Solitary pulmonary nodules: CT assessment. Radiology 1986; 160:307–12.
23 Siegelman SS, Zerhouni EA, Leo FP, Khouri NF, Stitik FP. CT of the solitary pulmonary nodule. Am J Roentgenol 1980; 135:1–13.
24 Zerhouni EA, Boukadoum M, Siddiky M, et al. A standard phantom for quantitative CT analysis of pulmonary nodules. Radiology 1983; 149:767–73.
25 Huston JI, Muhm JR. Solitary pulmonary nodules: evaluation with a CT reference phantom. Radiology 1989; 170:653–6.
26 Midthun DE, Swensen SJ, Jett JR. Approach to the solitary pulmonary nodule. Mayo Clin Proc 1993; 68:378–85.
27 Swensen SJ, Harms GF, Morin RL, Meyers JL. CT evaluation of solitary pulmonary nodules: value of 185-H reference phantom. Am J Roentgenol 1991; 156:925–9.
28 Higashi Y, Nakamura H, Matsumoto T, Nakanishi T. Dual-energy computed tomographic diagnosis of pulmonary nodules. J Thorac Imaging 1994; 9:31–4.
29 Bhalla M, Shepard JA, Nakamura K, Kazerooni EA. Dual kV CT to detect calcification in solitary pulmonary nodule. J Comput Assist Tomogr 1995; 19:44–7.

30 Swensen SJY, Yamashita K, McCollough CH, et al. Lung nodules: dual-kilovolt peak analysis with CT-multicenter study. Radiology 2000; 214:81–5.

31 O'Keefe ME, Good CA, McDonald JR. Calcification in solitary nodules of the lung. Am J Roentgenol 1957; 77:1023–33.

32 Seo JB, Im JG, Goo JM, Chung MJ, Kim MY. Atypical pulmonary metastases: spectrum of radiologic findings. Radiographics 2001; 21:403–17.

33 Winer-Muram HT. The solitary pulmonary nodule. Radiology 2006; 239:34–49.

34 Grewal RG, Austin JHM. CT demonstration of calcification in carcinoma of the lung. J Comput Assist Tomogr 1994; 18:867–71.

35 Mahoney MC, Shipley RT, Corcoran HL, Dickson BA. CT demonstration of calcification in carcinoma of the lung. Am J Roentgenol 1990; 154:255–8.

36 Woodring JH, Fried AM. Significance of wall thickness in solitary cavities of the lung: a follow-up study. Am J Roentgenol 1983; 140:473–4.

37 Woodring JH, Fried AM, Chuang VP. Solitary cavities of the lung: diagnostic implications of cavity wall thickness. Am J Roentgenol 1980; 135:1269–71.

38 Kui M, Templeton PA, White CS, Cai ZL, Bai YX, Cai YQ. Evaluation of the air bronchogram sign on CT in solitary pulmonary lesions. J Comput Assist Tomogr 1996; 20(6):983–6.

39 Lillington GA, Caskey CI. Evaluation and management of solitary multiple pulmonary nodules. Clin Chest Med 1993; 14:111–9.

40 Lillington GA. Disease-a-Month. St. Louis, MO: Mosby Year Book, 1991.

41 Good CA, Wilson TW. The solitary circumscribed pulmonary nodule. JAMA 1958; 166:210–5.

42 Good CA. Management of patient with solitary mass in lung. Chic Med Soc Bull 1953; 55:893–6.

43 Yankelevitz DF, Henschke CI. Does 2-year stability imply that pulmonary nodules are benign? Am J Roentgenol 1997; 168:325–8.

44 Hasegawa M, Sone S, Takashima S, et al. Growth rate of small lung cancers detected on mass CT screening. Br J Radiol 2000; 73:1252–9.

45 Cummings SR, Lillington GA, Richard RJ. Managing solitary pulmonary nodules. Am Rev Respir Dis 1986; 134:453–60.

46 Revel M-P, Bissery A, Bienvenu M, Aycard L, Lefort C, Frija G. Are two-dimensional CT measurements of small noncalcified pulmonary nodules reliable? Radiology 2004; 231:453–8.

47 Erasmus JJ, Gladish GW, Broemeling L, et al. Interobserver and intraobserver variability in measurement of non-small-cell carcinoma lung lesions: implications for assessment of tumor response. J Clin Oncol 2003; 21:2574–82.

48 Yankelevitz DF, Gupta R, Zhao B, Henschke CI. Small pulmonary nodules: evaluation with repeat CT—preliminary experience. Radiology 1999; 212:561–6.

49 Yankelevitz DF, Reeves AP, Kostis WJ, Zhao B, Henschke CI. Determination of malignancy in small pulmonary nodules based on volumetrically determined growth rates. Radiology 1998; 209(Suppl):375.

50 Revel M-P, Merlin A, Peyrard S, et al. Software volumetric evaluation of doubling times for differentiating benign versus malignant pulmonary nodules. AJR Am J Roentgenol 2006; 187:135–42.

51 Yamashita K, Matsunobe S, Tsuda T, et al. Solitary pulmonary nodule: preliminary study of evaluation with incremental dynamic CT. Radiology 1995; 194:399–405.

52 Zhang M, Kono M. Solitary pulmonary nodules: evaluation of blood flow patterns with dynamic CT. Radiology 1997; 205:471–8.

53 Swensen SJ, Viggiano RW, Midthun DE, et al. Lung nodule enhancement at CT: multicenter study. Radiology 2000; 214:73–80.

54 Shah SK, McNitt-Gray MF, Rogers SR, et al. Computer aided characterization of the solitary pulmonary nodule using volumetric and contrast enhancement features. Acad Radiol 2005; 12:1310–9.

55 Patz EF, Lowe VJ, Hoffman JM, et al. Focal pulmonary abnormalities: evaluation with F-18 fluorodeoxyglucose PET scanning. Radiology 1993; 188:487–90.

56 Gupta NC, Frank AR, Dewan NA, et al. Solitary pulmonary nodules: detection of malignancy with PET with 2-[F-18]-fluoro-2-deoxy-D-glucose. Radiology 1992; 184:441–4.

57 Dewan NA, Gupta NC, Redepenning LS, Phalen JJ, Frick MP. Diagnostic efficacy of PET-FDG imaging in solitary pulmonary nodules. Chest 1993; 104:997–1002.

58 Knight SB, Delbeke D, Stewart JR, Sandler MP. Evaluation of pulmonary lesions with FDG-PET. Chest 1996; 109:982–8.

59 Valk PE, Pounds TR, Hopkins DM, et al. Staging non-small cell lung cancer by whole-body positron emission tomographic imaging. Ann Thorac Surg 1995; 60:1573–81; discussion 81–2.

60 Scott WJ, Schwabe JL, Gupta NC, Dewan NA, Reeb SD, Sugimoto JT. Positron emission tomography of lung tumors and mediastinal lymph nodes using [^{18}F] fluorodeoxyglucose. Ann Thorac Surg 1994; 58:698–703.

61 Conti PS, Lilien DL, Hawley K, Keppler J, Grafton ST, Bading JR. PET and [^{18}F]-FDG in oncology: a clinical update. Nucl Med Biol 1996; 23:717–35.

62 Gupta NC, Maloof J, Gunel E. Probability of malignancy in solitary pulmonary nodules using fluorine-18-FDG and PET. J Nucl Med 1996; 37:943–8.

63 Hubner KF, Buonocore E, Gould HR, et al. Differentiating benign from malignant lung lesions using quantitative" parameters of FDG PET images. Clin Nucl Med 1996; 21:941–9.

64 Lewis P, Griffin S, Marsden P, et al. Whole-body ^{18}F-fluorodeoxyglucose positron emission tomography in preoperative evaluation of lung cancer. Lancet 1994; 344:1265–6.

65 Gould MK, Maclean CC, Kuschner WG, Rydzak CE, Owens DK. Accuracy of positron emission tomography for diagnosis of pulmonary nodules and mass lesions: a meta-analysis. JAMA 2001; 285:914–24.

66 Tan BB, Flaherty KR, Kazerooni EA, Iannettoni MD. American College of Chest P. The solitary pulmonary nodule. Chest 2003; 123(Suppl. 1):89S–96.

67 Nomori H, Watanabe K, Ohtsuka T, Naruke T, Suemasu K, Uno K. Evaluation of F-18 fluorodeoxyglucose (FDG)

PET scanning for pulmonary nodules less than 3 cm in diameter, with special reference to the CT images. Lung Cancer 2004; 45(1):19–27 [see comment].
68 Lowe VJ, Fletcher JW, Gobar L, et al. Prospective investigation of PET in lung nodules (PIOPILN). J Clin Oncol 1998; 16:1075–84.
69 Erasmus JJ, McAdams HP, Patz JEF, Coleman RE, Ahuja V, Goodman PC. Evaluation of primary pulmonary carcinoid tumors using FDG PET. Am J Roentgenol 1998; 170:1369–73.
70 Higashi K, Ueda Y, Seki H, et al. Fluorine-18-FDG PET imaging is negative in bronchioloalveolar lung carcinoma. J Nucl Med 1998; 39:1016–20.
71 Sabloff BS, Truong MT, Wistuba II, Erasmus JJ. Bronchioalveolar cell carcinoma: radiologic appearance and dilemmas in the assessment of response. Clin Lung Cancer 2004; 6:108–12.
72 Yi CA, Lee KS, Kim BT, et al. Tissue characterization of solitary pulmonary nodule: comparative study between helical dynamic CT and integrated PET/CT. J Nucl Med 2006; 47:443–50.
73 Cook GJR, Wegner EA, Fogelman I. Pitfalls and artifacts in 18FDG PET and PET/CT oncologic imaging. Semin Nucl Med 2004; 34:122–33.
74 Beyer T, Antoch G, Blodgett T, Freudenberg LF, Akhurst T, Mueller S. Dual-modality PET/CT imaging: the effect of respiratory motion on combined image quality in clinical oncology. Eur J Nucl Med Mol Imag 2003; 30:588–96.
75 Osman MM, Cohade C, Nakamoto Y, Wahl RL. Respiratory motion artifacts on PET emission images obtained using CT attenuation correction on PET-CT. Eur J Nucl Med Mol Imag 2003; 30:603–6.
76 Goerres GW, Kamel E, Heidelberg TN, Schwitter MR, Burger C, von Schulthess GK. PET-CT image co-registration in the thorax: influence of respiration. Eur J Nucl Med Mol Imag 2002; 29:351–60.
77 Goerres GW, Burger C, Kamel E, et al. Respiration-induced attenuation artifact at PET/CT: technical considerations. Radiology 2003; 226:906–10.
78 Pan T, Mawlawi O, Nehmeh SA, et al. Attenuation correction of PET images with respiration-averaged CT images in PET/CT. J Nucl Med 2005; 46:1481–7.
79 Truong MT, Pan T, Erasmus JJ. Pitfalls in integrated CT-PET of the thorax: implications in oncologic imaging. J Thorac Imag 2006;21:111–22.
80 Ost D, Fein AM, Feinsilver SH. Clinical practice. The solitary pulmonary nodule. N Eng J Med 2003; 348:2535–42 [see comment].

10

High-Resolution CT in the Multidetector CT Era

Prachi P. Agarwal and Ella A. Kazerooni
Division of Cardiothoracic Radiology, Department of Radiology, University of Michigan, Ann Arbor, Michigan, U.S.A.

INTRODUCTION

High-resolution CT (HRCT) of the lungs is aimed at resolving fine lung parenchymal anatomy to enable better assessment of the pattern and distribution of lung disease, with radiologic–pathologic correlation serving as the foundation of interpretation and differential diagnosis. It is the best in vivo way to evaluate both focal and diffuse lung disease, and to determine the distribution and severity of disease, the latter serving both prognostically for disease staging, as well as a method by which the impact of medical therapy can be judged. Thin-beam collimation (1–1.5 mm) combined with use of a high-spatial frequency reconstruction algorithm are the two most important technical factors that distinguish HRCT from conventional CT of the lungs.

Since the beginning, HRCT has used an incremental scanning technique, where the lung parenchyma was sampled at intervals ranging from as little as every 1 cm to as much as 6–10 cm apart when acquired as images at fixed anatomic landmarks of the aorta, carina, and just above the diaphragm. This provides valuable information on pattern and distribution of diffuse lung disease, but is less optimal in cases of focal disease, as only a portion of the lungs are actually imaged. Focal disease, such as lung nodules, which is common in patients with interstitial and obstructive lung disease that are at risk for cancer, cannot be followed for size and change using incremental HRCT techniques, requiring rescanning at thicker collimation continuously to include all the lungs, prior to the multidetector CT (MDCT) era (1,2). Furthermore, the noncontiguous incremental HRCT images provide an incomplete evaluation of the central tracheobronchial tree, where abnormalities can arise that present clinically with the same symptoms as lung disease, such as dyspnea. The MDCT scanners with 16 detector rows and higher have revolutionized thoracic imaging, with faster acquisition times that enable the entire lungs to be imaged using thin collimation in a single-breath hold. This was not consistently possible on MDCT scanners of fewer detectors, as the acquisition time was too long for patients to hold their breath, particularly for patients with shortness of breath. The MDCT scanners capable of generating isotropic volumetric high-resolution data sets now permit distortion free image reconstruction in any plane (2).

In this chapter, we (*i*) review the anatomical and technical aspects of image acquisition for HRCT, with an emphasis on MDCT; (*ii*) describe image interpretation and postprocessing tools, including two-dimensional reformation, such as multiplanar reformats, minimum intensity projection (MinIP), and maximum intensity projection (MIP); (*iii*) review the known artifacts; and (*iv*) discuss the applications of volumetric multidetector HRCT in specific clinical scenarios.

ANATOMICAL CONSIDERATIONS

The key to HRCT interpretation is a good understanding of the anatomy of the secondary pulmonary lobule (Fig. 1).

Secondary Pulmonary Lobule

The secondary pulmonary lobule is the smallest functional anatomic unit that can be defined on HRCT. It is a polyhedron measuring approximately 1–2.5 cm on each side and contains up to 12 pulmonary acini; the acinus is a portion of the lung supplied by the respiratory bronchiole. Lobules are marginated by interlobular septa, which contain pulmonary veins, connective tissue, and lymphatics (3). The center of the lobule consists of a centrilobular pulmonary arteriole and bronchiole which branch successively, producing intralobular arterioles and bronchioles and then acinar arterioles and respiratory bronchioles before terminating into the gas exchange units (4). The centrilobular arteriole and bronchiole measure approximately 1 mm in diameter (5). Secondary pulmonary lobules are best seen in the upper lobes, anterior and lateral portions of the middle lobe and lingula, and over the diaphragmatic surfaces of the lower lobes, where they are most developed (4). Axial incremental HRCT using a 1-mm beam collimation with a pixel size of 0.68 mm, a 35-cm scanning field of view (SFOV), and a 512 × 512 matrix

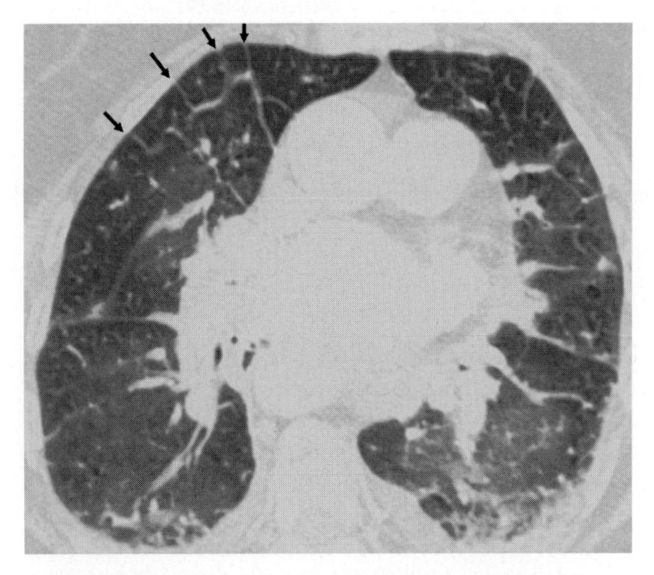

Figure 1 Axial helical CT demonstrates smooth thickening of interlobular septa (*arrows*) outlining secondary pulmonary lobules. Interlobular septa contain pulmonary veins, connective tissue, and lymphatics, and the center of the lobule consists of a centrilobular pulmonary arteriole.

can resolve structures down to 0.1 mm in diameter, provided their attenuation is significantly different from surrounding structures (6). Hence, centrilobular bronchioles measuring 1 mm in diameter with less than 0.1 mm walls cannot be visualized due to partial volume averaging of the air inside and outside the bronchioles with the thin walls (6). In contrast, acinar arteries measuring 0.3–0.5 mm are seen on HRCT approximately 3–5 mm from the interlobular septa (5,7,8). The centrilobular artery is routinely used to define the center of the pulmonary lobule (7).

Pulmonary Interstitium

The pulmonary interstitium consists of the central peribronchovascular interstitium investing the larger central bronchi and vessels and coursing peripherally, producing the peripheral centrilobular interstitium. It eventually merges with the subpleural interstitium located beneath the visceral pleura and extending into the lungs at various intervals as interlobular septa. The normal interlobular septa measure approximately 0.1 mm in thickness and can occasionally be visible in a normal lung (6). However, the even smaller intralobular septa is a fine web of connective tissue not visualized on HRCT unless abnormal.

HIGH-RESOLUTION CT TECHNIQUE

Thin collimation and a high-spatial frequency (sharp) algorithm for image reconstruction are the basic principles of HRCT technique. HRCT has been well proved to be more sensitive and specific than both plain radiographs and conventional CT for demonstrating normal and abnormal lung interstitium, and for accuracy of differential diagnosis (9,10,11). Important technical parameters for HRCT are discussed next.

Scan Collimation

The use of very thin collimation, generally 1–1.5 mm, is used to optimize spatial resolution and visualization of small structures by reducing volume averaging with the adjacent lung. Murata et al. (12) evaluated the optimal collimation for high-resolution chest CT and concluded that slight increase (ground-glass opacity) or decrease (emphysema) in lung attenuation was better-resolved using 1.5 mm collimation than 3 mm collimation. However, other findings, such as thickened interlobular septa, were equally well visualized with both techniques. When reviewing thin-collimation images, the vessels can appear nodular, as a smaller segment of the vessel lies in the plane, compared to a thicker collimation scan where vessels appear cylindrical/branching allowing for easy differentiation from nodules (13). This is particularly true for incremental images that are separated anatomically. In volumetric HRCT, the anatomic contiguity can be seen when scrolling on a workstation and can help prevent this misinterpretation. Scanners are now capable of submillimeter collimation of 0.5–0.625 mm. Nishimoto et al. compared the visibility of air cysts on CT images obtained at 0.5, 1.0, and 2.5 mm section thickness, using an inflation-fixed autopsied lung with idiopathic interstitial pneumonia in which the maximum diameters of the air cysts was measured under a stereomicroscope (14). Using contact radiographs as the gold standard, 341 air cysts were identified. The CT was performed on a 4-row detector scanner at 120 kVp, and 150 mAs, using a 70 mm field of view. About 60%, 34%, and 8% of the 1–2 mm cysts were identified on the 0.5, 1, and 2.5 mm slice thickness images, respectively. No cysts measuring less than 1 mm were seen at 2.5 mm slice thickness, while 28% and 22% of less than 1 mm cysts were seen using 0.5 and 1 mm slice thickness, respectively.

High-Spatial Frequency Reconstruction Algorithm

The HRCT uses a high-spatial frequency reconstruction algorithm, referred to on some scanners as a bone algorithm, which increases the spatial resolution and sharpness of the structures (Fig. 2). Mayo et al. demonstrated improved quantitative spatial resolution and better subjective image quality when scan data was reconstructed with a bone algorithm instead of standard algorithm (15). However, this improved detail comes at the expense of increased image noise. Image noise can be reduced by increasing mA or increasing the scan time to increase mAs; increasing scan time is generally not recommended as this increases motion related artifacts. Noise is more of a

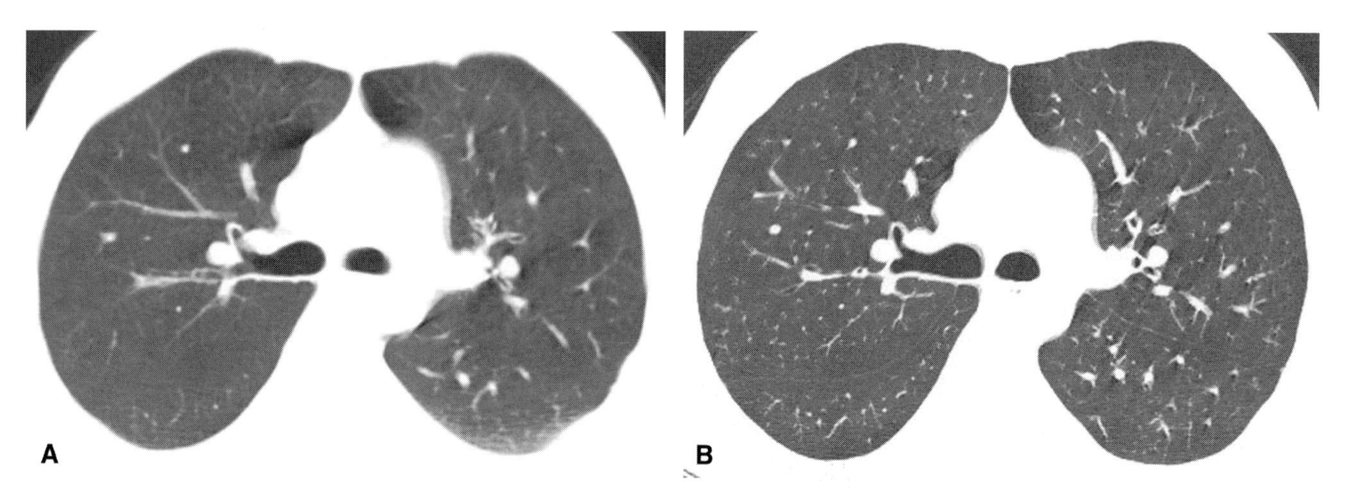

Figure 2 Volumetric CT scan obtained with 1.25 mm collimation and reconstructed using both a standard and a high-spatial frequency algorithm. Note the increased sharpness of the vessels and lung detail on the high-spatial frequency reconstruction algorithm image. (**A**) Standard algorithm; (**B**) High-spatial frequency "bone" algorithm.

concern in obese individuals due to attenuation of X-ray photons by the patient and is particularly marked in the paravertebral region, because of the photon attenuation by the spine. In these circumstances increased mA can be used, but it should be kept in mind that increasing the scan technique also increases radiation dose to the patient. This modification is not routinely necessary as diagnostic scans can be obtained in most individuals (13). Sometimes, even this provides suboptimal images in very obese patients, requiring an increase in collimation to 2–3 mm to reduce noise.

Zwirewich et al. (16) compared 10 mm standard lung CT images reconstructed using both high-spatial frequency and standard algorithms in 31 patients, recommending use of bone reconstruction algorithm for routine chest scans. They found that although the visible noise increased, the overall visual quality of the images was equal to or greater than the standard reconstruction algorithm in all of the lung images ($p < .001$) and in 85% of the mediastinal images ($p < .001$).

Matrix Size, Field of View, and Targeted Reconstruction

To reduce pixel size, the largest available matrix (usually 512 × 512) should be used. The field of view (FOV) should be large enough to include the thorax. Targeted reconstruction of a single lung instead of the entire thorax reduces the FOV and pixel size, thereby improving spatial resolution. It should however be remembered that the improvement in spatial resolution obtainable by retrospective targeting is limited by the resolution of the detectors and therefore, beyond a point, further reduction in FOV does not translate into improved spatial resolution (13). While targeted reconstructions improve spatial resolution, they are generally not used in routine clinical practice, due to the added reconstruction time, inability to compare one lung with the other, and lack of perceived or evaluated clinical benefit.

Incremental and Volumetric HRCT

Incremental HRCT

Individual images are obtained at spaced intervals during suspended respiration. Incremental HRCT therefore samples the lung and is most useful in the evaluation of diffuse interstitial lung disease. The HRCT in conjunction with a conventional CT may be needed depending on the clinical indication, particularly if the suspected abnormality has both a diffuse and focal component. Various scanning intervals have been used for HRCT, though a scan interval of 1 cm is commonly used. The scan spacing can vary with the clinical indication. Some have suggested that a limited HRCT obtained at three preselected levels may suffice for some forms of interstitial lung disease (17). Also, depending on the zonal predominance of the suspected disease or plain radiographic findings, more sections can be obtained in the abnormal region.

Two widely utilized supplementary HRCT techniques are prone imaging and imaging at end-expiration. Scanning with patient in prone position is necessary to differentiate early interstitial disease from atelectasis in dependent lung, known as dependent opacity. Unlike true interstitial disease, dependent opacity disappears on the prone images and can thus be easily differentiated (Fig. 3). It is most helpful in patients with normal lungs or subtle abnormalities to resolve the diagnostic dilemma of normal versus early interstitial disease. Volpe et al. (18) found that prone HRCT was helpful in confirming or excluding lung abnormality in 28% (10/36) of individuals with normal chest radiographs (CXR), 28% (5/18) with possibly abnormal radiographs, and 4% (2/46) with definitely abnormal CXR. Significantly, lower proportion of

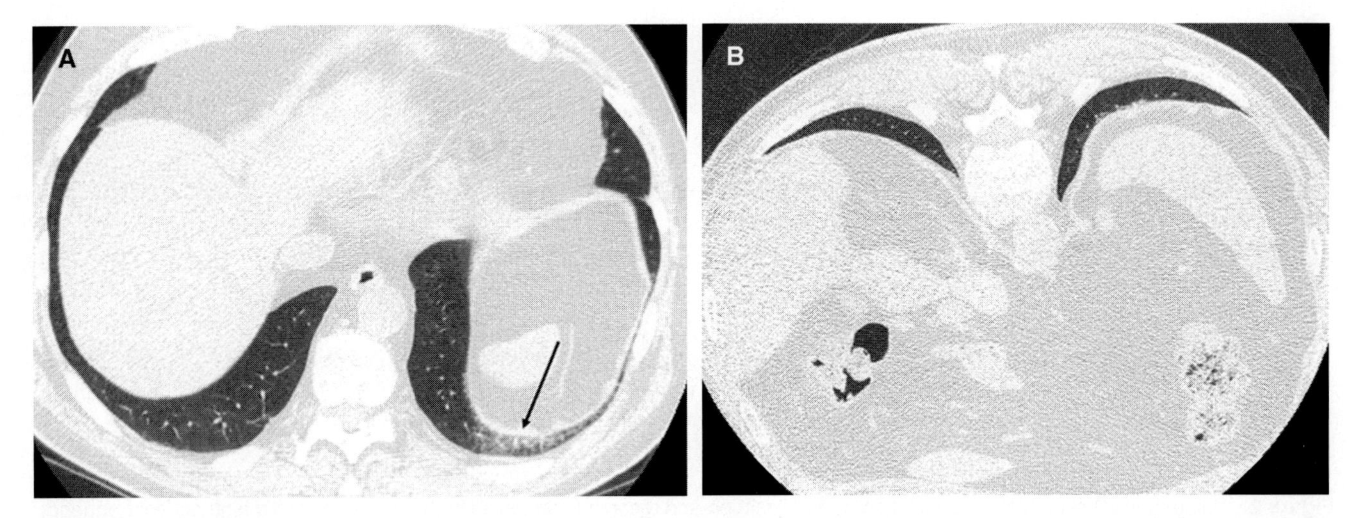

Figure 3 Volumetric HRCT with dependent atelectasis. The ground-glass opacity (*arrow*) in the left basilar region adjacent to the hemidiaphragm in the supine position disappears on the prone image, representing dependent atelectasis. Axial images in the (**A**) supine and (**B**) prone positions.

patients with definitely abnormal CXR benefited from prone scan compared to those with normal ($p = .008$) or possibly abnormal ($p = .02$) radio-graphs.

Expiratory HRCT images are useful to identify air trapping, which is a manifestation of small and large airway diseases, and emphysema. Areas showing air trapping fail to increase in attenuation on the expiratory images, while normal lung increases in attenuation with the reduction in air. Air trapping seen on expiratory images correlates with the degree of obstructive impairment in lung function in small airways disease (19). Also, expiratory images are useful in differentiating airway obstruction from infiltrative processes, both of which may produce a mosaic attenuation pattern on inspiratory images. Importantly, expiratory air trapping may be the only HRCT manifestation of small airway disease, such as asthma (Fig. 4) or bronchiolitis obliterans, and may be seen prior to the development of anatomic abnormalities, such as bronchiectasis or bronchial wall thickening (20). Expiratory imaging can be done at the end of a deep expiration with suspended respiration or trigger at a specific user selected lung volume based on spirometry (13).

In addition, fast multidetector scanners can acquire serial images during a forceful expiration, which increases the sensitivity for tracheomalacia. Boiselle et al. (21) recently showed the feasibility of cine imaging with 64-MDCT during a coughing maneuver for evaluating tracheomalacia. Seventeen patients with known or suspected benign central airway disease were scanned from the level of aortic arch to carina using a detector collimation of 0.5 mm × 64, 80 mA, 120 kVp, gantry rotation time of 0.4 s, and scan acquisition time of 7.2 s. The scan was performed in

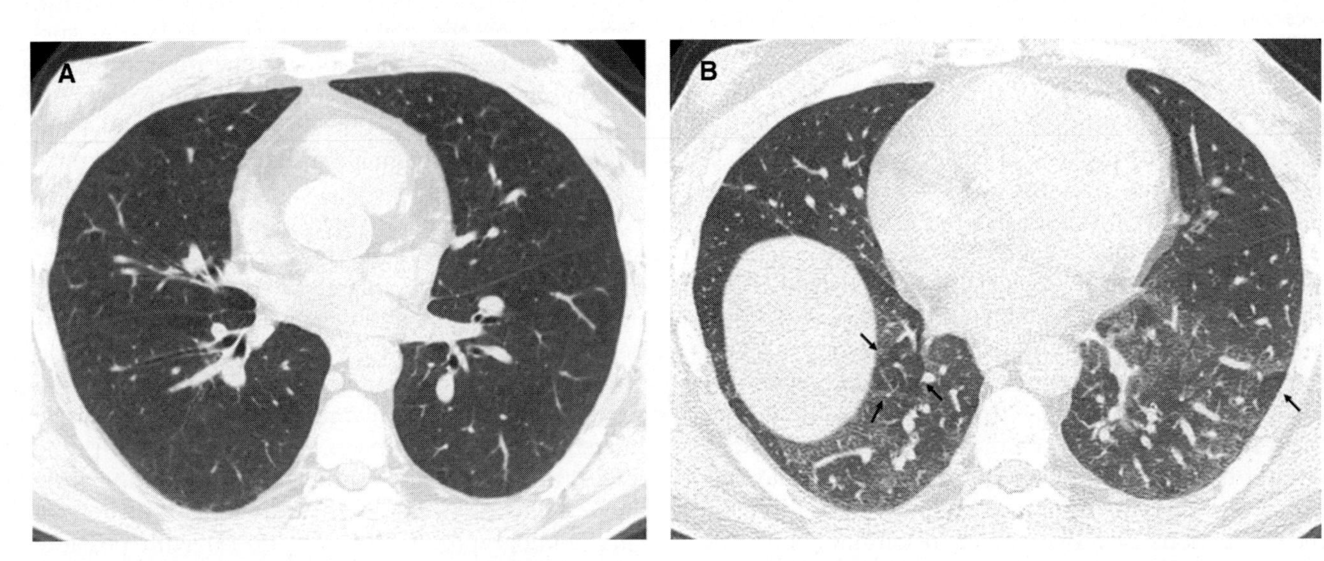

Figure 4 A 65-year-old female with asthma, a normal inspiratory HRCT, and abnormal expiratory HRCT. (**A**) Inspiratory image is normal. (**B**) Expiratory image reveals lobular air trapping (arrows).

cine mode beginning at end-inspiration and followed by repeated coughing maneuvers. More than 50% collapse during coughing was considered diagnostic of tracheomalacia. Sixteen of the 17 scanned patients were finally included in the study (1 patient had to be excluded due to technical error). Seventy-five percent (12/16) of patients met CT criteria for tracheomalacia. Of these 6 patients underwent bronchoscopy and the findings were concordant with those on CT. The estimated dose-length product (DLP) for the cine CT acquisition for a 70-kg patient was 220.8 mGy cm compared to a reference standard of 650 mGyy cm for a standard chest CT and 508.1 mGy cm for a dual phase helical (non cine) standard-dose inspiratory phase and low-dose expiratory CT scan of the trachea.

Volumetric HRCT

Multidetector volumetric HRCT allows contiguous visualization of the lung parenchyma with the ability to create three-dimensional images. It has several advantages over incremental HRCT, as listed below.

1. The entire lung is imaged with a volumetric HRCT. This ensures that important focal abnormalities, such as potential lung cancers, are not missed and is especially important in the context of diffuse diseases associated with an increased risk of bronchogenic cancer, such as emphysema (Fig. 5) and pulmonary fibrosis.
2. The ability to scroll through a stack of contiguous images allows for a better understanding of lung abnormalities and the relationship of findings to anatomic structures, including pulmonary vessels and airways. For example, dilated airways can be confidently differentiated from cysts by recognizing their tubular nature on adjacent images.
3. Volumetric 16-row and greater MDCT yields data sets with isotropic resolution, with the ability to generate distortion-free image reconstructions in any plane.
4. Both thin and thick sections can be reconstructed from the same data set. This makes it possible to assess both interstitial abnormalities using thin collimation, and nodules, focal abnormalities, and the central tracheobronchial tree using thicker collimation.
5. Multiplanar reconstructions allow rapid communication and demonstration of distribution and the pattern of diffuse lung disease to clinical colleagues who may be less facile with axial images (Figs. 6 and 7).

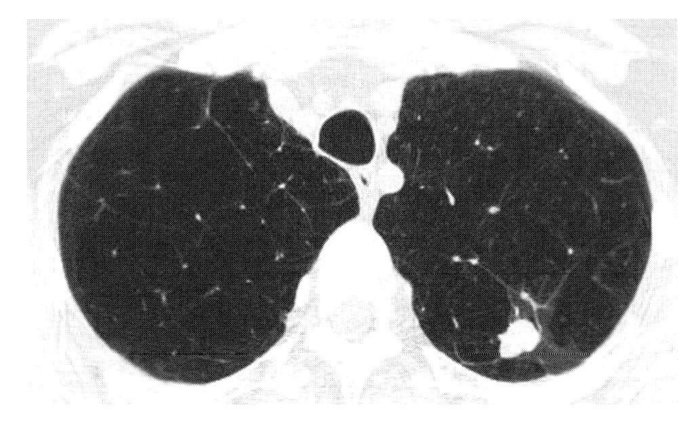

Figure 5 A 61-year-old female who underwent HRCT for the evaluation of emphysema. An unknown, incidental left upper lobe bronchogenic carcinoma was found.

The helical acquisition of multidetector HRCT results in a mild increase in effective slice thickness, due to the greater than one pitch used to acquire the data in a single-breath hold. This remains adequate for diagnostic purposes. For example, 16-row MDCT using a beam pitch of 1.375 (detector pitch 6) and detector collimations of 0.625 and 1.25 mm have an effective slice thickness of 0.8 and 1.50 mm, respectively (GE LightSpeed Qxi, technical specifications, GE Medical Systems, Milwaukee, Wisconsin, U.S.A.) (6).

The image quality of helical HRCT has been evaluated in several studies. Honda et al. (22) compared image quality and diagnostic efficacy of multidetector HRCT using six different MDCT parameters, as well as single-detector CT, using 11 cadaveric lungs. The image quality of multidetector HRCT using 1.25 mm × 4 mode was equal to single-detector HRCT, while the other modes were inferior. The parameters only mildly affected the diagnostic efficacy of multidetector HRCT, which was judged to be slightly worse when using 1.25 or 2.5 mm

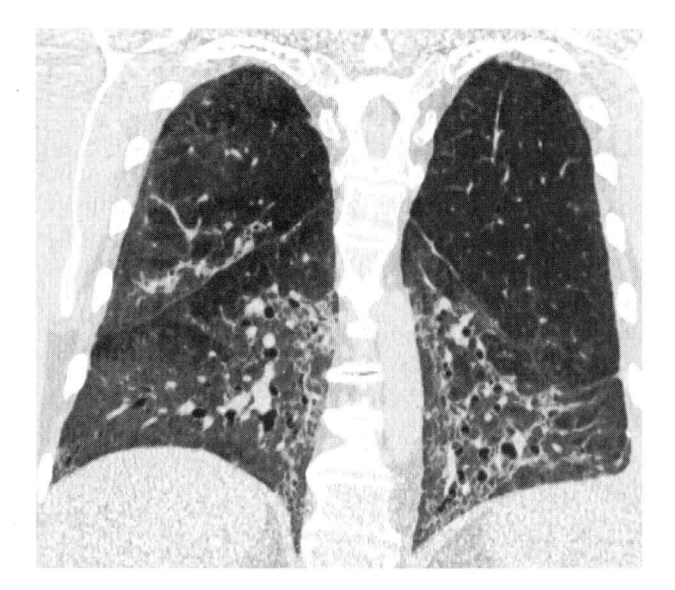

Figure 6 Volumetric HRCT of a 55-year-old male with nonspecific interstitial pneumonia (NSIP) diagnosed at surgical lung biopsy. Note the ground-glass opacity and traction bronchiectasis in a predominantly basilar distribution with relative sparing of the upper lungs, well illustrated on this coronal image.

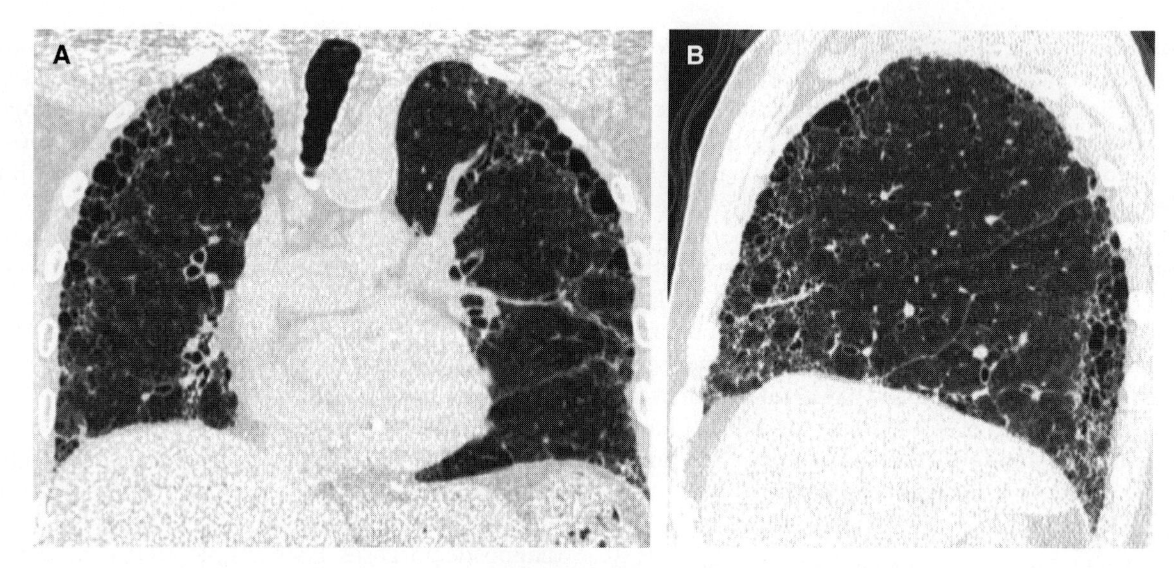

Figure 7 Volumetric HRCT of a 65-year-old male with usual interstitial pneumonitis. There is a subpleural and basilar predominant distribution of interlobular septal thickening and honeycombing on these (**A**) coronal and (**B**) sagittal images.

collimation with a pitch of 6, in one and four cases each, respectively. In these cases, they noted blurring of intralobular reticular opacities and vagueness of faint centrilobular nodules. In another study, Schoepf et al. randomly allocated 70 HRCT examinations in 67 patients to two groups (1). One group ($n = 35$) underwent MDCT using 1 mm collimation and a pitch of 6, and the other group ($n = 35$) underwent both conventional CT (5 mm collimation and pitch of 1.5) and standard axial HRCT (1 mm collimation at 10 mm intervals) on a single-detector CT scanner. They found no significant difference between the two sets of HRCT studies when rated for overall image quality, spatial resolution, depiction of bronchial walls, and presence of motion and streak artifacts. One potential limitation of this study was that comparison was made between two separate patient populations, rather than within the same patients; therefore, direct comparison was not possible. Similarly, Mehnert et al. showed equivalent image quality of multidetector HRCT to incremental HRCT images obtained on a single-detector CT scanner in 20 patients with diffuse lung disease (23). While sequential HRCT images were better than helically acquired multidetector HRCT images in terms of spatial resolution ($p = .02$), depiction of peripheral vessels ($p = .02$), and small bronchi ($p = .05$), multidetector HRCT was better for the depiction of interlobular septa ($p < .001$) and had three times less respiratory and cardiac motion artifact.

RECONSTRUCTIONS

Volumetric HRCT with isotropic resolution provides the radiologist a powerful tool enabling evaluation of lung parenchyma in all possible planes and orientations, as well as the tracheobronchial tree. Reconstruction of the axial data set in the coronal plane can reduce the number of individual images to be interpreted. Several studies have compared the quality of coronal reconstructions with direct coronal MDCT images. In the study by Honda et al. (24), 10 autopsy lung specimens were scanned using 4 protocols for axial scanning (0.5 mm collimation with 0.3 and 0.5 mm reconstruction intervals; 1 and 2 mm collimation with 0.5 and 1 mm reconstruction intervals); coronal reconstructions with 0.5 mm slice thickness were obtained from the axial data set. In addition, a direct coronal CT was acquired using 0.5 mm collimation, 0.3 mm reconstruction interval, 25.6 cm FOV, and a 512×512 matrix. There was equivalent image quality when comparing the coronal reconstructions obtained from the isotropic voxel data using 0.5 mm collimation, with or without overlap, to the direct coronal MDCT acquisition.

Remy-Jardin et al. compared the diagnostic accuracy of coronal images as an alternative to incremental HRCT in the diagnosis of interstitial lung disease (25). Volumetric 4×1 mm multidetector HRCT was obtained of the lungs in 50 patients with known or suspected interstitial lung disease. Both 1 mm coronal images and 1.25 mm axial images, each at 10 mm intervals, were reconstructed from the same volumetric data set. The mean number of coronal image reconstructions was significantly less than the axial image reconstructions, mean 19 versus 28 ($p < .01$). The quality of both image sets was rated high and sufficient for diagnostic purposes in suspected interstitial lung disease. Using axial HRCT as the reference standard, there was only one false negative result on the coronal image interpretations, yielding a sensitivity of 97% and specificity of 100%. In this case, mild ground-glass attenuation and bronchial dilatation were missed on the coronal images that were interpreted as normal; the findings could be appreciated in retrospect, and the false negative result thought to be due to the limited experience of the readers in interpreting coronal images in this case with mild disease that was limited to the lung bases. With respect to specific individual lung abnormalities, discrepancies between the two groups occurred in 4 patients (8%), with three false negative results on coronal images and one false positive, the latter felt to have been actually a false negative result from the axial images. Two of the three false-negative coronal image results were thought to be due to interpretative inexperience rather than a true limitation. In the third case of discordant interpretation small linear opacities perpendicular to the anterior chest wall were missed on coronal images. The single case attributed to actually being a false-negative case on the axial images was in a patient with sarcoidosis where abnormal interfaces were overlooked.

Newer Reconstruction Methods

Techniques such as MIP, sliding thin-slab maximum intensity projection (STS-MIP), and MinIP are readily available and their use can be tailored according to the specific clinical scenario.

Maximum Intensity Projection

The MIP images are achieved by displaying the highest attenuation value from the data encountered by a ray traced through the object of interest to the viewer (26). Because only the highest attenuation is displayed, MIP images represent less than 10% of the data (26). The STS-MIP reconstructions retain the high contrast resolution of thin section (1–3 mm) CT, while reducing partial volume effects within a sequence of overlapping thin slabs (27). These images viewed in sequence are less likely to obscure small structures in contrast to thick slab MIP images. There are ample studies in the literature that emphasize the role of STS-MIP image reconstructions for the detection of pulmonary nodules, due to improved visualization of peripheral vessels and greater distinction between nodules and vessels (Fig. 8A, B) (28,29,30). Coakley et al. evaluated MIP images and nodule detection, using 2 and 4 mm beads deployed in the peripheral airways to simulate 40 lung nodules in anesthetized dogs (28). CT was then performed with 5 mm collimation and a pitch of 2; MIP images were generated from overlapped slabs of seven consecutive 3 mm slices reconstructed at 2 mm intervals. MIP images increased the odds of pulmonary nodule detection by 2.18 ($p = .0002$), and increased reader confidence for nodule detection compared to axial image reconstructions ($p < .00001$). In a human study of 81 patients with suspected pneumoconiosis, sarcoidosis, smoker's bronchiolitis, and bronchiolitis of miscellaneous causes, 1 and 8 mm thick conventional CT images and focal helical CT were performed, the latter used to generate 3-mm, 5-mm, and 8-mm -thick MIP reconstructions (29). The sensitivity of MIP (3-mm-thick MIP, 94%; 5-mm-thick MIP, 100%; 8-mm-thick MIP, 92%) was significantly higher than conventional CT (8-mm-thick, 57%; 1-mm-thick, 73%) for the detection of micronodules ($p < .001$). The size of the detected micronodules was scored on a 3 point scale: 1 = rounded lesions <3 mm; 2 = rounded lesions 3–4 mm; 3 = rounded lesions 5–7 mm. In this study, all 36 patients with micronodular infiltration had micronodules <3 mm. Although MIPs did not demonstrate additional abnormalities when conventional CT findings were normal, they were useful when conventional axial CT was inconclusive by enabling detection of micronodules. When conventional axial CT did detect micronodules, MIPs better depicted their profusion and distribution. Gruden et al. studied the incremental effect of MIP image processing on the ability of junior and senior observers to detect small, <1 cm in diameter, central, and peripheral lung nodules on MDCT in 25 patients with metastatic disease and lung nodules ranging from 3 to 9 mm in diameter (31). CT examinations were obtained using 3.75 mm collimation, a pitch of 6, table speed of 15 mm/s, 140 kVp, and 180–210 mA, with MIP images reconstructed from the initial axial images at a slab thickness of 10 mm and reconstruction interval of 8 mm. Five reviewers, including three radiology residents and two radiology faculty members, independently interpreted both the axial and MIP images at two separate sessions. The reviewers cumulatively found a total of 122 nodules, 71 peripheral, and 51 central. The addition of MIP slabs significantly improved the detection of both central and peripheral nodules ($p < .001$). While the senior reviewers performed better than the junior reviewers in the detection of nodules of all types before the use of MIP processing ($p < .001$), the addition of MIP slabs reduced the effect of observer experience, and for peripheral nodules the significant difference in the number of lesions missed by senior and junior reviewers was eliminated. The addition of MIP slabs to the axial images improved the performance of the junior reviewers so that it was not statistically different from that of the senior reviewers interpreting axial images only.

Minimum Intensity Projection

These images are produced by displaying the lowest attenuation value encountered along a ray cast through an object toward the viewer's eye (26). These images are particularly useful for identifying areas and evaluating structures of low attenuation,

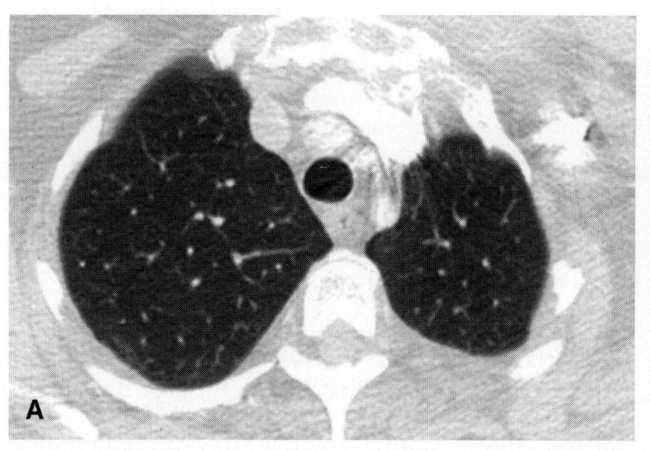

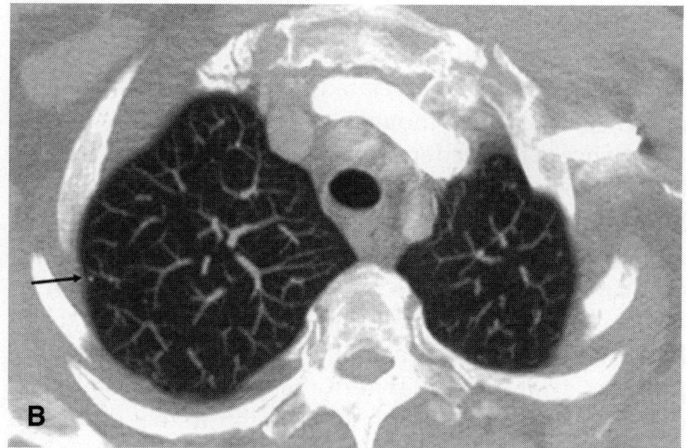

Figure 8 Impact of STS-MIP image reconstruction on the visualization of small pulmonary nodules. (**A**) A small pulmonary nodule is difficult to identify on a single thin slice image volumetric HRCT axial image. (**B**) On 5-mm-thick STS-MIP, the vessels appear cylindrical while the nodule (*arrow*) maintains its round shape, making detection easier.

such as emphysema, air trapping, the central tracheobronchial tree, and ground-glass opacities (30). In one study, the use of both MIP and MinIP techniques demonstrated additional findings not seen on conventional axial HRCT in 65% cases (13/20) (30). Remy Jardin et al. evaluated the role of MinIP in the diagnosis of emphysema in 29 patients undergoing lung resection, in which preoperative CT was performed with 1 mm collimation and 1 mm/s table speed (32). Three sets of sliding thin slab (STS) MinIP images were obtained with slab thickness of 3, 5, and 8 mm. The STS MinIP images had a higher sensitivity for emphysema detection compared to thin section CT of 81% versus 62%, while the specificity for both was 100%. In addition, emphysema was easier to detect on the 8 mm thick slabs.

RADIATION EXPOSURE

The high-spatial frequency reconstruction algorithm used in HRCT increases image noise. Increasing the mA can reduce noise, but at the same time also increases radiation dose to the patient. It is desirable to obtain the needed diagnostic information with the least possible radiation dose. Zwirewich et al. (33) evaluated the efficacy of low-dose HRCT in 31 patients using 1.5 mm collimation and 120 kVp at both 20 and 200 mA, at selected identical levels in the chest. The low-dose scan was equivalent to the conventional scan in the evaluation of vessels, lobar and segmental bronchi, anatomy of secondary pulmonary lobules, and in characterizing the extent and distribution of reticulation, honeycomb cysts, and thickened interlobular septa, but failed to demonstrate ground-glass opacity in two of 10 cases (20%) and emphysema in one of nine cases (11%) in which these findings were identified on the higher dose images. While these differences were not statistically significant and the two techniques were judged equally diagnostic in 97% of cases, this could be a result of the small sample size and low frequency of the abnormalities studied.

Although volumetric HRCT has several advantages over incremental HRCT, there is concern over increased radiation dose. Several studies have evaluated the image quality of volumetric HRCT obtained at varying mA levels. Jung et al. studied 12 patients with suspected bronchiectasis or lung cancer who underwent volumetric HRCT (120 kVp, 3 mm collimation, pitch 2, reconstruction interval 2 mm) at four different mA settings 150, 100, 70, and 40 mA, and incremental HRCT at 120 kVp, 170 mA, 1 mm collimation, and 10 mm intervals. There was no significant difference in the image quality at any of the four different mA levels ($p > .05$). The radiation dose for the 40 mA technique was 3.21 mGy, only slightly higher than the incremental HRCT at 2.17 mGy. The same authors evaluated the clinical applicability of volumetric HRCT in 52 patients with known or suspected small airway disease, with patients undergoing both incremental HRCT (120 kVp, 170 mA, 1 mm collimation at 10 mm intervals) and volumetric low-dose HRCT (120 kVp, 40 mA, 3 mm collimation, pitch 2; 24 s breath hold). Using the mean of positive interpretations for bronchiectasis by the five observers, volumetric HRCT identified more patients with bronchiectasis (47 vs. 44.5) and more bronchiectatic segments (193.5 vs. 152.5) than incremental HRCT. The authors concluded that low-dose HRCT at 40 mA has a greater diagnostic value than incremental HRCT for identifying bronchiectasis, with an acceptable image quality and only slightly higher radiation (34). Yi et al. (35) studied volumetric HRCT in 20 patients with suspected bronchiectasis, with acquisitions on a 4-row CT scanner using 120 kVp, 70 mA, 2.5 mm collimation, pitch 6, and six different mA settings (10, 20, 40, 70, 100, and 170 mA). The mean patient weight was 61 kg, which limits generalization to larger patients. The mean attenuation and standard deviation (SD) values were measured by placing regions of interest in the descending aorta, with SD values considered representative of image noise. Images of acceptable quality were obtained with tube current as low as 70 mA, while a further decrease to 40 mA abruptly increased the image noise and decreased image quality.

ARTIFACTS

Hurricane Artifact

Black and white linear opacities radiating out from objects with an attenuation value that is very different from adjacent structures on helical CT is called the hurricane artifact (36). This is believed to be due to a combination of several factors, such as data inconsistency between data acquisition and image reconstruction, partial volume averaging, and the cone beam effect. The artifact increases with an increase in table speed/slice collimation and is therefore more pronounced with MDCT than single-detector CT. Subtle abnormalities can be obscured by this artifact, therefore, low table speed/slice collimation is recommended. Black and white bands can be seen radiating from vessels filled with highly concentrated contrast in case of contrast enhanced MDCT, commonly seen on CT pulmonary angiograms. Although the exact mechanism of this artifact is unclear, it is attributed to absorption and attenuation of X-ray photons and motion artifact from rapidly moving contrast column (36,37). For these reasons, while CT pulmonary angiograms are obtained using similar collimation to HRCT examinations, it is not recommended that they be used to reconstruct an HRCT examination from the same contrast enhanced acquisition, as the artifacts make it difficult to evaluate for subtle interstitial lung disease and ground-glass opacity.

Motion Artifact

Motion artifacts are usually due to cardiac pulsation or respiration during image acquisition. These may manifest as a doubling artifact (Fig. 9), created an appearance of a duplicated fissure, vessels, or bronchi. Duplication of linear structures, particularly pulmonary vessels in the left lower lobe adjacent to the heart, may mimic bronchiectasis (Fig. 10), and knowledge of this artifact can prevent interpretive error. Pulsation artifacts or star artifacts are often seen adjacent to the heart and may manifest as streaks emanating from vessels resembling little stars (13).

Motion related artifacts can be reduced by using ECG gating (38), faster scanners (39), and spirometrically controlled respiration (40,41). Several studies have compared motion artifacts in high-resolution volumetric MDCT images obtained in a single-breath hold with incremental HRCT images obtained with several breath holds. There is no consensus as to which technique is associated with fewer artifacts. For example, Kelly et al. compared volumetric HRCT in the supine position with incremental HRCT acquired in the prone position in 47 patients with suspected interstitial disease; 40 studies were performed on 4-detector CT scanner and 7 on 16-detector CT scanner (42). Motion was graded at three anatomic levels on a scale of 0–3 (0, no motion; 1, mild motion; 2, moderate motion; 3, severe motion), and a total motion score derived by summing the scores from all three levels. The authors found significantly higher motion scores on volumetric HRCT images

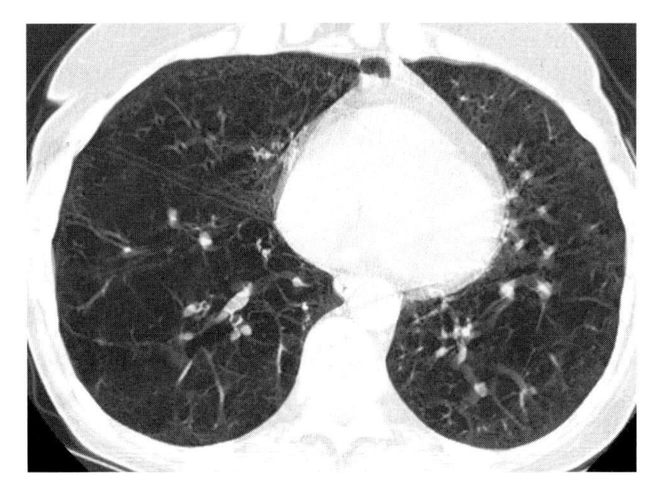

Figure 9 Volumetric HRCT with motion artifact creating a "doubling artifact" of the right major fissure and star artifacts around pulmonary vessels.

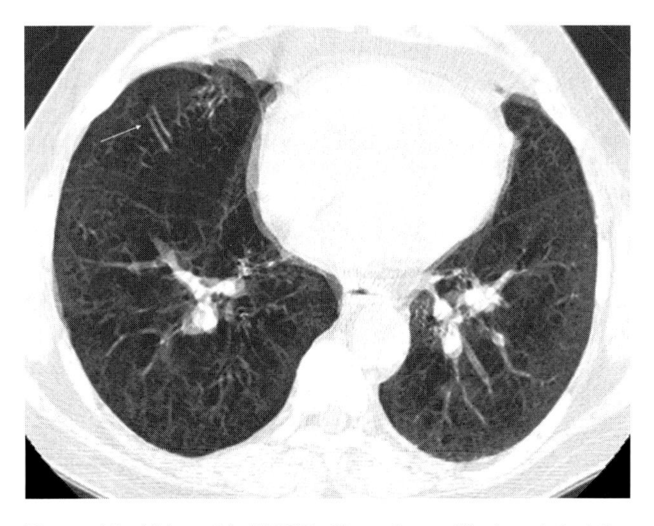

Figure 10 Volumetric HRCT with motion artifact and doubling of vessels (*arrow*) that can mimic bronchiectasis when close together.

compared to incremental HRCT images, with a median score of 3.0 versus 2.0 ($p = .02$). Mehnert et al. also evaluated the image quality of HRCT using spiral and incremental techniques, but in contrast found that breathing and heartbeat related motion artifacts were each three times higher using incremental HRCT technique ($p < .0001$) on a single-slice CT scanner compared to volumetric HRCT using 4-row detector scanner; overall image quality was not significantly different (23).

One important thing to remember is that volumetric MDCT can be problematic in dyspneic patients. This is because the entire helical scan is done in a single-breath hold, in contrast to an incremental HRCT, which is performed with a series of breath holds of 1 s or less. On 64-detector CT scanners, this is less of a problem, as the entire acquisition can be performed in approximately 5–8 s.

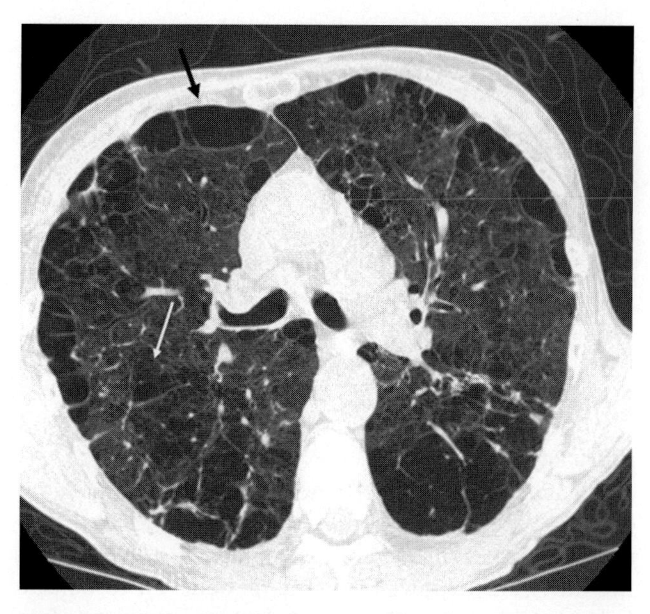

Figure 11 Volumetric HRCT in a 50-year-old male smoker with emphysema. Note the centrilobular emphysema seen as areas of abnormally low attenuation (*white arrow*) mainly surrounding the centrilobular artery branches, and paraseptal emphysema along the pleural surface (*black arrow*).

APPLICATION OF VOLUMETRIC CT IN SPECIFIC CLINICAL SCENARIOS

Evaluation of Emphysema

Emphysema is permanent abnormal enlargement of the airspaces distal to the terminal bronchiole, accompanied by destruction of their walls but without obvious fibrosis (43,44,45).

Emphysema is classified into three major subtypes, centrilobular, panlobular, and paraseptal. Centrilobular emphysema involves mainly the upper lungs, is commonly associated with cigarette smoking and is characterized on HRCT by multiple small round areas of abnormally low attenuation seen near the centers of secondary pulmonary lobules around the centrilobular artery branches (Fig. 11). In contrast, panlobular emphysema predominantly involves the lower lungs, is seen with α-1-antitrypsin deficiency, and appears on HRCT as uniform destruction of the pulmonary lobule and widespread areas of confluent low attenuation (Fig. 12). Paraseptal emphysema is subpleural or peripheral in location and involves the distal part of the secondary pulmonary lobule (Fig. 11). It may be an isolated finding or seen in association with centrilobular emphysema. Bullae are well demarcated areas of emphysema greater than 1 cm in diameter with wall thickness of less than 1 mm, and can accompany any form of emphysema. If significantly large, referred to as giant bullae, they can lead to respiratory compromise.

HRCT is invaluable in detection of emphysema, differentiating cystic lung disease from emphysema by demonstrating the absence of definable walls, and in quantifying emphysema. In addition, since emphysema patients are at risk for lung cancer, both on the basis of emphysema and cigarette smoking independently, CT detects and characterizes lung nodules. In the past, incremental HRCT in conjunction with a helical CT had to be performed for a comprehensive evaluation of emphysema and lung nodules at the same time. With the advent of volumetric HRCT all of the needed clinical information can be obtained from a single-helical inspiratory acquisition. The same data set is reconstructed at narrow collimation using a high-spatial frequency

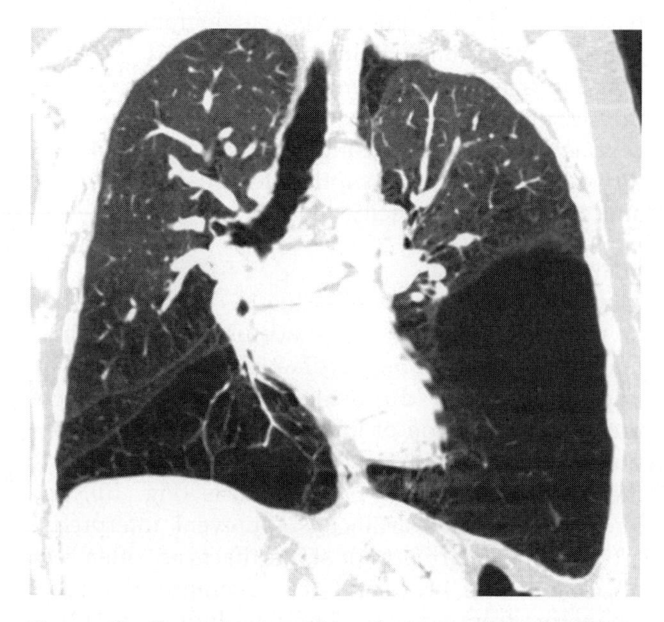

Figure 12 Coronal reformation of a volumetric HRCT in a 40-year-old female with α-1-antitrypsin deficiency. Note the panlobular emphysema in a lower lung predominant distribution.

reconstruction algorithm to evaluate the lung parenchyma, and thicker contiguous slice reconstructions with a standard algorithm to identify, characterize, and follow lung nodules. The role of CT in assessment of patients before surgery for emphysema such as bullectomy, lung transplant, and lung volume reduction surgery (LVRS) is detailed below.

Bullectomy

CT helps in preoperative evaluation by demonstrating the extent of bullous disease, degree of compression of adjacent lung, and severity of emphysema in remaining lung. Studies have shown that surgical treatment for bullous emphysema is most effective when bullae are larger than one-third of a hemithorax, with evidence of compression of adjacent lung tissue and an FEV1 of less than 50% predicted (46). Surgery is generally avoided in the presence of associated extensive emphysema (13).

Lung Transplantation

There are stringent selection criteria for lung transplantation. CT helps to determine the more abnormal lung and therefore the one chosen for single transplantation, which is performed more commonly than bilateral transplantation. Markedly abnormal pleura may also direct the surgeon to transplant the contralateral side (13). In a study of 190 transplant candidates in which both CXR and CT scans were reviewed, CT changed the determination of the more abnormal lung in 16% patients (27/169) from the CXR interpretation. Subsequently, 45 patients underwent transplantation and the decision regarding the side of transplant based on radiographs was changed in four patients (9%) due to the information provided from CT. In addition, three bronchogenic carcinomas were found on pretransplant imaging, of which two were occult on the CXR (47). This further emphasizes the need to be able to get lung parenchymal detail of HRCT with volumetric data in the evaluation of lung nodules, now possible with multidetector HRCT.

Lung Volume Reduction Surgery

Lung volume reduction surgery (LVRS) is based on the premise that removal of emphysematous poorly functioning lung parenchyma improves elastic recoil and reduces thoracic volume thereby resulting in improved chest wall excursion and tidal volume (48). It can be performed as both a unilateral or bilateral procedure, and either by video-assisted thoracoscopic surgery (VATS), sternotomy, or thoracotomy (48). The clinical outcome after LVRS depends on the regional distribution of emphysema (49–55). Patients with heterogeneous or focal emphysema have a better prognosis after LVRS compared than patients with diffuse emphysema (Fig. 12). An estimate of emphysema distribution and severity can be obtained from CT by visual scoring or quantitative analysis based on attenuation thresholds (Fig. 13). There is excellent correlation between the determination of emphysema severity by CT using both visual and quantitative methods with pathological specimens (56). Müller et al. used the density mask technique with 10 mm thick sections and found a good correlation ($r = .89$) with emphysema scores measured on inflation-fixed lung specimens using a modification of Thurlbeck et al. picture grading system (57). Similarly, there was good correlation between the visual score with the pathology score (0.9). The sensitivity for emphysema detection using visual score was 71% and 86% by two readers and 86% for the density mask method. Quantitative measurement is performed on inspiratory images to avoid any inaccuracy resulting from air trapping on expiration (48).

Because of the risk of lung cancer in emphysema patients, a standard HRCT should be supplemented by a contiguous CT to maximize detection and evaluation of lung nodules. Volumetric HRCT accomplishes both the above mentioned objectives (evaluation of emphysema as well as detection of lung nodules) in a single scan. There is an approximately 5% incidence of incidentally detected lung cancer in emphysema patients being evaluated for either LVRS or lung transplant, most of which are first detected on CT and are occult on CXRs (47,58). However, a significant proportion of noncalcified lung nodules in these patients do not turn out to be cancers. It has been estimated that about 11–26% have one or more noncalcified nodule (47,58,59). In one series, only 22% of the detected nodules were greater than 1 cm in size (60). The location of nodule is important to identify with respect to the proposed area of lung resection in LVRS candidates. If needed, a combined LVRS and nodule resection can be performed in selected patients. Though this procedure is associated with little morbidity and mortality (59), the postoperative outcome in these patients has been reported to be less satisfactory than those of patients undergoing LVRS alone (61).

Evaluation of Diffuse Interstitial Lung Disease

Incremental HRCT samples the lung at intervals with each image being obtained independently during a separate breath hold. These images are samples of the lung parenchyma, and are useful in evaluating the presence, pattern, and severity of diffuse interstitial lung disease. However, there is also an increased risk of lung cancer in usual interstitial pneumonitis (UIP) and with an estimated incidence of 4.4–9.8% (62–64). UIP is thought to be an independent risk factor for

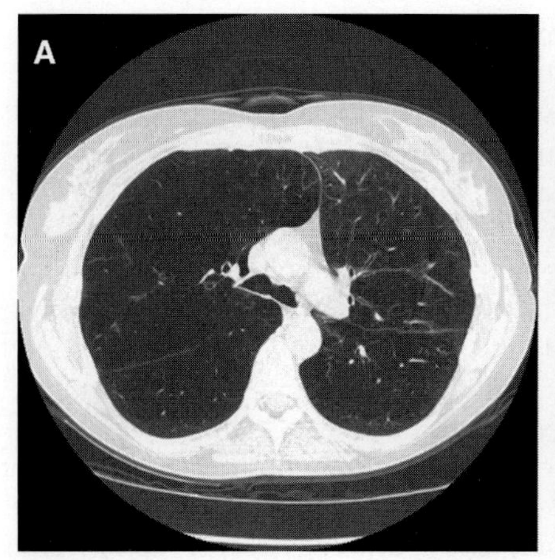

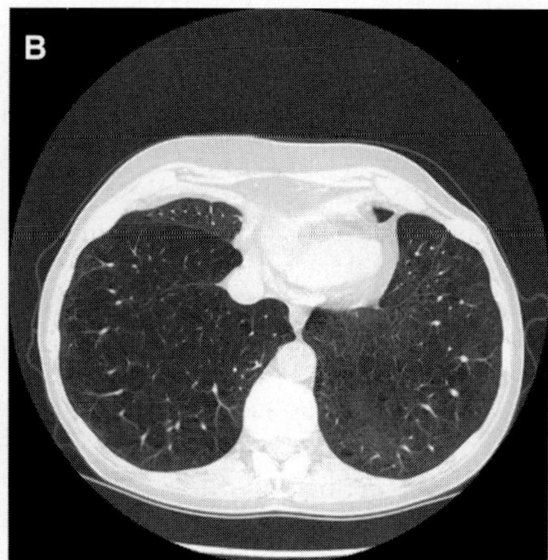

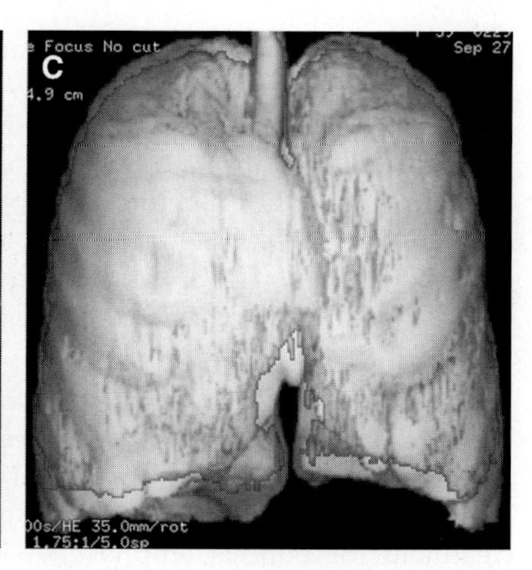

Figure 13 Volumetric HRCT in a 58-year-old male being evaluated as a candidate for LVRS. Axial sections at (**A**) the level of carina and (**B**) through the lower lobes show diffuse severe emphysema. (**C**) Three-dimensional shaded surface display using the density mask technique demonstrates diffuse severe emphysema.

lung cancer, with an independent relative risk of approximately 7.3 (63,64). Squamous cell carcinoma is the predominant type. These cancers often occur in areas of fibrosis, with up to 50% of the cancers first identified as incidental findings on imaging done for another reason (65,66). Volumetric HRCT is therefore preferable as it allows a comprehensive evaluation of both the interstitial process and lung nodules. Another advantage of MDCT is the ability to reconstruct the data in any desired plane, thereby permitting a better depiction of the distribution of disease. For interstitial diseases with a predominantly nodular distribution, MIP images improve the detection of nodules, their profusion, and their distribution relative to the secondary pulmonary lobule (2). Similarly, subtle ground-glass attenuation not easily visualized on the routine axial images, appears more pronounced, and easier to recognize on MinIP as an abnormal contrast between endobronchial air and lung parenchyma (2). Multiplanar reformats are useful in differentiating lung cysts from cystic bronchiectasis by demonstrating lack of connection between the air filled structure and bronchi in the former (Fig. 14). Also, volumetric CT allows the reader to scroll through a stack of contiguous images and hence the tubular nature of dilated bronchi is easily differentiated from lung cysts. This is particularly useful in cases of Langerhans cell histiocytosis that may present with bizarre, irregular cysts closely mimicking bronchiectasis. Similarly, traction bronchiolectasis can be differentiated from honeycombing in usual interstitial pneumonitis.

While computer aided diagnosis (CAD) is being aggressively developed for lung nodule detection, characterization, and growth on CT images, CAD is also being applied to interstitial diseases. The assessment of lung fibrosis holds promise (67). Best et al. evaluated quantitative CT indexes in idiopathic pulmonary fibrosis and studied its relationship with physiologic impairment. The authors used measurements of skewness, kurtosis, and mean lung attenuation on HRCT histograms in 144 patients with idiopathic pulmonary fibrosis and found moderate correlation with pulmonary function tests (68).

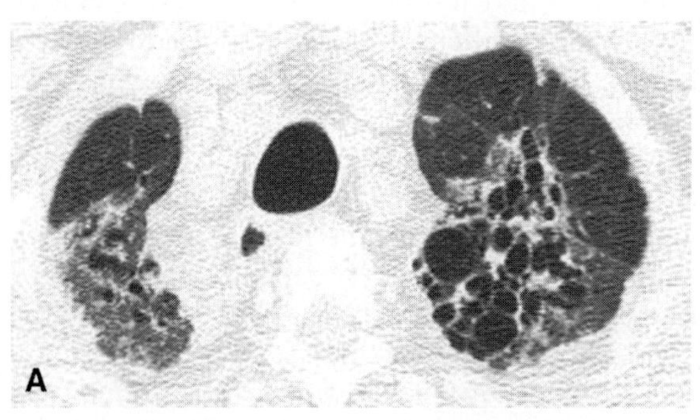

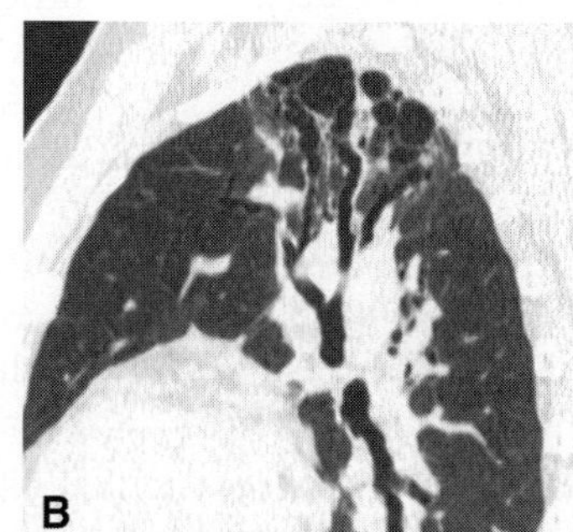

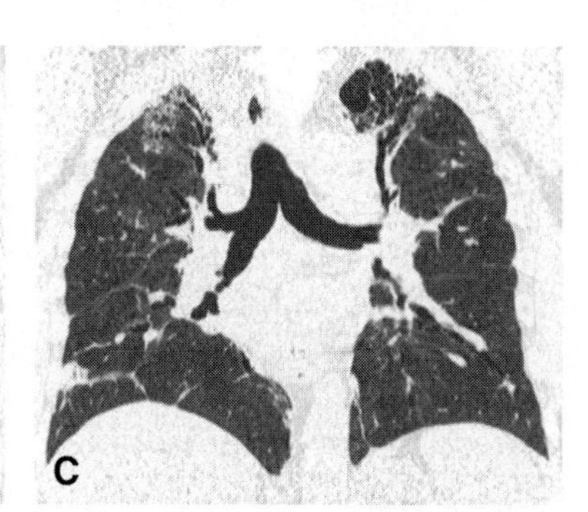

Figure 14 Volumetric HRCT in a 56-year-old female patient with suspected interstitial lung disease. Axial section through the lung apices (**A**) demonstrates multiple cystic spaces in cross section at the left apex that could be interpreted as honeycombing. (**B**) Sagittal and (**C**) coronal reformatted images clearly show dilated bronchi leading to the cysts and communicating with them, differentiating bronchiectasis from cystic lung disease.

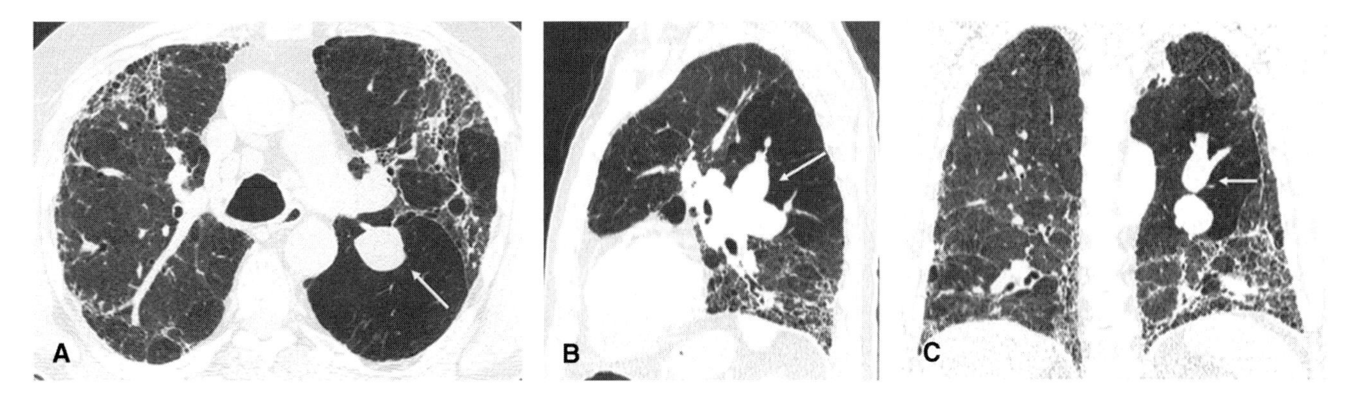

Figure 15 Volumetric HRCT in a 53-year-old female patient with usual interstitial pneumonitis (UIP) and a lung mass. (**A**) Axial image demonstrates a mass (*arrow*) in the superior segment of left lower lobe with surrounding lucency. (**B**) Sagittal and (**C**) coronal reformats clearly demonstrate the branching and tubular nature of this lesion (*arrow*) with surrounding parenchymal low attenuation compatible with bronchocele due to bronchial atresia. The ability to scroll through contiguous images and make multiplanar reformats from a multidetector HRCT helps to confidently differentiate it from a malignant mass.

IMAGING OF THE AIRWAYS

Incremental HRCT has several inherent disadvantages because of interscan gaps. These include difficulty in identifying the lack of normal tapering in cases of bronchiectasis, especially of the small distal airways, a possibility of missing airway pathology in the "skip" regions, and confusing mucoid impaction with pulmonary masses (Fig. 15). Studies have compared incremental HRCT with volumetric CT in the evaluation of bronchiectasis and substantiated the superiority of the latter in this context (34). The ability to reconstruct coronal images and analyze them in conjunction with axial images has been shown to improve both the detection rate and reader confidence in identifying the distribution and type of bronchiectasis (69). Sung et al. evaluated the effectiveness of additional coronal images in the diagnosis of bronchiectasis using low-milliamperage MDCT (69). Volumetric CT scans (2.5 mm collimation, table speed of 15 mm/s, table rotation time of 1 s, 120 kVp, 70 mA) were obtained in 110 patients with suspected bronchiectasis, with coronal images reconstructed at 1.3–2 mm section thickness. Two independent observers first assessed only the axial images, and then both axial and coronal images together. Using axial images alone, bronchiectasis was detected in 97% of patients (213/220 patients, $k = 0.888$), versus 100% (220/220 patients, $k = 1.000$) ($p = .0001$) when using both the axial and coronal images, and reader confidence for the distribution of bronchiectasis was also higher ($p = .008$).

In addition to the smaller airways and lung parenchyma, multidetector HRCT allows detailed evaluation of the central tracheobronchial tree. One important clinical application is the evaluation of patients with hemoptysis, which may be caused by various conditions including neoplasia, bronchiectasis, pneumonia, and bronchitis (70). Fiberoptic bronchoscopy (FOB) is most useful in older patients with a smoking history and a focally abnormal CXR (71). The diagnostic yield of FOB is lower when the CXR is normal, in which case malignancy is found in approximately 6% of smokers over 40 years of age (72). In this latter scenario, CT can identify the cause of hemoptysis in a significant number of individuals. For example, in a study by Millar et al., CT identified the cause of hemoptysis in 20 of 40 patients with a normal CXR, normal FOB, and normal sputum examination (73). For this indication, incremental HRCT would need to be supplemented with an additional helical scan. However, using volumetric HRCT, the evaluation for both bronchiectasis and central airway disease can be accomplished from one acquisition.

Not only can a volumetric scan identify central airway tumors, it can also assess the locoregional spread and the craniocaudal extent (Fig. 16). The relationship of the tumor with adjacent tissue and mediastinal lode enlargement is well demonstrated with this technique. In a study of 44 patients with known malignancy, 4×1.25 mm MDCT with virtual bronchoscopy had a sensitivity of 83% and specificity of 100% for identifying endobronchial lesions (74).

Regarding the evaluation of stenoses, multiplanar reconstructions (MPR) are very useful. Slight variations in caliber of airways can be difficult to appreciate on axial images alone, causing webs and focal strictures to be missed. MPRs enable detection of these abnormalities and accurate measurement of their craniocaudal extent. Quint et al. evaluated the accuracy of helical CT with MPRs for detecting central airway stenosis in 27 lung transplant recipients and 17 other patients using CT performed at 3 mm collimation with a pitch ratio of 1, 3 mm/s table speed, 280 mA and 120 kVp (75). In transplant recipients, images were obtained from approximately 2 cm above

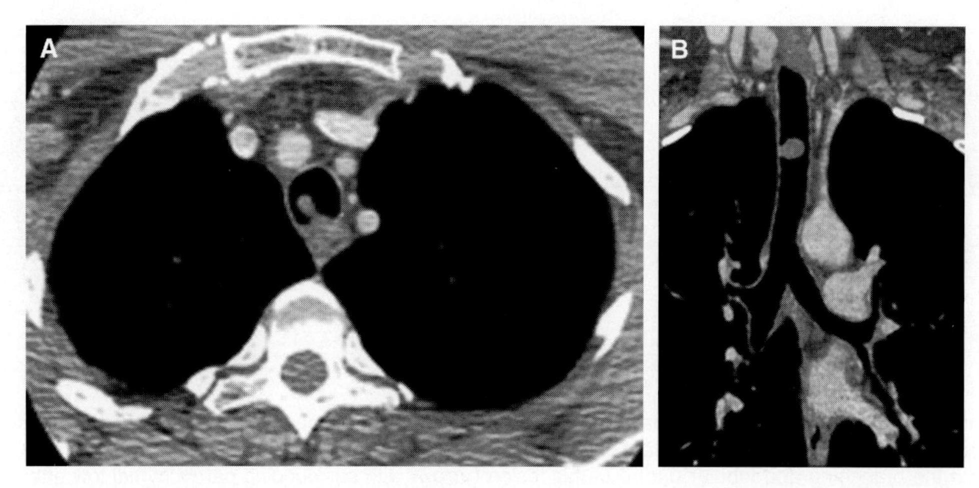

Figure 16 Volumetric HRCT of a 45-year-old female with tracheal leiomyoma. (**A**) Axial image demonstrates a polypoid lesion arising from the trachea posteriorly. (**B**) The coronal image demonstrates the craniocaudal extent and relationship to the carina.

the carina to approximately 7 cm below the carina, while for the other patients imaging was done from the epiglottis to the level of the left upper lobe of the bronchus. CT data was reconstructed in the axial plane at 1.5 mm intervals and used to create 1-pixel-thick angled coronal and sagittal MPRs oriented along the long axis of the airway being studied. CT findings were compared to bronchoscopy and conventional tomography. In transplant recipients, axial CT alone was 91% accurate, CT with MPRs was 94% accurate, and conventional tomography 89% accurate in the evaluation of bronchial anastomosis. For stenosis in non-transplant patients, axial CT alone and CT scans with MPRs were both 91% accurate, with the single false negative finding being focal tracheomalacia at bronchoscopy.

CT can be used to evaluate the airway distal to a stenosis or mass that is not passable with a bronchoscope. A limitation of MDCT is its inability to identify the subtle mucosal changes of early malignancies recognized by direct visualization with bronchoscopy (74). A study of 20 patients comparing MDCT with flexible bronchoscopy reported sensitivity and specificity of 90% and 96.6% for central airway stenoses and 90% and 95.6% for segmental strictures, respectively (76).

EVALUATION OF CANCER PATIENTS WITH RESPIRATORY SYMPTOMS

Dyspnea is a frequent symptom in cancer patients and can be due to various reasons, including lymphangitic

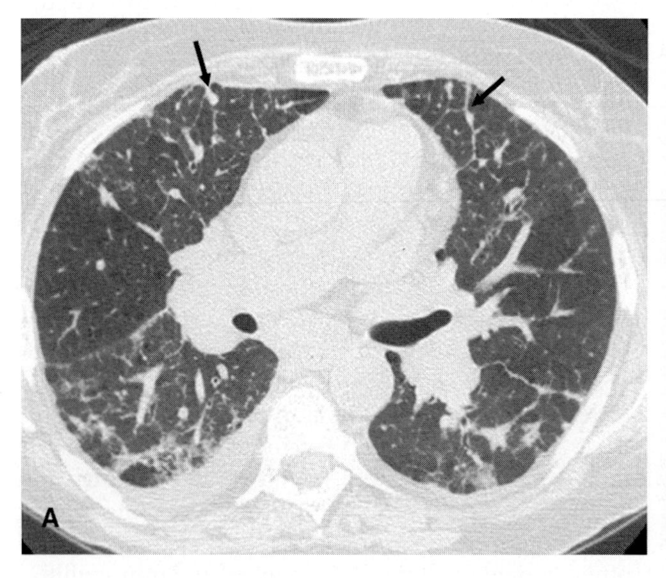

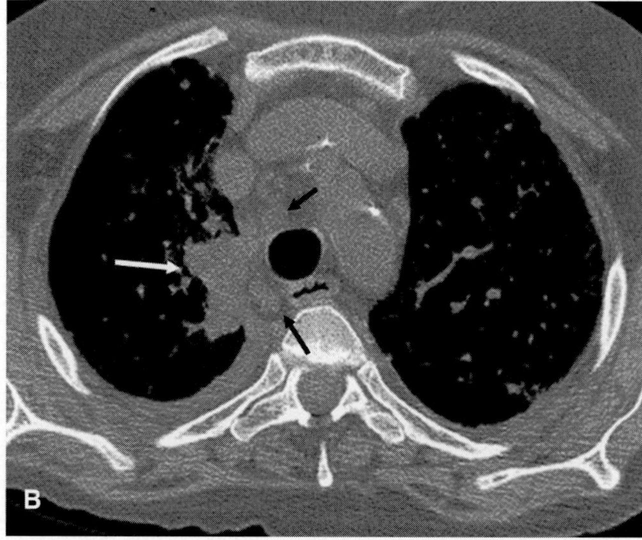

Figure 17 Volumetric HRCT in a 69-year-old female with lung cancer who presents with dyspnea. Multidetector HRCT allows a comprehensive evaluation of the lung for possible lymphangitic spread as well as the tumor extent. (**A**) Note the nodular interlobular septal thickening (*arrows*) consistent with lymphangitic carcinomatosis. (**B**) The right upper lobe primary bronchogenic cancer (*white arrow*) along with enlarged mediastinal nodes (*black arrows*) and tiny right pleural effusion is also seen.

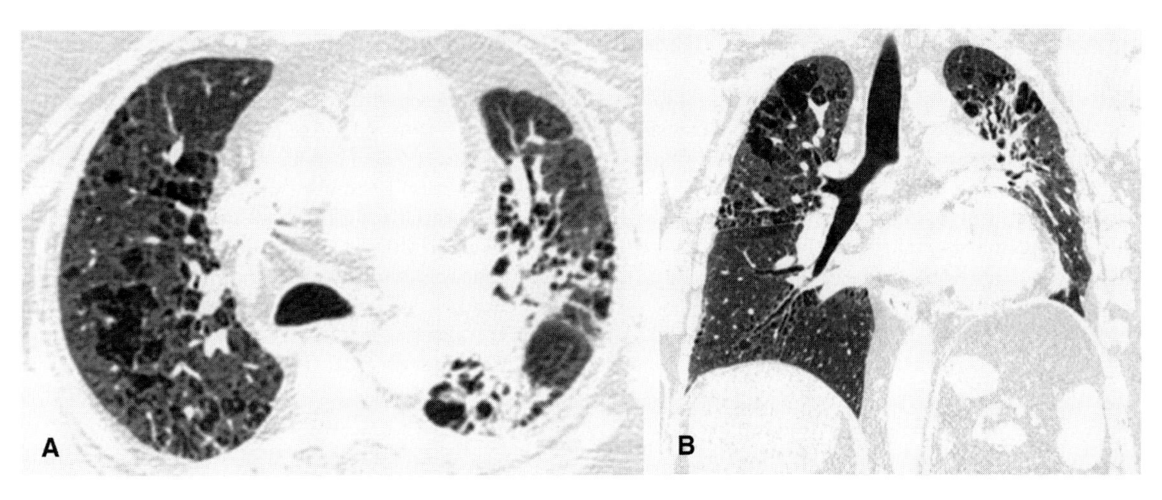

Figure 18 Postradiation changes in a patient with lung cancer. Note the air space disease with bronchiectasis in a left paramediastinal location with straight margins on the axial image (**A**) better evaluated on the coronal reformat (**B**).

spread of tumor, hematogenous lung metastases, postobstructive atelectasis due to tumor obstructing a bronchus, pleural effusions, radiation lung injury, and drug-induced lung toxicity (6). Additionally, these patients are predisposed to developing venous thromboembolic disease and infection, and may have other comorbid conditions such as chronic obstructive pulmonary disease (COPD), all of which can present with shortness of breath (77,78).

Lymphangitic carcinomatosis refers to tumor growth in the lymphatic system of the lungs. HRCT is the test of choice and exquisitely demonstrates smooth and nodular thickening of the peribronchovascular interstitium, interlobular septa, and subpleural interstitium with preservation of the normal lung architecture forming a polygon appearance (Fig. 17). However, since oncology patients often have more than one cause of dyspnea, an incremental HRCT alone cannot provide all the information because of interscan gaps. Thus, a comprehensive evaluation necessitates an additional helical scan to fully evaluate the extent of tumor, presence of lung metastases, and effect of the tumor on airways. Multidetector HRCT serves the dual purpose in a single acquisition and can be used to evaluate the fine parenchymal details of lymphangitic carcinomatosis as well as tumor extent. Sometimes dyspnea may be a result of therapy (e.g., radiotherapy and chemotherapeutic drugs) itself. Radiation related lung injury is confined to the treatment field, and can be recognized by its temporal progression and course. In the acute stage, radiation pneumonitis presents as diffuse ground-glass opacities in the treatment field, which develop into patchy airspace disease. The onset of these findings is varied and can develop within 1 week of therapy, usually peaking 3–4 months after therapy (79,80,81). Radiation fibrosis may develop within 3 months of treatment, or many years later, but is typically stable after 1–2 years, and has a characteristic appearance of architectural distortion and traction bronchiectasis with straight boundaries conforming to the radiation field (Fig. 18) (80,81).

SUMMARY

Volumetric HRCT has several advantages over a standard incremental HRCT, and is useful in specific clinical scenarios where evaluation of both focal and diffuse components of a disease process and/or the central tracheobronchial tree is needed. Attention to radiation dose is important, and can be managed using low-dose volumetric HRCT techniques.

REFERENCES

1 Schoepf UJ, Bruening RD, Hong C, et al. Multislice helical CT of focal and diffuse lung disease: comprehensive diagnosis with reconstruction of contiguous and high-resolution CT sections from a single thin-collimation scan. Am J Roentgenol 2001; 177:179–84.
2 Beigelman-Aubry C, Hill C, Guibal A, Savatovsky J, Grenier PA. Multi-detector row CT and postprocessing techniques in the assessment of diffuse lung disease. RadioGraphics 2005; 25:1639–52.
3 Pipavath S, Godwin JD. Imaging of interstitial lung disease. Clin Chest Med 2004; 25:455–65, v–vi.
4 Gotway MB, Reddy GP, Webb WR, Elicker BM, Leung JW. High-resolution CT of the lung: patterns of disease and differential diagnoses. Radiol Clin North Am 2005; 43:513–42, viii.
5 Webb WR. Thin-section CT of the secondary pulmonary lobule: anatomy and the image—the 2004 Fleischner lecture. Radiology 2006; 239:322–38.
6 Bhartia B, Kazerooni EA. Multislice CT in the investigation of interstitial lung disease. In: Multislice CT: Principles and Protocols. Knollman F, Coakley FV, eds. Philadelphia, PA: Saunders/Elsevier, 2006:60–77.

7 Webb WR, Stein MG, Finkbeiner WE, et al. Normal and diseased isolated lungs: high resolution CT. Radiology 1988; 166:81–87.
8 Murata K, Itoh H, Todo G, et al. Centrilobular lesions of the lung: demonstration by high resolution CT and pathologic correlation. Radiology 1986; 161:641–5.
9 Schurawitzki H, Stiglbauer R, Graninger W, et al. Interstitial lung disease in progressive systemic sclerosis: high-resolution CT versus radiography. Radiology 1990; 176:755–9.
10 Remy-Jardin M, Remy J, Deffontaines C, Duhamel A. Assessment of diffuse infiltrative lung disease: comparison of conventional CT and high-resolution CT. Radiology 1991; 181:157–62.
11 Mathieson JR, Mayo JR, Staples CA, Muller NL. Chronic diffuse infiltrative lung disease: comparison of diagnostic accuracy of CT and chest radiography. Radiology 1989; 171:111–6.
12 Murata K, Khan A, Rojas KA, Herman PG. Optimization of computed tomography technique to demonstrate the fine structure of the lung. Invest Radiol 1988; 23:170–5.
13 Webb WR, Muller NL, Naidich DP. Technical aspects of high resolution computed tomography. In: Webb WR, Muller NL, Naidich DP, eds. High Resolution CT of the lung. 3rd ed. Philadelphia: Lippincott Williams and Wilkins, 2001:1–47.
14 Nishimoto Y, Takahashi M, Murata K, et al. Honeycombing cysts in an inflated and fixed lung specimen: the effect of CT section thickness. Korean J Radiol 2005; 6:17–21.
15 Mayo JR, Webb WR, Gould R, et al. High-resolution CT of the lungs: an optimal approach. Radiology 1987; 163:507–10.
16 Zwirewich CV, Terriff B, Muller NL. High-spatial-frequency (bone) algorithm improves quality of standard CT of the thorax. AJR Am J Roentgenol 1989; 153:1169–2273.
17 Kazerooni EA, Martinez FJ, Flint A, et al. Thin-section CT obtained at 10-mm increments versus limited three-level thin-section CT for idiopathic pulmonary fibrosis: correlation with pathologic scoring. AJR Am J Roentgenol 1997; 169:977–83.
18 Volpe J, Storto ML, Lee K, et al. High-resolution CT of the lung: determination of the usefulness of CT scans obtained with the patient prone based on plain radiographic findings. AJR Am J Roentgenol 1997; 169: 369–74.
19 Arakawa H, Webb WR, McCowin M, Katsou G, Lee KN, Seitz RF. Inhomogeneous lung attenuation at thin-section CT: diagnostic value of expiratory scans. Radiology 1998; 206:89–94.
20 Arakawa H, Webb WR. Air trapping on expiratory high-resolution CT scans in the absence of inspiratory scan abnormalities: correlation with pulmonary function tests and differential diagnosis. AJR Am J Roentgenol 1998; 170:1349–53.
21 Boiselle PM, Lee KS, Lin S, Raptopoulos V. Cine CT during coughing for assessment of tracheomalacia: preliminary experience with 64-MDCT. AJR Am J Roentgenol 2006 Aug; 187:W175–7.
22 Honda O, Johkoh T, Tomiyama N, et al. High-resolution CT using multidetector CT equipment: evaluation of image quality in 11 cadaveric lungs and a phantom. AJR Am J Roentgenol 2001; 177:875–9.
23 Mehnert F, Pereira PL, Dammann F, et al. High resolution multislice CT of the lung: comparison with sequential HRCT slices. Rofo Fortschr Geb Rontgenstr Neuen Bildgeb Verfahr 2000; 172:972–7.
24 Honda O, Johkoh T, Yamamoto S, et al. Comparison of quality of multiplanar reconstructions and direct coronal multidetector CT scans of the lung. AJR Am J Roentgenol 2002; 179:875–9.
25 Remy-Jardin M, Campistron P, Amara A, et al. Usefulness of coronal reformations in the diagnostic evaluation of infiltrative lung disease. J Comput Assist Tomogr 2003; 27:266–73.
26 Dalrymple NC, Prasad SR, Freckleton MW, Chintapalli KN. Informatics in radiology (infoRAD): introduction to the language of three-dimensional imaging with multidetector CT. RadioGraphics 2005; 25:1409–28.
27 Napel S, Rubin GD, Jeffrey RB Jr. STS-MIP: a new reconstruction technique for CT of the chest. J Comput Assist Tomogr 1993; 17:832–8.
28 Coakley FV, Cohen MD, Johnson MS, Gonin R, Hanna MP. Maximum intensity projection images in the detection of simulated pulmonary nodules by spiral CT. Br J Radiol 1998; 71:135–40.
29 Remy-Jardin M, Remy J, Artaud D, Deschildre F, Duhamel A. Diffuse infiltrative lung disease: clinical value of sliding-thin-slab maximum intensity projection CT scans in the detection of mild micronodular patterns. Radiology 1996; 200:333–9.
30 Bhalla M, Naidich DP, McGuinness G, Gruden JF, Leitman BS, McCauley DI. Diffuse lung disease: assessment with helical CT—preliminary observations of the role of maximum and minimum intensity projection images. Radiology 1996; 200:341–7.
31 Gruden JF, Ouanounou S, Tigges S, et al. Incremental benefit of maximum-intensity-projection images on observer detection of small pulmonary nodules revealed by multidetector CT. AJR Am J Roentgenol 2002; 179:149–57.
32 Remy-Jardin M, Remy J, Gosselin B, Copin MC, Wurtz A, Duhamel A. Sliding thin slab, minimum intensity projection technique in the diagnosis of emphysema: histopathologic-CT correlation. Radiology 1996; 200:665–71.
33 Zwirewich CV, Mayo JR, Muller NL. Low-dose high-resolution CT of lung parenchyma. Radiology 1991; 180:413–7.
34 Jung KJ, Lee KS, Kim SY, Kim TS, Pyeun YS, Lee JY. Low-dose, volumetric helical CT: image quality, radiation dose, and usefulness for evaluation of bronchiectasis. Invest Radiol 2000; 35:557–63.
35 Yi CA, Lee KS, Kim TS, Han D, Sung YM, Kim S. Multidetector CT of bronchiectasis: effect of radiation dose on image quality. AJR Am J Roentgenol 2003; 181:501–5.
36 Johkoh T, Honda O, Mihara N, et al. Pitfalls in the interpretation of multidetector-row helical CT images at window width and level setting for lung parenchyma. Radiat Med 2001; 19:181–4.

37 Rubin GD, Lane MJ, Bloch DA, et al. Optimization of contrast enhanced thoracic spiral CT. Radiology 1996; 201:785–91.
38 Schoepf UJ, Becker CR, Bruening RD et al. electrocardiographically gated thin section CT of the lung. Radiology 1999; 212:649–54.
39 Stern EJ, Webb WR. Dynamic imaging of lung morphology with ultrafast high resolution computed tomography. JTI 1993; 8:273–82.
40 Robinson TE, Leung AN, Moss RB, et al. Standardized high resolution CT of the lung using a spirometer-triggered electron beam CT scanner. AJR Am J Roentgenol 1999; 172:1636–8.
41 Long FR, Castile RG, Brody AS, et al. Lungs in infant and young children: improved thin section CT with a noninvasive controlled ventilation technique-initial experience. Radiology 1999; 212:588–93.
42 Kelly DM, Hasegawa I, Borders R, Hatabu H, Boiselle PM. High-resolution CT using MDCT: comparison of degree of motion artifact between volumetric and axial methods. AJR Am J Roentgenol 2004; 182: 757–9.
43 Snider GL. Pathogenesis and terminology of emphysema. Am J Resp Crit Care Med 1994; 149:1382–3.
44 Thurlbeck WM, Muller NL. Emphysema: definition, imaging and quantification. AJR Am J Roentgenol 1994; 163:1017–25.
45 Snider GL, Kleinerman J, Thurlbeck WM, et al. The definition of emphysema: report of a national Heart, Lung and Blood institute, Division of Lung diseases workshop. Am Rev Resp Dis 1985; 132:182–5.
46 Snider GL. Reduction pneumoplasty for giant bullous emphysema: implications for surgical treatment of nonbullous emphysema. Chest 1996; 109:540–8.
47 Kazerooni EA, Chow LC, Whyte RI, et al. Preoperative examination of lung transplant candidates: value of chest CT compared with chest radiography. AJR Am J Roentgenol 1995; 165:1343–8.
48 Kazerooni EA. Pre and post operative imaging in lung volume reduction surgery. In: Grainger RG, Allison DJ, Adam A, Dixon AK, eds. Grainger and Allison's Diagnostic Radiology: A Textbook of Medical Imaging. Vol. 1, 4th ed. New York: Churchill Livingstone, 2001:563–76.
49 McKenna RJ Jr, Brenner M, Fischel RJ, et al. Patient selection criteria for lung volume reduction surgery. J Thorac Cardiovasc Surg 1997; 114:957–64.
50 Bae K, Slone R, Gierada D, et al. Patients with emphysema: quantitative CT analysis before and after lung volume reduction surgery. Work in progress. Radiology 1997; 203:705–14.
51 Slone RM, Gierada DS. Radiology of pulmonary emphysema and lung volume reduction surgery. Semin Thorac Cardiovasc Surg 1996; 8:61–82.
52 Slone RM, Pilgram TK, Gierada DS, et al. Lung volume reduction surgery: comparison of preoperative radiologic features and clinical outcome. Radiology 1997; 204:685–93.
53 Gierada DS, Slone RM, Bae KT, et al. Pulmonary emphysema: comparison of preoperative quantitative CT and physiologic index values with clinical outcome after lung-volume reduction surgery. Radiology 1997; 205: 235–42.
54 Suga K, Nishigauchi K, Matsunaga N, et al. Three-dimensional surface displays of perfusion SPET in the evaluation of patients with pulmonary emphysema for thoracoscopic lung volume reduction surgery. Nucl Med Commun 1997; 18:719–27.
55 Suga K, Nishigauchi K, Matsunaga N, et al. Preliminary application of dynamic pulmonary xenon-133 single-photon emission tomography in the evaluation of patients with pulmonary emphysema for thoracoscopic lung volume reduction surgery. Eur J Nucl Med 1998; 25:410–6.
56 Bankier AA, De Maertelaer V, Keyzer C, et al. Pulmonary emphysema: subjective visual grading versus objective quantification with macroscopic morphometry and thin-section CT densitometry. Radiology 1999; 211:851–8.
57 Muller NL, Staples CA, Miller RR, et al. Density mask. An objective method to quantitate emphysema using computed tomography. Chest 1988; 94:782–7.
58 Rozenshtein A, White CS, Austin JH, et al. Incidental lung carcinoma detected at CT in patients selected for lung volume reduction surgery to treat severe pulmonary emphysema. Radiology 1998; 207:487–90.
59 McKenna RJ Jr, Fischel RJ, Brenner M, Gelb AF. Combined operations for lung volume reduction surgery and lung cancer. Chest 1996; 110:885–8.
60 Adusumilli S, Kazerooni EA, Ojo T. Screening CT for lung cancer: a study of emphysema patients being evaluated for lung volume reduction surgery. Radiology 1998; 209 Suppl:222–3.
61 Swensen SJ, Viggiano RW, Midthun DE, et al. Lung nodule enhancement at CT: multicenter study. Radiology 2000; 214:73–80.
62 Kusajima K, Murata Y, Ohshi F, et al. Characteristics of chronic interstitial pneumonia seen in the lung operated for lung cancer. Nihon Kyobu Shikkan Gakkai Zasshi 1992; 30:1673–81.
63 Hubbard R, Venn A, Lewis S, Britton J. Lung cancer and cryptogenic fibrosing alveolitis. A population-based cohort study. Am J Respir Crit Care Med 2000; 161:5–8.
64 Turner-Warwick M, Lebowitz M, Burrows B, Johnson A. Cryptogenic fibrosing alveolitis and lung cancer. Thorax 1980; 35:496–9.
65 Kawasaki H, Nagai K, Yokose T, et al. Clinicopathological characteristics of surgically resected lung cancer associated with idiopathic pulmonary fibrosis. J Surg Oncol 2001; 76:53–57.
66 Aubry MC, Myers JL, Douglas WW, et al. Primary pulmonary carcinoma in patients with idiopathic pulmonary fibrosis. Mayo Clin Proc 2002; 77:763–70.
67 Ko JP, Naidich DP. Computer-aided diagnosis and the evaluation of lung disease. J Thorac Imaging 2004; 19:136–55.
68 Best AC, Lynch AM, Bozic CM, et al. Quantitative CT indexes in idiopathic pulmonary fibrosis: relationship with physiologic impairment. Radiology 2003; 228:407–14.
69 Sung YM, Yi CA, Yoon YC, et al. Additional coronal images using low-milliamperage multidetector row

CT: effectiveness in the diagnosis of bronchiectasis. J Comput Assist Tomogr 2003; 27:490–5.

70 Hirshberg B, Biran I, Glazer M, Kramer MR. Hemoptysis: etiology, evaluation, and outcome in a tertiary referral hospital. Chest 1997; 112:440–4.

71 Weaver LJ, Solliday N, Cugell DW. Selection of patients with hemoptysis for fiberoptic bronchoscopy. Chest 1979; 76:7–10.

72 Lederle FA, Nichol KL, Parenti CM. Bronchoscopy to evaluate hemoptysis in older men with nonsuspicious chest roentgenograms. Chest 1989; 95:1043–7.

73 Millar AB, Boothroyd AE, Edwards D, Hetzel MR. The role of computed tomography (CT) in the investigation of unexplained haemoptysis. Respir Med 1992; 86:39–44.

74 Finkelstein SE, Schrump DS, Nguyen DM, Hewitt SM, Kunst TF, Summers RM. Comparative evaluation of super high-resolution CT scan and virtual bronchoscopy for the detection of tracheobronchial malignancies. Chest 2003; 124:1834–40.

75 Quint LE, Whyte RI, Kazerooni EA, et al. Stenosis of the central airways: evaluation by using helical CT with multiplanar reconstructions. Radiology 1995; 194:871–7.

76 Hoppe H, Dinkel HP, Walder B, von Allmen G, Gugger M, Vock P. Grading airway stenosis down to the segmental level using virtual bronchoscopy. Chest 2004; 125:704–11.

77 Reuben DB, Mor V. Dyspnea in terminally ill cancer patients. Chest 1986; 89:234–236.

78 Kvale PA, Simoff M, Prakash UB. Lung cancer. Palliative care. Chest 2003; 123:284S–311.

79 Ikezoe J, Takashima S, Morimoto S, et al. CT appearance of acute radiation-induced injury in the lung. AJR Am J Roentgenol 1988; 150:765–70.

80 Libshitz HI. Radiation changes in the lung. Semin Roentgenol 1993; 28:303–20.

81 Libshitz HI, Shuman LS. Radiation-induced pulmonary change: CT findings. J Comput Assist Tomogr 1984; 8:15–19.

11

Lung Cancer Screening: Past, Present, and Future

Charles S. White
Department of Diagnostic Radiology, University of Maryland Medical Center, Baltimore, Maryland, U.S.A.

Phillip M. Boiselle
Department of Radiology, Beth Israel Deaconess Medical Center and Harvard Medical School, Boston, Massachusetts, U.S.A.

INTRODUCTION

Lung cancer remains the leading cause of mortality from cancer. In 2007, it is estimated that over 213,000 new cases of lung cancer will be diagnosed in the United States alone (1). The 5-year survival rate from the disease is 14% and has increased only slightly since the early 1970s, despite an extensive and costly research effort to find effective therapy. The disparity in survival between early- and late-stage lung cancer is substantial, with a 5-year survival rate of approximately 70% in Stage IA disease compared to less than 5% in Stage IV disease, according to the recently revised Lung Cancer Staging criteria (2). Unfortunately, as many as 60% of patients present with advanced-stage lung cancer.

The disproportionately high prevalence and mortality of advanced lung cancer has encouraged attempts to detect early lung cancer with screening programs aimed at smokers. Smokers have an incidence rate of lung cancer that is 10 times that of nonsmokers and account for greater than 80% of lung cancer cases in the United States (3). Until recently, two main approaches have been used to screen for lung cancer: chest radiography and sputum cytology. The first section of this chapter describes the evolution and results of screening studies using these techniques and the controversies that developed surrounding the results of these studies. The following section describes several emerging technologies for early lung cancer detection, with a special emphasis on low-dose spiral CT.

LUNG CANCER SCREENING: A HISTORICAL PERSPECTIVE

Screening studies for lung cancer date to the 1950s and 1960s, when several studies were undertaken using a variety of screening protocols that combined chest radiography and sputum analysis. The protocols employed different screening time intervals and the study design was either uncontrolled or controlled but nonrandomized. The most widely publicized study was the Philadelphia Pulmonary Neoplasm Research Project, in which only 6 of 94 patients with lung cancer detected at screening survived more than 5 years (4). No study showed an advantage for lung cancer screening.

The subsequent development of more sophisticated techniques of chest radiography and sputum analysis in the 1960s and the methodologic limitations of the early studies led to the concept that lung cancer screening might prove efficacious if a more rigorous study design was used. In that context, three large randomized controlled studies (National Cancer Institute Cooperative Early Lung Cancer Group) were initiated among male smokers in the 1970s at the Mayo Clinic, Memorial Sloan-Kettering Cancer Center, and the Johns Hopkins Medical Institutions.

In the Mayo Lung Project, 10,933 men who were 45 years of age or older and who smoked more than a pack of cigarettes daily were assessed with chest radiographs and sputum cytology (5). Lung cancers found in these patients were designated as "prevalence cases." The 9,211 men with negative chest radiographs and sputum cytology were randomized into two groups. The control group of 4,593 patients was given the standard Mayo Clinic recommendation at that time, a yearly chest radiograph and sputum cytologic examination, but no individualized follow-up was pursued. The study group of 4618 patients was scheduled once every 4 months for a chest radiograph and a sputum container was sent to collect a 3-day pooled sputum sample, which was returned to the Mayo Clinic. All patients were contacted yearly to assess their status. Approximately 75% of men in the study group complied with the every 4 month protocol.

When the study ended in 1983, lung cancer had been detected in 206 patients in the study group and 160 patients in the control group (5). Resectability was higher in the study group than in the control group (46% vs. 32%) but this advantage was not reflected in mortality rates. The death rates in the two groups were statistically similar: 3.2 per 1,000 person-years in the study group compared to 3.0 per 1,000 person-years in the control group.

A closer analysis of the data reveals that the every-4-month screening protocol detected a higher proportion of lung cancer at an early stage (42%) than in the control group (25%) and a corresponding 5-year survival benefit was found (6). However, despite these apparent advantages, no mortality benefit was demonstrated from screening.

Several explanations for the difference between the survival and mortality data have been postulated, including lead-time bias, overdiagnosis, and control group contamination (3). Lead-time bias occurs if the lung cancer is detected at an early stage in its natural history but the ultimate time of death is unchanged. In the Mayo Clinic study, the lung cancers in the screened population were detected at an earlier stage than in the control group, resulting in longer survival and apparent 5-year survival benefit. However, assuming the eventual time of death remained unchanged, no mortality benefit would be observed.

Overdiagnosis occurs if cancers that are indolent are disproportionately detected by lung cancer screening. Patients with slow-growing tumors would have a prolonged disease course that would favorably affect 5-year survival data. Indolent cancers would not be as likely to be detected in the control group because they would remain asymptomatic for an extended period of time and the patient might succumb to other illness. If such indolent cancers were disproportionately found in the screened population, a survival advantage but no mortality benefit would be shown for this population. Length-time bias is a related bias but describes detection of indolent cancer over a more limited time frame than overdiagnosis.

Prostate cancer is an example of a disease in which overdiagnosis might occur. Two-thirds of men over 60 years of age that die of other causes have undiagnosed, presumably indolent prostate cancer at autopsy. As for prostate cancer, it was suggested that overdiagnosis of lung cancer might account for the difference between survival and mortality data (3).

Contamination of the control group may also have been problematic in the Mayo Clinic study (5). Investigators estimated that approximately 50% of control patients in fact, underwent chest radiography during the course of the study and thus took on some characteristics of the screened population (contamination). One-third of the lung cancer in the control group was detected as a result of such "nonstudy" chest radiographs.

The Memorial Sloan-Kettering Cancer Center and the Johns Hopkins Medical Institutions studies used similar protocols that were substantively different than that of the Mayo Clinic project (7,8). These studies were designed to determine any advantage gained by the addition of yearly sputum samples to annual chest radiographs. Because chest radiography was used in both the study and the control populations, the trials were not useful to evaluate the efficacy of annual chest radiographs.

The Memorial Sloan-Kettering Cancer Center study consisted of 10,040 men over 45 years of age that smoked at least one pack of cigarettes (7). Patients were randomly assigned to two groups. The control group, composed of 5,072 men, underwent annual chest radiography. The screened population of 4,985 received an annual chest radiograph and pooled sputum cytology every 4 months. The 288 lung cancers found in these groups were evenly split between the two groups. There was no significant difference in the operability, 5-year survival, or mortality between the screened and control populations.

The Johns Hopkins study employed a protocol that was nearly identical to that of the Memorial Sloan-Kettering Cancer Center study (8). Similar numbers of lung cancers were detected in the screened and control populations, and the survival and mortality data were not significantly different in the two groups. Thus, neither study demonstrated an advantage for annual screening sputum cytology.

Two other studies have been reported from Europe that assessed the screening potential of chest radiography for lung cancer (9–11). A randomized controlled study from Czechoslovakia reported in the mid-1980s, evaluated 6,364 male smokers between the ages of 40 and 64 (9,10). Both screened and control groups were followed over a 3-year period. The screened group ($n=3172$) underwent both chest radiograph and sputum cytology every 6 months for the duration of the study. The control group ($n=3174$) received only a chest radiograph at the end of the 3-year period. Thirty-nine cancers were detected in the screened group compared to 27 in the control group. However, no clear advantage in mortality was demonstrated in the screened group.

A case-controlled study reported from Germany in the late 1980s assessed the rate of lung cancer detection among patients who had undergone biannual surveillance for tuberculosis with chest radiography (11). The 130 men in this screening program who died of lung cancer were matched with an aged-match control group consisting of men from the same district. No mortality benefit was found for the patients who participated in the screening program.

The failure of these studies to demonstrate a mortality advantage for lung cancer screening with either chest radiography or sputum cytology led most organizations to recommend that routine screening not be undertaken. The American Cancer Society noted that, "the Society did not feel it would be responsible to advocate screening for a large group of people... without better evidence that they would derive some benefit" (12). Based on the evidence, the view that "screening for lung cancer...is not recommended" has been widely professed (3). At present, no major organization advocates routine screening for lung cancer.

Over the past several years, several investigators have proposed a reassessment of the data from the four randomized lung cancer trials (13,14). Strauss et al. noted that although the Johns Hopkins Institute and Memorial Sloan-Kettering Cancer Center studies were not designed specifically to assess the efficacy of chest radiographic screening, both control and screened populations achieved survival rates approximately three times greater than prevailing norms. They suggested that the use of an annual chest radiographic screening protocol might have led to an improved outcome even if a mortality benefit was not shown (13).

Strauss et al. also contended that the improved resectability, lower stage, and better survival in the Mayo and Czech studies could not be adequately explained on the basis of lead-time bias or overdiagnosis. With respect to overdiagnosis, they cited evidence from an autopsy study that suggests indolent lung cancer occurs only rarely (15). Based on evaluation of the Mayo Lung Project data, they also noted that patients in that trial with early lung cancer who either were medically unsuitable or refused surgical resection had a much lower rate of survival than those who underwent surgical treatment (10% vs. 70%) (16). Strauss et al. suggested that the behavior of lung cancer is almost always aggressive even when detected at an early stage and, thus, overdiagnosis is unlikely to be a substantial confounding factor (13). In the view of the authors, the increases in survival and other parameters of the screened group in the Mayo and Czech studies could not be explained by study design biases. They speculated that the screening protocol itself might have led to a better outcome. They recommended a reappraisal of the role of chest radiographs in early lung cancer detection.

Other methodologic criticisms of the Mayo Lung Project have been raised. The contamination that occurred because 50% of the patients in the control group underwent chest radiographs decreased the distinctiveness of the screened and control group, leading to greater difficulty in detecting a difference between populations. A larger trial might, therefore, be required to show a difference (14).

Miettinen has suggested that the nine-year period over which cumulative mortality rate was calculated in the Mayo Lung Project is excessive (17). He has stated that this period of time likely underestimated the maximum effect of screening. Based on his analysis of the data, the time between 3 and 7 years after completion of prevalence screening is optimal because it "represents a compromise between one that is narrow enough to address the full effect, and one that is wide enough to show a meaningful number of deaths from the disease." He believes that if the more appropriate timing of cumulative mortality rates is used, the Mayo Lung data cannot be interpreted as providing direct evidence against screening.

The lingering questions with respect to the major lung cancer screening trials of the 1970s and 1980s, in combination with the development of potent new imaging and nonimaging techniques, engendered renewed interest in lung cancer screening throughout the 1990s. The remainder of this chapter describes early results using these newer technologies.

LUNG CANCER SCREENING: ANOTHER LOOK WITH NEW LENSES

In recent years, a wealth of new technologies has emerged that are capable of detecting lung cancer at an early, potentially treatable stage. These technologies include low-dose spiral CT (LDCT), digital radiography, advanced sputum analysis, and autofluorescence (AF) and virtual bronchoscopy (VB). In the following paragraphs, the potential contributions and challenges of these emerging technologies are discussed, with a special emphasis on LDCT.

Low-Dose Spiral Computed Tomography

CT plays an established role in the assessment of patients with clinically suspected and proven bronchogenic carcinoma. Recently, LDCT has been explored as a tool for detecting early lung cancer in asymptomatic individuals at risk for this disease, with encouraging preliminary results (18–20).

The first large-scale LDCT screening studies that were published in the English literature were performed by Kaneko et al. (18) and Sone et al. (19). Both of these studies were performed in Japan, a country with a rich history of cancer screening. More recently, Henschke et al. (20) reported their experience with LDCT screening at two large teaching hospitals in New York. The promising results of these preliminary studies have led many researchers, clinicians, health-care policy officials, and lung cancer patient advocates to revisit the topic of lung cancer screening (21).

In 1996, Kaneko et al. reported the use of biannual chest radiographs and spiral CT scans in screening 1369 Japanese adults at high risk for developing lung cancer (18). Peripheral lung cancer was detected in 15 (1%) subjects by CT but in only 4 (0.3%) by chest radiography. A vast majority (93%) of detected cancers were classified as Stage I.

In 1998, Sone et al. published their experience in screening 5483 Japanese adults between the ages of 40 and 74 years, including smokers and nonsmokers, using LDCT and miniature fluorophotography (19). Nineteen patients (prevalence 0.48%) were diagnosed with lung cancer, including 84% with Stage I disease. Miniature fluorophotography was interpreted as negative for malignancy in 18 of the 19 patients with lung cancer. In retrospect, however, judgment errors were present in three cases, in which positive findings were erroneously attributed to benign etiologies. Conventional chest radiographs obtained prior to surgery showed no evidence of a lung mass in 10 of 19 patients. There was one false-negative CT scan in a patient with an endobronchial lesion.

In 1999, Henschke et al. reported the results of baseline screening using LDCT and chest radiography in the Early Lung Cancer Action Project (ELCAP), which began in 1993 (20). In this study, 1000 asymptomatic patients greater than 60 years of age with a positive smoking history (>10 pack-years) underwent screening with both LDCT and chest radiography. LDCT was performed with the following parameters: single breath-hold, spiral acquisition; 140 kVp, 40 mA; 10 mm collimation; 2:1 pitch; 5 mm reconstruction interval; and high-resolution (bone) algorithm. Only the lung windows (width 1500, level 650) were provided for interpretation, and each study was interpreted separately by two board-certified radiologists, with a third expert radiologist available for cases that lacked consensus readings.

In order to guide the evaluation of noncalcified pulmonary nodules that were detected in the ELCAP study, the following algorithm was proposed: nodules <5 mm in diameter (average of length and width) were followed by serial CT scans to assess for interval growth over a 2-year period (3, 6, 12, and 24 months), nodules between 5 and 10 mm in diameter were either followed or biopsied, and nodules >10 mm in diameter were biopsied. Patients with more than six noncalcified nodules, diffuse bronchiectasis, ground-glass opacities, or any combinations of these features were classified as having diffuse disease and were not evaluated by this algorithm. As reviewed later in this chapter, these algorithms have recently changed for smaller lung nodules in response to growing knowledge about the high rate of benignancy among very small lung nodules and the difficulty in detecting growth of small nodules during short-term intervals.

In the original ELCAP study, 27 of 1000 (2.7%) subjects were found to have lung cancer by LDCT versus 7 (0.7%) by chest radiography. With regard to the cancers detected by CT, 26 (96%) were resectable and 23 (85%) were Stage I neoplasms. In contrast, chest radiography detected only 4 (17%) of 23 cases of Stage I disease. The results of the Japanese and ELCAP studies clearly show that LDCT is superior to conventional chest radiography in the detection of early lung cancer. Indeed, a review of the Japanese experience with screening by Kaneko (22) reports that the average peripheral lesion detected by chest radiography was 3.0 cm compared to 1.6 cm for spiral CT (Figs. 1 and 2).

Notably, these early screening studies were performed using single-detector CT with relatively thick sections. More recently, the advent of multi-detector-row CT (MDCT) scanners has improved the ability of CT to detect small lung nodules by providing faster scanning times and allowing routine use of thinner slice sections. The first large-scale screening study performed using MDCT was performed by Swensen et al. at the Mayo Clinic (23). These investigators used low-dose MDCT to screen 1520 participants >50 years of age with a $\geq$20 pack-year history of cigarette smoking. Each participant underwent five annual CT examinations (baseline and four subsequent annual scans). At the end of five

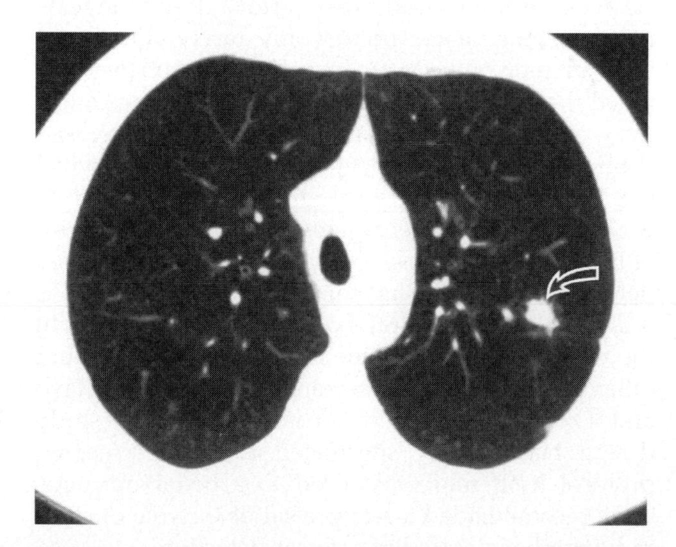

Figure 1 Early lung cancer detection by CT. Computed tomography image (lung windows) reveals an approximately 1.5 cm diameter spiculated peripheral lung nodule (*arrow*) in the left upper lobe, which proved to represent an adenocarcinoma. This is the typical size of a lung cancer detected with screening spiral CT scans in the Japanese experience. Median tumor size in the recent International ELCAP study was slightly smaller (13 mm baseline, 9 mm on annual CT). Also note the presence of centrilobular emphysema.

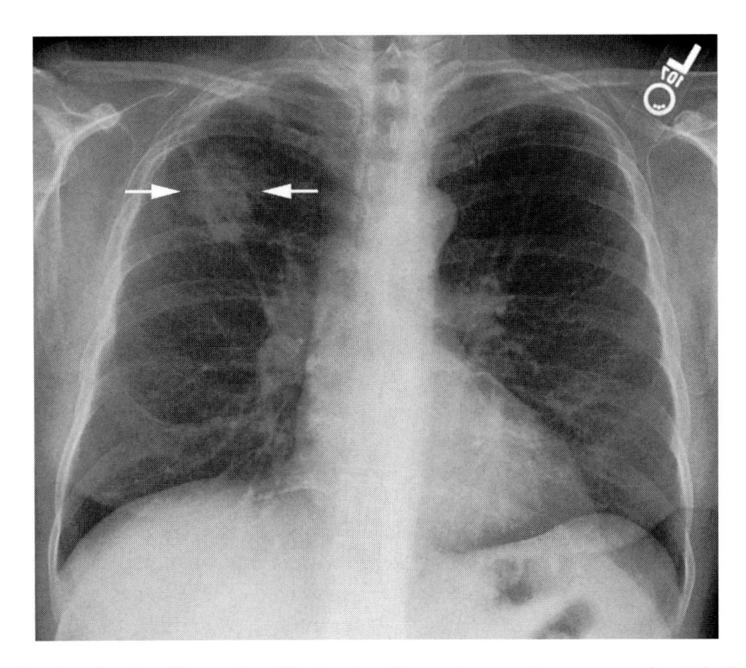

Figure 2 Lung cancer detection by chest radiography. PA chest radiograph reveals an approximately 3-cm-diameter right upper lobe spiculated lung nodule (*arrows*), which proved to represent an adenocarcinoma. This is the typical size of a lung cancer detected with screening chest radiographs in the Japanese experience.

annual CT examinations, 3356 noncalcified nodules were detected in 1118 (74%) of 1520 participants, and a total of 68 lung cancers were diagnosed (31 initial, 34 subsequent, and 3 interval cancers). Approximately 60% of the cancers detected in this trial were Stage I lesions. Notably, 13 participants underwent a total of 15 surgeries for benign disease, but there were no surgical mortalities. Based upon their findings, these investigators concluded that CT can detect early-stage lung cancers, but the rate of benign nodule detection is high.

More recently, Henschke et al. have published the results of a large, international, collaborative screening effort by the International ELCAP investigators (24). This study reported the results of CT screening among a cohort of over 31,000 asymptomatic persons at risk for lung cancer. This cohort was imaged between 1993 and 2005, using a variety of different CT scanners in both academic hospitals and community-based practice settings. In this study, 484 (1.5%) of 31,567 participants were diagnosed with lung cancer at either baseline screening ($n=405$) or annual screening ($n=74$). The estimated 10-year survival rate for all participants with lung cancer diagnosed at CT (regardless of stage at diagnosis or treatment) was 80%. For those who underwent resection within 1 month after diagnosis, the estimated 10-year survival rate was 92%, whereas all 8 patients with untreated lung cancer died within 5 years after diagnosis.

In combination, the studies reviewed in Table 1 demonstrate the consistent ability of LDCT to detect lung cancer at an early, potentially curable stage. Although it may seem intuitive that early detection should result in a decrease in lung cancer mortality, it is important to note that the impact of LDCT on disease-specific mortality has yet to be determined. Unlike other outcome measures (such as patient survival), mortality is not affected by several biases, including lead-time bias, length-time bias, and overdiagnosis (21,25,26). Mortality is thus considered the ultimate outcome measure of a screening study, and a significant reduction in disease-specific mortality is widely regarded as a requisite for a screening study to be adopted as standard care (21,25,26).

The National Lung Screening Trial (NLST), the largest lung cancer specific screening trial ever conducted, has been designed in order to address the important outstanding question of whether screening

Table 1 LDCT Screening Studies

Study	Screening population	Lung cancer prevalence	% Stage I
Henschke et al. (20)	$n=1000>10$ pk-yrs >60 y/o	27 (2.7%)	85
Sone et al. (19)	$n=5483\pm$ smoking 40–74 y/o	19 (0.48%)	84
Kaneko et al. (18)	$n=1369>20$ pk-yrs[a] >50 y/o[a]	15 (1%)	93
Swensen et al. (23)	$n=1520\geq$ 20 pk-yrs	68 (4%)	60
Henschke et al. (24)	$n=31{,}567\pm$ smoking 40–86 y/o	484 (1.5%)	85

[a]Most but not all patients met these criteria.
Abbreviations: LDCT, low-dose spiral CT; pk-yrs, pack-years of cigarette smoking; y/o, years old.
Source: From Refs. 18–20,23,24.

with low-dose CT reduces lung cancer specific mortality in comparison to screening with chest radiography (27). Participants in this trial are healthy individuals aged 55 to 74 with heavy (≥30 pack-year) present or former smoking histories who were recruited from across the United States at over 30 institutions. Each subject has been randomized to receive either low-dose MDCT or chest radiography at baseline and annually for two additional years. The end point of the trial is lung cancer specific mortality, which will be determined by following participants for 5 to 7 years after entry into the trial. The trial was launched in 2002 and completed accrual of over 53,000 subjects in 2004 (27). At the time of this publication, the imaging phase of the trial has been completed. However, data regarding mortality will not be available until after 2009, reflecting the long time interval required to assess this important end point.

In addition to the lack of mortality data, there are currently several important potential limitations of this technique (Table 2). First, it is important to note the relatively high false-positive rate of this method, particularly when one considers a noncalcified nodule of any size as a positive screening result. For example, using this criterion for a positive result, at baseline screening in the original ELCAP trial, 233 of 1000 patients (23.3%) were found to have 1 to 6 noncalcified nodules at LDCT, but only 27 of these nodules proved to be malignant (20). Notably, 74% of subjects in the Mayo Clinic trial had one or more noncalcified nodules at baseline and/or annual incidence CT screening, resulting in false-positive rates on a per-nodule basis of >90% (23). The higher prevalence of noncalcified nodules in the Mayo Clinic trial compared to the original ELCAP study is likely related to both geographical (higher prevalence of granulomatous exposure in the Mayo Clinic population) and technical factors. Regarding technical factors, the Mayo Clinic investigators used more up-to-date technology compared to the original ELCAP study, including multidetector rather than single-detector CT scanners, narrower slice collimation (5 vs. 10 mm), and cine viewing rather than film viewing. Each of these technical factors is known to enhance the detection rate of small nodules.

Table 2 Current Challenges of LDCT

Current challenges	Potential solutions
Relatively high false-positive rate	Expected decrease at annual repeat screen Use of threshold nodule size (4 or 5 mm) for positive result to reduce false-positive rate
High cost for follow-up CT scans of false positives	Additional noninvasive imaging methods (PET, C+CT) may decrease the number of follow-up studies Further study of malignant growth rates of small nodules may allow for fewer follow-up studies
Difficulty in detecting malignant growth rate in small nodules	Computer-aided volumetric measurements are more accurate
Bias toward detecting adenocarcinomas	Combine LDCT with advanced sputum analysis in order to detect more squamous cell lesions
Potential for "overdiagnosis"	Further study of this subject is required

Abbreviations: LDCT, low-dose spiral CT; PET, positron emission tomography; C+CT, CT nodule contrast enhancement.

Although the original ELCAP study reported only one recommended biopsy for a nodule that eventually proved benign (20), the Mayo Clinic trial reported 13 patients who underwent surgical resection for nodules that proved benign (23). Thus, individuals undergoing lung cancer screening should be aware of the potential risks of biopsy or surgery for lesions that may prove benign.

Even when intervention is avoided, the potential costs of performing serial follow-up CT scans in such a high percentage of patients has important financial implications for using LDCT as a mass screening tool, leading some experts to question whether this screening technique can be cost-effective (28). Moreover, in addition to financial costs, there are also psychological costs to consider for patients with false-positive nodules. Such patients must wait 2 years before receiving a final assurance that a nodule is benign. It is likely that some patients are better suited to a "watch and wait" approach than others. In order to gauge the magnitude of these issues, the NLST is measuring the "psychological" costs associated with the screening process among its participants.

Compared to baseline prevalence screening, one would anticipate a lower false-positive rate at repeat yearly screening (21). Henschke et al. have reported their findings from the first annual repeat LDCT exam in the ELCAP screening population (29). At annual repeat screening, 31 of 623 patients (5%) had truly new or growing nodules compared to baseline screening LDCT. Nine of these nodules proved to be negative or demonstrated benign calcifications on additional high-resolution CT imaging. Of the remaining nodules, eight were larger than 5 mm in diameter and were biopsied and seven of these nodules were proven malignant. In this study, the overall detection rate of nonsmall-cell lung cancer on first annual repeat spiral CT was 1%, and 83% were Stage IA neoplasms.

The recent introduction of a size threshold for a positive screening result has markedly reduced the reported rate of false-positive screening results using LDCT (24). Whereas initial screening studies considered any noncalcified nodule as a fully positive screening result requiring follow-up several months after detection, a growing body of data from lung cancer screening trials has shown that nodules <4–5 mm in diameter do not require follow-up prior to the next annual screening CT scans. For example, based upon an analysis of baseline and first-year annual screening CT scans in nearly 3000 subjects, Henschke et al. have concluded that "in CT screening for lung cancer, the detection of noncalcified nodules of less than 5.0 mm in diameter on the initial CT images at baseline need not be taken to imply a fully positive result of that test; that is, it need not give rise to further diagnostic work-up prior to the first annual repeat screening" (30). However, these investigators emphasize that such small nodules do need to be reexamined at the first annual screening CT to determine whether growth has occurred. Henschke et al. have emphasized that the use of a nodule size threshold for a fully positive result is only employed for the baseline screening CT (24). At annual screening, any newly identified noncalcified nodule is considered a positive result, regardless of size (24).

In its study design, the NLST trial has employed a slightly smaller threshold value of ≥4 mm as a positive screening result. Similarly, the recently published Fleischner Society guidelines for management of noncalcified nodules incidentally detected at CT in the nonscreening population recommends that nodules ≤4 mm be reassessed in 1 year when detected in an individual at high risk for lung cancer (31). Thus, current practice patterns for addressing small, noncalcified pulmonary nodules are changing in both screening and nonscreening settings.

A second potential limitation of LDCT relates to the difficulty of reliably detecting a malignant growth rate in small <1 cm nodules (32). For example, if a 5 mm nodule doubles in volume over a 6-month period, its diameter will increase by only 1.25–6.25 mm (32), a difference that may be difficult to accurately detect using conventional methods of measurement (Fig. 3). More sophisticated methods of nodule measurement will be required to meet the challenge of accurately measuring growth of small nodules. Recent advances in computer-aided three-dimensional nodule measurement using sophisticated software programs (Fig. 4) have led to improvements in detecting growth of small pulmonary nodules (33–35). Such programs are now commercially available for use on standard three-dimensional imaging workstations. However, to date, the prevalence with which such tools are being used in daily practice is uncertain. Improved integration of three-dimensional processing methods with image display on clinical workstations will likely enhance the accessibility and use of such tools in the near future.

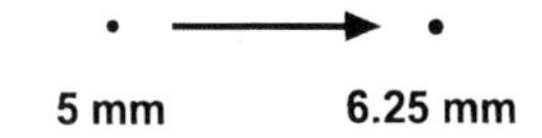

Figure 3 Difficulty in measuring growth of small nodules. Doubling the volume of a 5 mm diameter nodule results in a diameter increase of only 1.25 mm, a difference that may be difficult to detect with conventional methods of measurement on axial CT images.

When following lung nodules for potential growth, it is important to be aware of the broad spectrum of growth rates that may be encountered among lung cancers (Fig. 5). For example, in a retrospective review of 34 patients with surgically resected peripheral adenocarcinomas less than 3 cm who underwent preoperative CT, Aoki et al. (36) found that lung nodule doubling time ranged between 42 and 1486 days. These authors concluded that that there are two main types of peripheral adenocarcinoma. One starts as a localized ground-glass opacity on CT with a slow growth pattern (usually representing bronchoalveolar cell carcinoma) and the other starts as a solid attenuation with relatively rapid growth (usually representing invasive adenocarcinoma). Purely ground-glass nodules should thus be followed at longer time intervals than

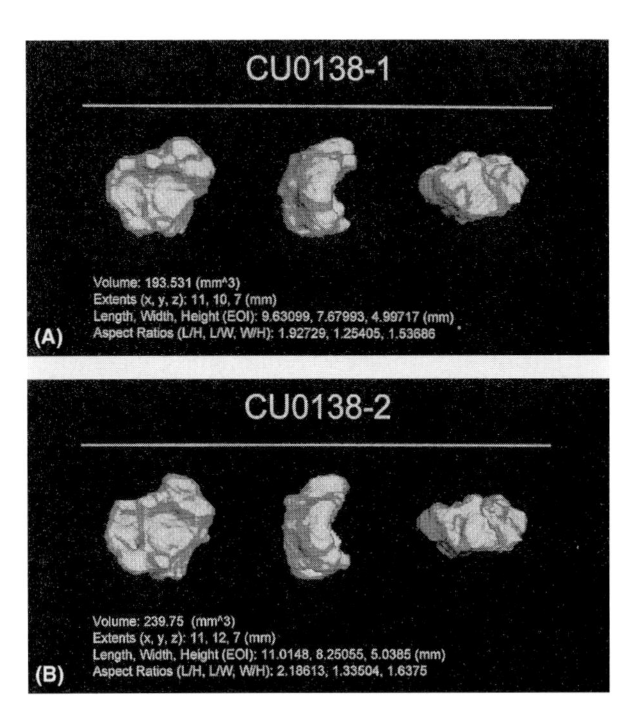

Figure 4 Three-dimensional volumetric analysis of lung nodule showing early detection of malignant growth rate in proven nonsmall-cell lung cancer. (**A**) Three-dimensional volumetric reconstruction images of a small left apical lung nodule with a volume measurement of 193.531 mm^3. (**B**) Follow-up 3D volumetric reconstruction images of the same nodule performed 4 months later reveals interval increase in volume to 239.75 mm^3. Interval growth of the nodule was not readily apparent on axial high-resolution CT images. *Source*: Courtesy of David Yankelevitz, from Ref. 79.

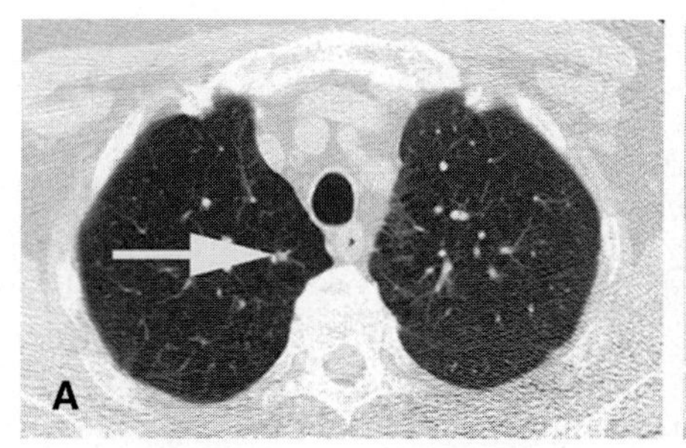

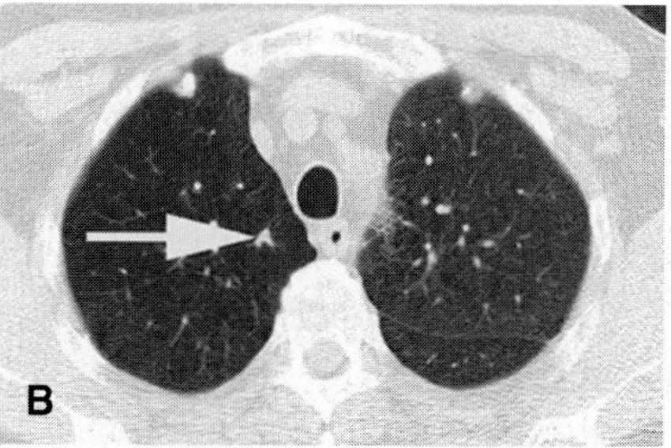

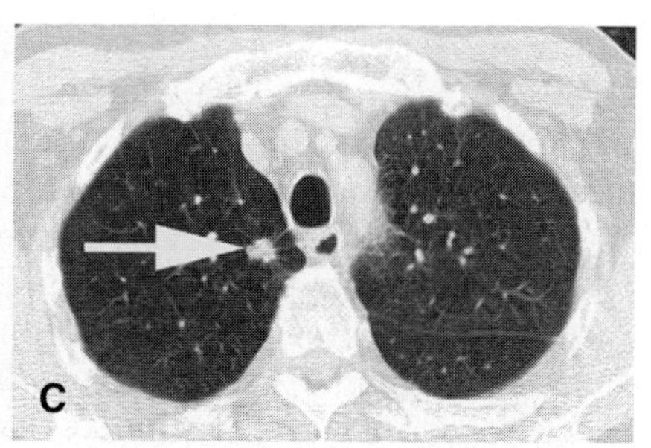

Figure 5 Slowly growing lung cancer. Serial CT scans over a 2-year period demonstrate progressive, slow interval growth of a small right apical lung nodule, which proved to represent a squamous cell carcinoma at pathology following eventual surgical resection (**A** = baseline, **B** = 1 year later, **C** = 2 years after baseline CT).

solid nodules and may also require follow-up for more than 2 years.

A third potential limitation of LDCT screening is its bias toward detecting adenocarcinomas, which comprise the vast majority of peripheral lung cancers (21,37). In the ELCAP baseline study, over 90% of neoplasms were characterized as an adenocarcinoma cell type; a majority were pure adenocarcinomas and a minority were bronchoalveolar cell carcinomas and adenosquamous subtypes (20). In the larger, international ELCAP study, slightly greater than 70% of lung cancers were adenocarcinomas (24). This bias could potentially be reduced by pairing LDCT with a complementary tool for detecting central neoplasms such as advanced sputum analysis techniques (21). These techniques are discussed below.

A fourth potential limitation of LDCT concerns the possible "overdiagnosis" of lung cancer (21). With regard to lung cancer screening, the detection of bronchioloalveolar cell adenomas, a benign lesion that may have malignant potential (38,39), is an example of potential overdiagnosis. This is a controversial subject that requires further study.

Finally, as with any screening study, there will be false-negative cases. Kakinuma et al. (40) reported seven cases of lung cancer that were initially missed at screening LDCT and subsequently detected on repeat LDCT screening studies performed 6–18 months later. Missed nodules were retrospectively categorized as either conspicuous (mean diameter = 11 mm; $n = 3$) or inconspicuous (mean diameter = 6 mm; $n = 4$). In order to reduce the number of false-negative cases, these authors emphasize the importance of examining noncalcified nodules with thin-section CT, even when adjacent lesions of prior tuberculosis exist. They also caution that one should carefully inspect pulmonary vessels in order to distinguish them from small pulmonary nodules. Despite an initial "missed" diagnosis, six of seven lesions were Stage I neoplasms at the time of diagnosis. Li et al. (41) retrospectively assessed 32 lung cancers that were initially missed on 39 low-dose CT screening examinations (some cancers were missed on more than one exam). Among the 39 missed diagnoses at CT, 23 were classified as detection errors and 19 as interpretation errors. Contributing factors included subtle "ground-glass" nodule density and overlap of nodules with adjacent normal structures for cancers missed due to detection errors, and location within a complex background of other pulmonary disease (e.g., emphysema, fibrosis) for cancers missed due to interpretation errors. Interestingly, despite a substantial delay of at least one year before eventual diagnosis, a vast majority of lesions (28 of 32) were Stage I at the time of diagnosis (including 26 Stage IA lesions).

The ELCAP investigators reported an analysis of missed lung nodules on screening LDCT that were subsequently identified on follow-up diagnostic CT scans (42). Among the 163 patients who underwent diagnostic CT imaging, 36 (22%) had additional nodules, which were not detected on LDCT. The majority (85%) of missed nodules measured 5 mm in

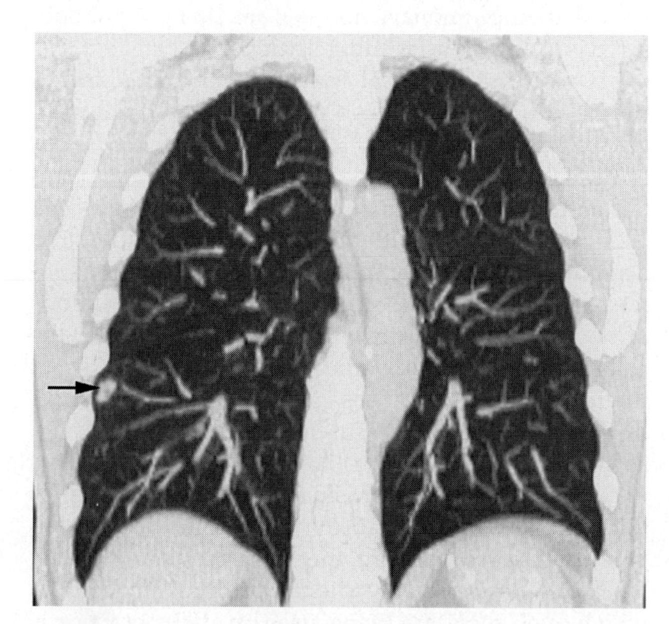

Figure 6 Coronal reformation, maximal intensity projection CT image displays small peripheral lung cancer (*arrow*), which is easily differentiated from adjacent vessels due to continous display of vascular structures with this reformation method compared to traditional axial CT images.

diameter or less and none were greater than 10 mm in diameter. Thus, small size appears to be the most important factor related to missed nodules on LDCT. Interestingly, a majority of missed nodules were located peripherally.

Recent advances in technology will likely improve the ability of LDCT to detect and accurately characterize lung nodules (33–35,43–46). These advances include the use of MDCT scanners, cine-based viewing, computerized detection methods, and multiplanar reformation (Fig. 6) and three-dimensional reconstruction methods. For example, Armato et al. (47) evaluated the performance of a fully automated computerized method for detecting lung nodules among a group of cases that included 38 of the 39 screening CT scans of initially "missed" lung cancers from the study reported by Li et al. (41). Using this technique, 84% of the cancers that were initially missed were correctly detected.

In addition to computer-aided detection, the addition of more specific noninvasive methods of imaging evaluation such as CT nodule enhancement (48) and FDG-PET imaging (49–52) may help to reduce the number of cases requiring close follow-up or biopsy (21). These techniques are discussed further in Chapter 9.

In summary, although nonrandomized studies published to date have consistently shown the ability of low-dose CT to detect lung cancer at an early stage, the impact of screening upon lung cancer specific mortality has yet to be determined and will await the results of the ongoing NLST. This trial will also provide important information regarding financial and psychological costs of screening and biomarker analysis to assist risk stratification.

Table 3 Consensus Statement[a] of the Society of Thoracic Radiology

- Lung cancer is the most common cause of cancer death in both men and women in the industrialized world. It is a major public health problem.
- Screening for lung cancer with chest radiography has not been shown to lower disease-specific mortality. CT screening offers hope for earlier detection that could lower disease-specific mortality; it is unproven.
- Concerns have been raised regarding false-positive diagnoses, overdiagnosis, cost, and morbidity and mortality related to intervention.
- Promotion of CT screening to the general population by medical professionals with a financial interest in an enterprise is inappropriate.
- There is insufficient evidence to justify recommending CT screening for lung cancer to patients, including those at high risk for lung cancer.

[a]This consensus statement was published in conjunction with a minority, dissenting opinion for points 2–5 (54).
Source: From Ref. 53.

The Society of Thoracic Radiology has recently constructed a revised consensus statement on the topic of screening for lung cancer with LDCT. Excerpts from this statement are provided in Table 3 (53,54).

Digital Chest Radiography

The results of the LDCT studies described in the previous section have clearly shown the limited ability of conventional chest radiography to detect early lung cancer. Emerging technological advancements in digital chest radiography, including computer-aided diagnosis, temporal subtraction, and dual-energy subtraction methods, may significantly improve the ability of chest radiography to detect small lung nodules (55–57). Once this technology matures, future studies will be necessary to address the ability of digital chest radiography to detect early lung cancer (21).

Sputum Cytology and Advanced Sputum Analysis Techniques

In screening studies, the sensitivity of sputum cytology for detecting lung cancer is approximately 20–30% and the specificity is approximately 98% (6,58,59). Improvement in sensitivity can be achieved by adherence to proper techniques for collection, processing, and interpretation of samples (59). Sputum cytology demonstrates the highest sensitivity for squamous cell carcinoma and the lowest yield for adenocarcinoma (21).

Of the various CT screening studies for lung cancer, only the Mayo Clinic study has employed routine sputum assessment in conjunction with CT screening. In this study of 1520 participants, 2 (3%) of 68 primary lung cancers were detected by sputum alone (one incidence case and one baseline case) (21). Thus, the addition of traditional sputum cytology has only a modest impact upon lung cancer detection rate.

Table 4 Biomarkers

Biomarker	Analysis	Biological role	Application
HnRNP A2/B1	Protein I in sputum cells	mRNA processing	Early detection/ monitoring
K-ras	DNA in sputum homogenates	Cell-cycle regulation	Early detection/ risk assessment
Genomic instability	DNA in sputum homogenates	Chromosomal integrity	Early detection/ risk assessment

Source: Ref. 63.

In recent years, there have been several exciting advances in sputum analysis techniques, most notably the development of automated analysis of sputum specimens for biomarkers (60–67). This technology capitalizes on advances in our understanding of the molecular events that lead to lung cancer. In the future, it is likely that a panel of biomarkers (Table 4) will be used to identify the early clonal phase of lung cancer, thus allowing detection of lung cancers at a very early stage (63). Importantly, biomarker characterization may also allow for targeted treatment of early lung cancer (63).

Conventional, Autofluorescence, and Virtual Bronchoscopy

Conventional bronchoscopy is a valuable technique for localizing preinvasive lung cancer within the airways. In general, conventional bronchoscopy can detect nodular or polypoid lesions >2 mm in size and flat or superficially spreading lesions >2 cm in diameter (21,67). With regard to carcinoma in situ, 75% of lesions are superficial or flat and 25% are nodular or polypoid (21,67).

AF is a recently developed optical imaging method that is designed to improve the detection of small preinvasive lesions that are not visible by conventional, "white light" bronchoscopy (67–72). AF involves illuminating the bronchial surface with violet or blue light (400–440 nm) in order to distinguish normal from abnormal tissues. Upon such illumination, dysplastic lesions and carcinoma in situ will show a diminution in the intensity of AF.

The light-induced fluorescence endoscopy (LIFE) device, which was designed to capitalize on differences in AF properties in order to aid in the detection and localization of preinvasive lung cancer, has been approved by the FDA for the detection of early lung cancer (67,68). Except for differences in the illuminating light and the addition of a special camera, the LIFE device is similar to conventional bronchoscopy (68,69). In the hands of a bronchoscopist who has received extensive training in using this device, it adds only a few minutes to a conventional bronchoscopic procedure. A recent multicenter trial using LIFE showed that it improved the detection rate of preinvasive lung cancer by severalfold compared to conventional fiber-optic bronchoscopy alone (68).

Recently, Bard et al. (72) have reported that the combined use of AF with various methods of optical spectroscopy (AF spectroscopy, diffuse reflectance spectroscopy, and differential path length spectroscopy) facilitate an increased positive predictive value of AF for detecting endobronchial tumors. The best results were achieved when all three spectroscopic techniques were combined.

Because of its invasive nature and high cost, screening with AF should currently be reserved for patients with a very high pretest probability of lung cancer (21). For widespread screening, AF should ideally be coupled with a noninvasive, first-line study that selects patients with a high pretest probability of harboring early lung cancer (21). For example, a study by Phillips et al. describes the use of a breathalyzer to identify volatile organic compounds that may serve as potential markers for lung cancer (73). Similarly, Machado et al. (74) have shown the potential feasibility of clinical monitoring of volatile organic compounds in exhaled breath using a multisensor "electronic nose" device as a relatively convenient and noninvasive test in patients with suspected lung cancer. Carpagnano et al. (75) have recently shown that DNA in exhaled breath condensate can be analyzed for the presence of microsatellite alterations, which have been proposed as an early marker in lung carcinogenesis. Future studies are needed to determine the precise role of these exciting new technologies in the detection of early lung cancer.

VB is a novel noninvasive method for assessing the airways, which combines helical CT data and virtual reality computing in order to create three-dimensional endobronchial simulations (76–78). This technique is described in detail in Chapter 9. A recent preliminary investigation by Summers et al. assessed the computer-assisted detection of polypoid airway lesions on VB images (77). This technique was associated with a relatively high sensitivity (90%) for lesions >5 mm in diameter, but was limited by a poor specificity.

Current limitations of VB include its labor-intensive nature, the limited experience of most radiologists with this technique, and its inability to differentiate malignant from benign lesions (21,76–78). Future technological advances will hopefully overcome many of these obstacles.

LUNG CANCER SCREENING: FUTURE DIRECTIONS

The current wealth of emerging technologies for the early detection of lung cancer provides hope that we may be able to reduce the burden of disease in the near future (21). To date, LDCT is the most promising emerging technology for lung cancer screening, but ongoing advances in other techniques may change this perspective in the future. Biomarkers will likely be the ultimate method of early lung cancer detection in the future.

Important questions to answer before proceeding to mass screening include the effect of screening on lung cancer mortality, the cost-effectiveness of widespread screening, the optimal screening tools to use, and the subsets of present and former smokers who are most likely to benefit from screening. Ongoing research studies are being performed to answer these questions.

REFERENCES

1 Jemal A, Siegel R, Ward E, et al. Cancer statistics, 2007. Cancer J Clin 2007; 57:143–66.
2 Mountain CF. Revisions in the international system for staging lung cancer. Chest 1997; 111:1710–7.
3 Eddy DM. Screening for lung cancer. Ann Intern Med 1989; 111:232–7.
4 Boucot KR, Weiss W. Is curable lung cancer detected by semi-annual screening? J Am Med Assoc 1973; 224:1361–5.
5 Fontana RS, Sanderson DR, Woolner LB, Taylor WF, Miller WE, Muhm JR. Lung cancer screening: the Mayo program. J Occup Med 1986; 28:746–50.
6 Fontana RS, Sanderson DR, Taylor WF, et al. Early lung cancer detection: results of the initial (prevalence) radiologic and cytologic screening in the Mayo Clinic study. Am Rev Resp Dis 1984; 130:561–5.
7 Melamed MR, Flehinger BJ, Zaman MB, Heelan RT, Perchick WA, Martini N. Screening for early lung cancer: results of the Memorial Sloan-Kettering study in New York. Chest 1984; 86:44–53.
8 Tockman MS. Survival and mortality from lung cancer in a screened population: the Johns Hopkins Study. Chest 1986; 89(Suppl):324S–5.
9 Kubik A, Polak J. Lung cancer detection: results of a randomized prospective study in Czechoslovakia. Cancer 1986; 57:2427–37.
10 Kubik A, Haerting J. Survival and mortality in a randomized study of lung cancer detection. Neoplasma 1990; 37:467–75.
11 Ebeling K, Nischan P. Screening for lung cancer—results from a case-control study. Int J Cancer 1987; 40:141–4.
12 American Cancer Society. Guidelines for the cancer related checkup. Cancer 1980; 30:199–207.
13 Strauss GM, Gleason RE, Sugarbaker DJ. Chest X-ray screening improves outcome in lung cancer: a reappraisal of randomized trials on lung cancer screening. Chest 1995; 107(Suppl):270S–9.
14 Henschke CI, Yankelevitz DF. Screening for lung cancer. J Thorac Imag 2000; 15:21–7.
15 McFarlane MJ, Feinstein AR, Wells CK. Clinical features of lung cancer discovered as a post-mortem "surprise." Chest 1986; 90:520–3.
16 Flehinger BJ, Kimmel M, Melamed MR. The effect of surgical treatment on survival from early lung cancer: implications for screening. Chest 1992; 101:1013–8.
17 Miettinen OS. Screening for lung cancer. Radiol Clin North Am 2000; 38:479–86.
18 Kaneko M, Eguchi K, Ohmatsu H, et al. Peripheral lung cancer: screening and detection with low-dose spiral CT versus radiography. Radiology 1996; 201:798–802.
19 Sone S, Takashima S, Li F, et al. Mass screening for lung cancer with mobile spiral computed tomography scanner. Lancet 1998; 351:1242–5.
20 Henschke CI, McCauley DI, Yankelevitz DF, et al. Early Lung Cancer Action Project: overall design and findings from baseline screening. Lancet 1999; 54:99–105.
21 Boiselle PM, Ernst A, Karp DD. Lung cancer detection in the 21st century: potential contributions and challenges of emerging technologies. Am J Radiol 2000; 175:1215–21.
22 Kaneko M. CT scanning for lung cancer in Japan: International Conference on Prevention and Early Diagnosis of Lung Cancer, Varese, Italy, December 9–10, 1998, Cancer 2000; 89:2485–588.
23 Swensen SJ, Jett JR, Hartman TE, et al. CT screening for lung cancer: five-year prospective experience. Radiology 2005; 235:259–65.
24 The International Early Lung Cancer Action Program Investigators. Survival of patients with stage I lung cancer detected on CT screening. N Eng J Med 2006; 355:1763–71.
25 Riegelman RK, Hirsch RP. Screening. In: Riegelman RK, Hirsch RP, eds. Studying a Study and Testing a Test: How to Read the Health Science Literature. 3rd ed. Boston, MA: Little, Brown, 1996:183–91.
26 Strauss GM, Gleason RE, Sugarbaker DJ. Screening for lung cancer: another look; a different view. Chest 1997; 111:754–68.
27 Aberle DR, Chiles C, Gatsonis C, et al. Imaging and cancer: research strategy of the American College of Radiology Imaging Network. Radiology 2005; 235:741–51.
28 Mahadevia PJ, Fleisher LA, Frick KD, et al. Lung cancer screening with helical computed tomography in older adult smokers: a decision and cost-effectiveness analysis. JAMA 2003; 289:313–22.
29 Henschke CI, Naidich DP, Yankelevitz DF, et al. Results of Early Lung Cancer Action Program (ELCAP): first-annual repeat low-dose CT screening in high risk subjects (abstract). Radiology 1999; 213:303.
30 Henschke CI, Yankelevitz DF, Naidich DP, et al. CT screening for lung cancer: suspiciousness of nodules according to size on baseline scans. Radiology 2004; 231:164–8.
31 MacMahon H, Austin JH, Gamsu G, et al. Guidelines for management of small pulmonary nodules detected on CT scans: a statement from the Fleischner Society. Radiology 2005; 237:395–400.
32 Erasmus JF, Connolly JE, Me Adams HP, Roggli VL. Solitary pulmonary nodules: part II. Evaluation of the indeterminate nodule. RadioGraphics 2000; 20: 59–66.
33 Wyckoff N, McNitt-Gray MF, Goldin JG, Sayre JW, Aberle DR. The use of contrast-enhancement, texture and three-dimensional size and shape features for classification of solitary pulmonary nodules (abstract). Radiology 1999; 213:172.
34 Zhao B, Yankelevitz DF, Reeves A, Henschke CI. Two-dimensional multi-criterion segmentation of pulmonary nodules on helical CT images. Med Phys 1999; 6:889–95.
35 Yankelevitz DF, Gupta R, Zhao B, Henschke CI. Small pulmonary nodules: evaluation with repeat

CT—preliminary experience. Radiology 1999; 212: 561–6.
36 Aoki T, Nakata H, Watanabe H, et al. Evolution of peripheral lung adenocarcinomas: CT findings correlated with histology and tumor doubling time. Am J Roentgenol 2000; 74:763–8.
37 Jett J, Feins R, Kvale P, et al. Pretreatment evaluation of non-small-cell lung cancer. Am J Respir Crit Care Med 1997; 156:320–2.
38 Logan PM, Miller RR, Evans K, Miiller NL. Bronchogenic carcinoma and coexistent bronchioloalveolar cell adenomas: assessment of radiology detection and follow-up in 28 patients. Chest 1996; 109:713–7.
39 Miller RR. Bronchioloalveolar cell adenoma. Am J Surg Pathol 1990; 14:904–12.
40 Kakinuma R, Ohmatsu H, Kaneko M, et al. Detection failures in spiral CT screening for lung cancer: analysis of CT findings. Radiology 1999; 212:61–6.
41 Li F, Sone S, Abe H, et al. Lung cancers missed at low-dose helical CT screening in a general population: comparison of clinical, histopathologic, and imaging findings. Radiology 2002; 225:673–83.
42 Naidich DP, Yankelevitz DF, McGuinness G, et al. Noncalcified nodules missed on low-dose helical CT (abstract). Radiology 1999; 213(p):303.
43 Liang Y, Kruger RA. Dual-slice versus single-slice spiral scanning: comparison of the physical performance of two computed tomography scanners. Med Phys 1996; 23:205–20.
44 Seltzer SE, Judy PF, Adams DF, et al. Spiral CT of the chest: comparison of cine and film-based viewing. Radiology 1995; 197:73–8.
45 Tillich M, Kammerhuber F, Reittner P, et al. Detection of pulmonary nodules with helical CT: comparison of cine and film-based viewing. Am J Radiol 1997; 169:1611–4.
46 Armato SG III, Giger ML, Moran CJ, et al. Computerized detection of pulmonary nodules on CT scans. RadioGraphics 1999; 19:1303–11.
47 Armato SG III, Li F, Giger ML, et al. Lung cancer: performance of automated lung nodule detection applied to cancers missed in a CT screening program. Radiology 2002; 225:685–92.
48 Swensen SJ, Viggiano RW, Midthun DE, et al. Lung nodule enhancement at CT: multicenter study. Radiology 2000; 214:273–80.
49 Al-Sugair A, Coleman RE. Applications of PET in lung cancer. Semin Nucl Med 1998; 28:303–19.
50 Coleman RE. PET in lung cancer. J Nucl Med 1999; 40:814–20.
51 Patz EF, Lowe VJ, Hoffman JM, et al. Focal pulmonary abnormalities: evaluation with ^{18}F fluorodeoxyglucose PET scanning. Radiology 1993; 188:487–90.
52 Gupta NC, Maloof J, Gunel E. Probability of malignancy in solitary pulmonary nodules using fluorine-18-FDG and PET. J Nucl Med 1996; 37:943–8.
53 Swensen S, Aberle DR, Kazerooni EA, et al. Consensus statement: CT screening for lung cancer. J Thorac Imag 2005; 20:321.
54 Henschke CI, Austin JH, Berlin N, et al. Minority opinion: CT screening for lung cancer. J Thorac Imag 2005; 20:324–5.
55 Kobayashi T, Xu XW, MacMahon H, et al. Effect of a computer-aided diagnosis scheme on radiologists' performance in detection of lung nodules on radiographs. Radiology 1996; 199:843–8.
56 Kido S, Ikozoe J, Naito H, et al. Clinical evaluation of pulmonary nodules with single-exposure dual-energy subtraction chest radiography with an iterative noise-reduction algorithm. Radiology 1995; 194:407–12.
57 MacMahon H, Engelmann RM, Behlen FM, et al. Computer-aided diagnosis of pulmonary nodules: results of a large-scale observer test. Radiology 1999; 213:723–6.
58 Frost JK, Ball WC Jr, Levin ML. Early lung cancer detection: results of the initial (prevalence) radiologic and cytologic screening in the Johns Hopkins study. Am Rev Respir Dis 1984; 130:549–54.
59 Kennedy TC, Proudfoot SP, Franklin WA, et al. Cytopathological analysis of sputum in patients with airflow obstruction and significant smoking histories. Cancer Res 1996; 56:4673–768.
60 Field JK. Selection and validation of new lung cancer markers for the molecular-pathological assessment of individuals with a high risk of developing lung cancer. In: Brambilla C, Brambilla E, eds. Lung Tumors: Fundamental Biology and Clinical Management. New York: Marcel Dekker, 1999:287–302.
61 Tockman MS, Mulshine JL, Piantadosi S, et al. Prospective detection of preclinical lung cancer: results from two studies of heterogeneous nuclear ribonucleoprotein A2/B1 overexpression. Clin Cancer Res 1997; 3:2237–46.
62 Gazdar AF, Minna JD. Molecular detection of early lung cancer (editorial). J Natl Cancer Inst 1999; 91:299–301.
63 Mulshine JL, Henschke CI. Prospects for lung cancer screening (commentary). Lancet 1999; 355:592–3.
64 Ahrendt SA, Chow JT, Xu LH, et al. Molecular detection of tumor cells in bronchoalveolar lavage fluid from patients with early stage lung cancer. J Natl Cancer Inst 1999; 91:332–9.
65 Hibi K, Westra WH, Borges M, Goodman S, Sidransky D, Jen J. PGP9.5 as a candidate tumor marker for non-small-cell lung cancer. Am J Pathol 1999; 155:711–5.
66 Payne PW, Sebo TJ, Doudkine A, et al. Sputum screening by quantitative microscopy: reexamination of a portion of the National Cancer Institute cooperative early lung cancer study. Mayo Clin Proc 1997; 72:697–704.
67 Lam S, Shibuya H. Early diagnosis of lung cancer. Clin Chest Med 1999; 20:53–61.
68 Lam S, Kennedy T, Unger M, et al. Localization of bronchial intraepithelial neoplastic lesions by fluorescence bronchoscopy. Chest 1998; 113:696–702.
69 Vermylen P, Pierard P, Roufosse C, et al. Detection of bronchial preneoplastic lesions and early lung cancer with fluorescence bronchoscopy: a study about its ambulatory feasibility under local anaesthesia. Lung Cancer 1999; 25:161–8.
70 Alexander W. Autofluorescence for bronchial imaging. J Clin Laser Med Surg 1991; 9:331–3.
71 Prakash UBS. Advances in bronchoscopic procedures. Chest 1999; 116:1403–8.

72 Bard MPL, Amelink A, Skurcichina M, et al. Optical Spectroscopy for the Classification of Malignant Lesions of the Bronchial Tree. Chest 2006; 129:995–1001.
73 Phillips M, Gleeson K, Hughes JM, et al. Volatile organic compounds in breath as markers of lung cancer: a cross-sectional study. Lancet 1999; 353:1930–3.
74 Machado RF, Laskowski D, Deffenderfer O, et al. Detection of lung cancer by sensor array analyses of exhaled breath. Am J Respir Crit Care Med 2005; 171:1286–91.
75 Carpagnano F, Stea G, Susca A, et al. 3p microsatellite alterations in exhaled breath condensate from patients with non-small cell lung cancer. Am J Respir Crit Care Med 2005; 172:738–44.
76 Vining DJ, Liu K, Choplin RH, Haaponik EF. Virtual bronchoscopy: relationships of virtual reality endobronchial simulations to actual bronchoscopic findings. Chest 1996; 109:549–53.
77 Summers RM, Selbie WS, Malley JD, et al. Polypoid lesions of airways: early experience with computer-assisted detection by using virtual bronchoscopy and surface curvature. Radiology 1998; 208:331–7.
78 Fleiter R, Merkle EM, Aschoff AJ, et al. Comparison of real-time virtual and fiberoptic bronchoscopy in patients with bronchial carcinoma: opportunities and limitations. Am J Radiol 1997; 169:1591–5.
79 Henschke CI, Yankelevitz DI. CT screening for lung cancer. Radiol Clin North Am 2000; 38:487–95.

12

Tracheomalacia: Functional Imaging of the Large Airways with Multidetector-Row CT

Phillip M. Boiselle
Department of Radiology, Beth Israel Deaconess Medical Center and Harvard Medical School, Boston, Massachusetts, U.S.A.

INTRODUCTION

The trachea is a compliant structure that normally dilates slightly with inspiration and narrows during expiration as a reflection of the difference between intrathoracic and intraluminal pressures (Fig. 1) (1). Tracheomalacia refers to weakness of the airway walls and/or supporting cartilage and is characterized by an accentuation of this physiological process, resulting in excessive expiratory collapse (Fig. 2) (1–4). Although the earliest reports of this condition date to the 1930s and 1940s, tracheomalacia has only recently been recognized as a relatively common and potentially treatable cause of chronic cough, dyspnea, and recurrent infections (3).

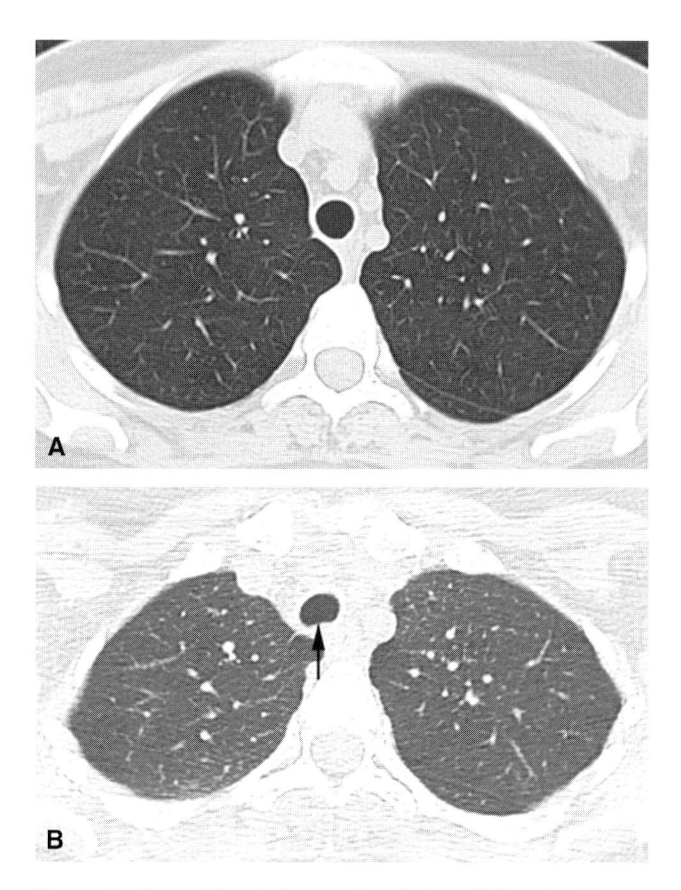

Figure 1 Normal inspiratory and expiratory CT tracheal lumen changes in 36-year-old woman. (**A**) End-inspiratory CT scan demonstrates a round shape of the tracheal lumen. (**B**) Dynamic-expiratory CT scan demonstrates normal degree of expiratory tracheal luminal narrowing with slight anterior bowing of posterior membranous wall. *Source*: From Ref. 24.

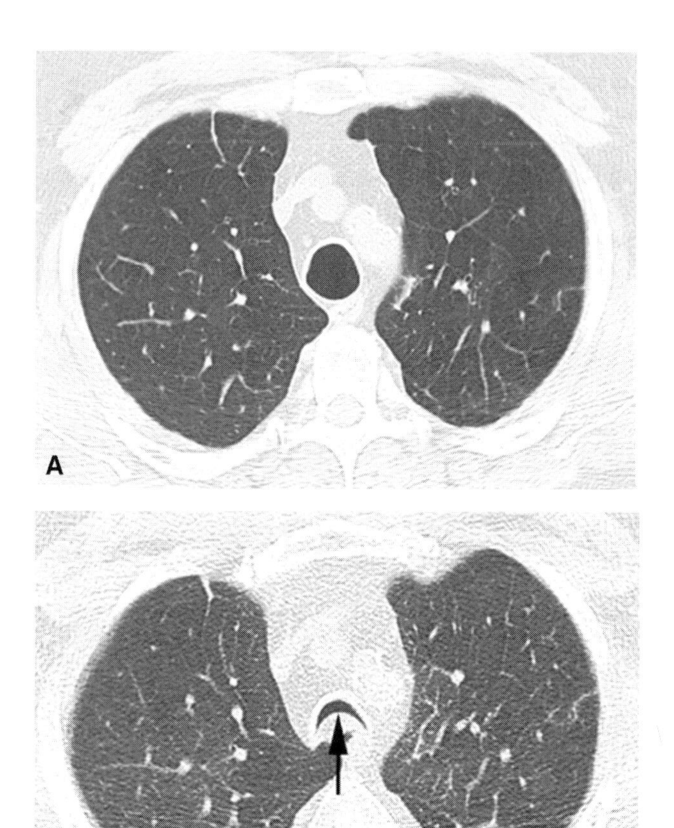

Figure 2 Tracheomalacia in 51-year-old man with chronic cough. (**A**) End-inspiratory CT scan demonstrates a normal oval shape of the tracheal lumen. (**B**) Dynamic-expiratory CT scan demonstrates excessive expiratory collapse, consistent with tracheomalacia. Note frown-like, crescenteric configuration of tracheal lumen (*arrow*). *Source*: From Ref. 24.

Table 1 Risk Factors for Acquired Tracheomalacia

Chronic obstructive lung disease
Posttraumatic and iatrogenic
Postintubation
Posttracheostomy
Radiation therapy
External chest trauma
Postlung transplantation
Chronic infection/bronchitis
Chronic inflammation
Relapsing polychondritis
Chronic external compression of the trachea
Paratracheal neoplasms (benign and malignant)
Paratracheal masses (e.g., goiter, congenital cyst)
Aortic aneurysms and vascular rings
Skeletal abnormalities (e.g., pectus, scoliosis)

Tracheomalacia may be either congenital or acquired. The acquired form is associated with a variety of risk factors and comorbidities, most notably chronic obstructive pulmonary disease (Table 1) (1–3). Because tracheomalacia cannot be detected with routine end-inspiratory imaging studies, it is widely considered an underdiagnosed condition. For example, bronchoscopic series report a prevalence ranging from 4.5% to 23% (3,5,6). Recent CT studies also support the concept that this is an underdiagnosed condition (7,8).

Although bronchoscopy with functional maneuvers can reliably detect tracheomalacia, it is not clinically feasible or desirable to perform this invasive test in all patients who present with chronic cough and other nonspecific respiratory symptoms. Fortunately, recent advances in multidetector-row CT (MDCT) imaging afford the opportunity to noninvasively diagnose tracheomalacia with similar sensitivity to conventional bronchoscopy (9–11). In this chapter, we review the technical aspects of performing and interpreting functional imaging studies of the large airways using MDCT.

TECHNICAL ASPECTS

Historical Perspective: Evolving Diagnostic Imaging Methods

During the past few decades, a variety of noninvasive imaging methods have been applied to the diagnosis of tracheomalacia. Historically, cine-fluoroscopy was employed, but this method was limited by several factors, including a relatively poor display of anatomic detail, the subjective and operator-dependent nature of this technique, an inability to simultaneously display the anteroposterior and lateral walls of the trachea, and a tendency to underestimate the degree of collapse compared to bronchoscopy (5). With the advent of CT imaging, it became possible to obtain a more objective and reproducible display of the airways and to quantitatively measure the degree of collapse. The introduction of helical CT technology further improved imaged quality, but early single-detector helical scanners were limited by a relatively long acquisition time, an important drawback for functional imaging. The advent of electron-beam CT, which acquired images with a temporal resolution of 50–100 ms per slice, made it possible to obtain "real-time" cross-sectional images of the airways during dynamic breathing and coughing (12–14). However, this technique was limited by its relatively low-spatial resolution, limited z-axis coverage, and restricted availability.

More recently, the advent of MDCT has overcome the limitations of previous CT technologies by providing a successful combination of fast speed, high-spatial resolution, and large anatomic coverage. These factors have facilitated the ability to acquire a helical data set of the entire airways during a single-expiratory maneuver (dynamic expiratory CT) (4,8–11).

Provocative Maneuvers for Functional Airway Imaging: Physiological Correlations

Unlike traditional anatomical imaging, in which the airways are evaluated at maximal end-inspiration, functional imaging requires obtaining CT data during or after provocative maneuvers such as expiration and coughing.

When considering these provocative maneuvers, it is important to review the relationship of tracheal collapse to intrathoracic pressures. Changes in size of malacic trachea and bronchi depend on the difference between the intraluminal pressure inside the airways and the pleural (intrathoracic) pressure outside (1,15). Pleural pressure depends mostly on respiratory muscles, and is high during expiratory efforts. In contrast, intraluminal pressures are highly variable, and depend on airflow. When airflow is zero, intraluminal pressure equals alveolar pressure and differs from pleural pressure only by the elastic recoil pressure of the lung, which depends on lung volume. At maximal lung volume with no flow (end-inspiration), the intraluminal pressure is 20–30 cm H_2O greater than pleural pressure, and the pressure difference expands the trachea. At low lung volumes with no flow (end-expiration), the intraluminal pressure is nearly equal to pleural pressure, and the trachea is unstressed. The trachea is most compressed during cough and dynamic expiration at low lung volume, when pleural pressure is high ($\sim$100 cm H_2O), and expiratory flow limitation in the small airways prevents transmission of the high alveolar pressures to the central airways. Under these conditions, intraluminal pressure is nearly atmospheric, and the large transmural pressure causes tracheal collapse (16).

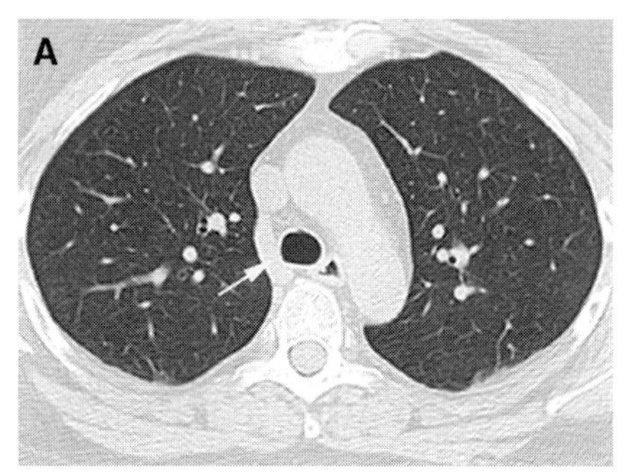

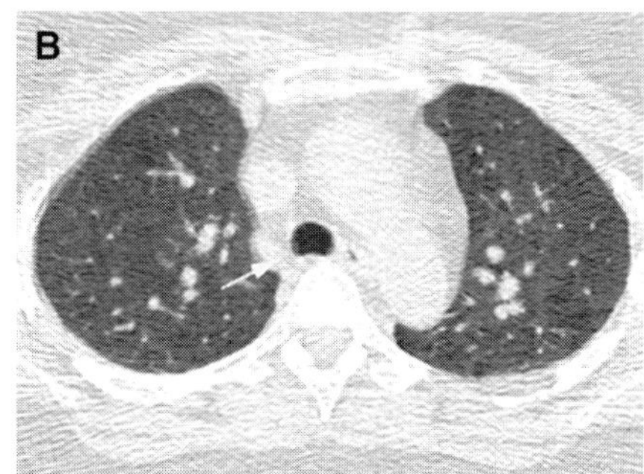

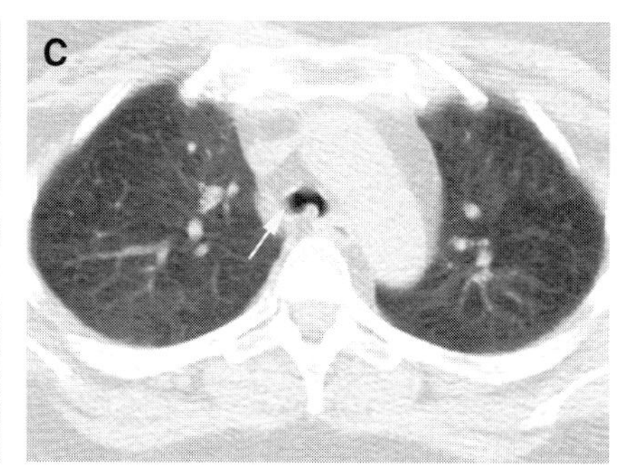

Figure 3 Comparison of airway collapse during different expiratory maneuvers. These images show normal tracheal appearance at the level of aortic arch at end-inspiration (**A**), with small degree of collapse at end-expiration (**B**) and significant (>50%) collapse during dynamic-expiration (**C**). *Source*: From Ref. 15.

Baroni et al. directly compared the ability of end-expiratory and dynamic expiratory CT imaging methods to elicit tracheomalacia (15). Consistent with the principles of respiratory physiology, this study showed that dynamic expiratory CT elicited a significantly greater degree of tracheal collapse than end-expiratory CT (Fig. 3). In this study, the mean percentages of airway collapse measured with the two techniques at three levels were: (*i*) aortic arch: dynamic-expiration = 53.9% versus end-expiration = 35.7% ($p = .0046$); (*ii*) carina: dynamic-expiration = 53.6% versus end-expiration = 30.9 % ($p < .001$); and (*iii*) bronchus intermedius: dynamic-expiration = 57.5% versus end-expiration = 28.6% ($p = .0022$).

It is known that cough elicits an even higher level of intrathoracic–extratracheal pressure than forced exhalation. Thus, imaging during coughing should theoretically be the most sensitive method for eliciting tracheal collapse in patients with malacia. In an early study of 8 adult patients with suspected tracheomalacia evaluated with electron-beam CT, Hein et al. elicited a much higher average percentage of collapse during coughing (71%) than at end-expiration (36%) (17). However, this method was limited to imaging a single slice of the trachea during each cine sequence. This resulted in a "sampling" of the trachea, with the need for repeated acquisitions, resulting in a relatively high radiation exposure and long exam time.

More recently, the advent of 64-slice MDCT has helped to overcome the limitations of electron-beam CT due to its high spatial and temporal resolution, combined with its large anatomic coverage capability. During a single-cine acquisition, 64-slice MDCT provides anatomic coverage of 3–4 cm in the *z*-axis, allowing simultaneous assessment of portions of the trachea and proximal main bronchi. The author's group recently reported our preliminary clinical experience with this method showing that it is both technically feasible and highly sensitive for detecting malacia (18).

At present, cine 64-MDCT is still somewhat limited in its *z*-axis coverage, resulting in either a single "sampling" of the trachea or the need for several acquisitions to provide complete anatomical coverage. Fortunately, future advances in CT imaging will soon provide greater coverage, allowing simultaneous cine evaluation of the entire intrathoracic airways during a single-imaging acquisition (18).

Diagnostic Criterion: A Moving Target?

The vast majority of studies reported in the literature support the use of a threshold of greater than or equal to 50% collapse as diagnostic of tracheomalacia when using either bronchoscopy or CT. However, it is important to note that several studies have advocated the adoption of different threshold values. For example, Stern et al. obtained a degree of tracheal collapse greater than 50% at end-expiration in 4 of 10 healthy young adult male volunteers scanned with an electron-beam CT (19). Based upon their findings, these authors recommended a more conservative threshold of 70% of collapse as indicative of tracheomalacia. Similarly, Heussel et al. have reported that healthy volunteers can sometimes exceed the standard diagnostic criterion (14). On the other hand, Aquino et al. studied 23 normal subjects and 10 patients with bronchoscopically-proven acquired tracheobronchomalacia using end-expiratory CT scans, and obtained a positive-predictive value of 89–100% using a threshold of >18% collapse for the upper trachea, and >28% for the midtrachea (20). Although the use of a lower threshold when imaging at end-expiration fits well with physiological principles, the low threshold values of 18% and 28% likely overlap substantially with those of normal subjects and will require further validation. In contrast, based upon a review of our preliminary experience with 64-MDCT "cine" imaging during coughing, we have suggested that a higher threshold value of 70% should be considered when using this robust provocative maneuver to elicit tracheal collapse (18).

Based upon these studies, it seems reasonable that the recommended threshold criterion of collapse for diagnosing tracheomalacia will vary depending upon which provocative maneuver has been employed. However, the precise values for accurate diagnosis have yet to be validated in large studies. Thus, there is a need to obtain normative data regarding the range of tracheal collapse using different provocative maneuvers among patients of varying ages, ethnicities, and both genders, both with and without coexistent pulmonary disease. Until this data has been published, it seems reasonable to employ a diagnostic threshold of >50% reduction for dynamic expiration and >70% reduction during coughing. However, one should keep in mind that there is likely overlap with normal at the lower range of positive.

Protocols: How to Perform a Functional MDCT Study

In order to ensure a high-quality study, technologists should be trained to coach and monitor patients as they perform the respiratory techniques (end-inspiration, dynamic expiration, coughing) that are included in the functional imaging protocol that is being employed. Technologists should also be trained to recognize the characteristic appearance of inspiratory and expiratory CT scans in order to ensure that the imaging sequences have been successfully performed during the appropriate respiratory maneuvers. For centers that are just beginning to use this technique, it is recommended that the radiologist observe and monitor cases until the technologists have become comfortable coaching patients with these maneuvers.

In the following paragraphs, functional airway imaging protocols from the author's institution are reviewed, including paired inspiratory–dynamic expiratory CT and cine CT during coughing. The end-expiratory imaging technique is not reviewed because it has been supplanted by the more effective dynamic expiratory imaging method.

Paired inspiratory–dynamic expiratory CT includes imaging during two different phases of respiration: end-inspiratory (imaging during suspended end inspiration) and continuous dynamic expiratory (imaging during forceful exhalation). This protocol can be successfully performed with any type of MDCT scanner. However, in the author's experience, the best results are produced with scanner configurations of eight or more detector rows. Prior to helical scanning, initial scout topographic images are obtained to determine the area of coverage, which extends from the proximal trachea through the main bronchi, corresponding to a length of approximately 10–12 cm. Helical scanning is performed in the craniocaudal dimension for both end-inspiratory and dynamic-expiratory scans. The end-inspiratory scan is performed first (170 mAs, 120 kVp, 2.5 mm collimation, pitch equivalent of 1.5). Following the end-inspiratory scan, patients are subsequently coached with instructions for the dynamic-expiratory component of the scan (40 mAs, 120 kVp, 2.5 mm collimation, high-speed mode, with pitch equivalent of 1.5). For this sequence, patients are instructed to take a deep breath in and to blow it out during the CT acquisition, which is coordinated to begin with the onset of the patient's forced expiratory effort.

Cine CT during coughing requires use of a 64-MDCT scanner. At the author's institution this protocol is performed with detector collimation 0.5 mm x 64; mAs = 80; kVp = 120; gantry rotation = 0.4 s.

An initial scout topographic image is obtained to determine the area of coverage, which extends 3.2 cm in craniocaudal length. In order to "sample" the trachea and proximal main bronchi within a single acquisition, the inferior aspect of the acquisition is set at the level of the carina, and the superior aspect of the acquisition is set 3.2 cm above this level, which corresponds to approximately the level of the aortic arch. A 5 s acquisition is acquired in cine mode beginning at end-inspiration and followed by repeated coughing maneuvers. Images are reconstructed at 8 mm collimation in a standard algorithm, creating four contiguous cine data sets from a single acquisition.

This protocol can also be modified for use with 64-MDCT scanners from other vendors. Depending upon the scanner configuration, there is a potential to increase the z-axis coverage (e.g., 0.625 x 64 = 4.0 cm z-axis coverage).

Radiation Exposure: Avoiding a "Double-Dose" CT

Because paired inspiratory–dynamic expiratory CT requires imaging during two phases of respiration, it has the potential to result in a "double dose" compared to a traditional single-phase CT scan unless methods for dose reduction are employed. Similarly, there is a potential for high radiation exposure using cine techniques unless dose reduction methods are used.

Fortunately, the high inherent contrast between the air-filled trachea and soft-tissue structures allows for significant reductions in dose without negatively influencing image quality for assessing luminal dimensions of the airway (4,10). For example, a clinical study by Zhang et al. (10) showed no difference between standard (240–260 mAs) and low-dose (40–80 mAs) images for assessing the tracheal lumen during dynamic expiration in the evaluation of suspected malacia.

As reviewed in the previous section on protocols, the author employs a low-dose (30–40 mAs) technique when imaging during coughing or expiration. In contrast, a standard-dose technique is employed for the end-inspiratory scan. The estimated radiation dose (expressed as dose-length product) for a dual-phase study (standard dose end-inspiratory sequence +

low-dose dynamic expiratory sequence) for a 70 kg patient is approximately 500 mGy cm, which is comparable to a routine chest CT (reference value 600 mGy cm) (21). By comparison, the estimated dose for a low-dose cine CT is approximately 200–220 mGy. cm. However, unlike the dual-phase scan, which covers the entirety of the central airways, a single-cine acquisition only covers 3.2–4.0 cm in the *z*-axis (depending upon the scanner configuration). If repeated at multiple levels to provide similar coverage to the dual-phase CT, the total dose for serial cine acquisitions would be greater than the dual-phase technique.

Beyond the Axial Plane: Role for Multiplanar Reformations and 3D Reconstructions

Volumetric data acquisition using MDCT allows for the creation of three-dimensional (3D) reconstructions and multiplanar reformations (MPR), which have the potential to aid diagnosis and preoperative planning (4,9,22,23). Virtual bronchoscopic images, which provide an intraluminal perspective similar to conventional bronchoscopy, are particularly helpful for assessing dynamic changes in the lumen of the main bronchi, which course obliquely to the axial plane and are not optimally evaluated by traditional axial CT images (Fig. 4). Paired inspiratory and dynamic-expiratory sagittal reformation images along the axis of the trachea are helpful for displaying the craniocaudal extent of excessive tracheal collapse during expiration and may aid planning for stent placement or corrective tracheoplasty procedures (Fig. 5) (4,22,23).

INTERPRETATION

Making the Diagnosis

Interpretation of CT images for the diagnosis of tracheomalacia requires careful review and comparison of both end-inspiratory and dynamic-expiratory images. End-inspiratory images provide important anatomical information about the tracheal size and shape, the thickness of the tracheal wall, and the presence or absence of extrinsic masses compressing the trachea. A previous study by this author has shown that the tracheal lumen is almost always normal in appearance on end-inspiration CT (24). Notable exceptions include: (1) patients with relapsing polychondritis (Fig. 6), who may demonstrate characteristic wall thickening and calcification that spares the posterior membranous wall of the trachea; (2) patients with lunate tracheal shape (coronal > sagittal dimension), which is frequently associated with tracheomalacia (Fig. 7); and (3) patients with extrinsic tracheal compression from adjacent vascular anomalies or thyroid masses, in whom long-standing compression has been complicated by tracheomalacia.

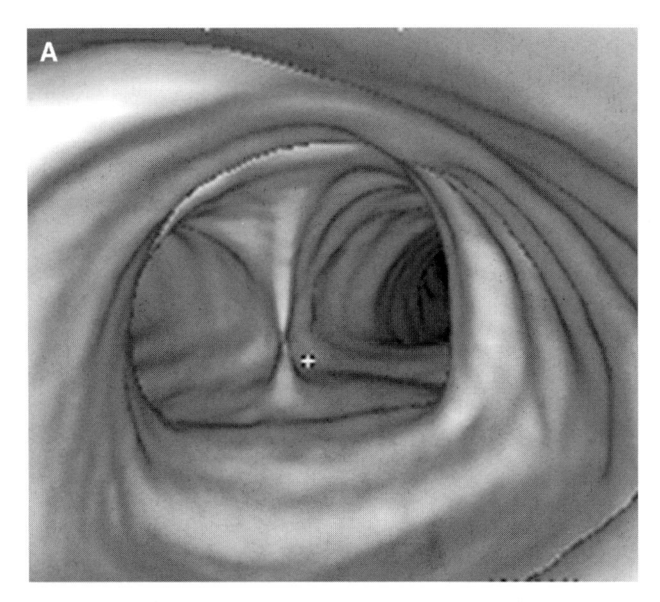

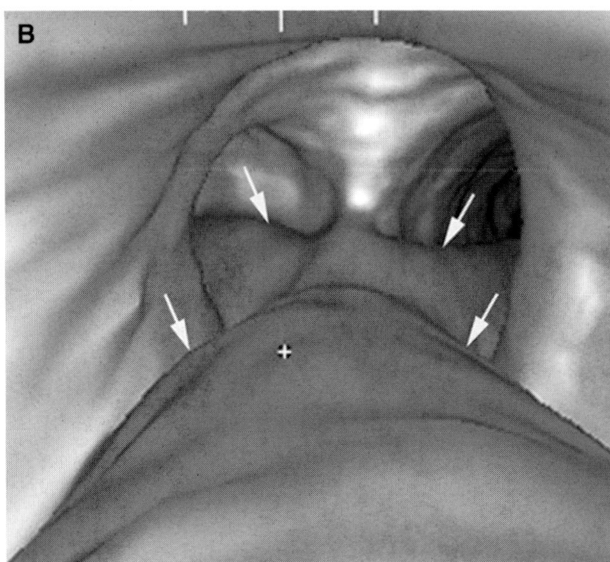

Figure 4 Virtual bronchoscopic assessment of tracheobronchomalacia. Virtual-bronchoscopy images at carinal level obtained at end-inspiration (**A**) and dynamic-expiration (**B**) show excessive anterior protrusion of the posterior wall of the distal trachea, carina and main bronchi at expiration (*arrows* in **B**), significantly reducing the airway caliber.

The most accurate means for diagnosing malacia on CT is to use an electronic tracing tool to calculate the cross-sectional area of the airway lumen on images at the same anatomic level obtained at inspiration and dynamic expiration (Fig. 8) (4). Such tools can be found on commercially available picture archiving and communication system (PACS) stations as well as with 3D workstations. As described in the previous section, >50% expiratory reduction in cross-sectional area is considered diagnostic. Care should be taken to ensure that the same anatomical level is compared between the two sequences by comparing vascular structures and other anatomical landmarks.

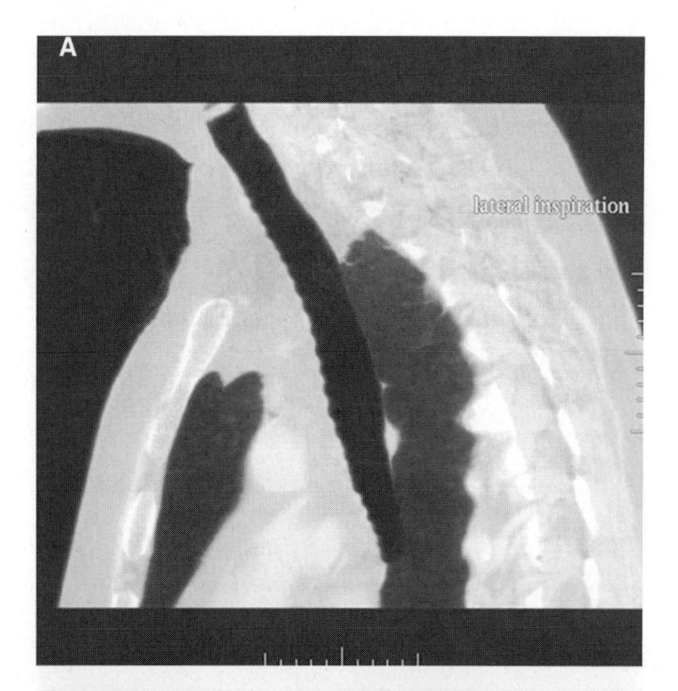

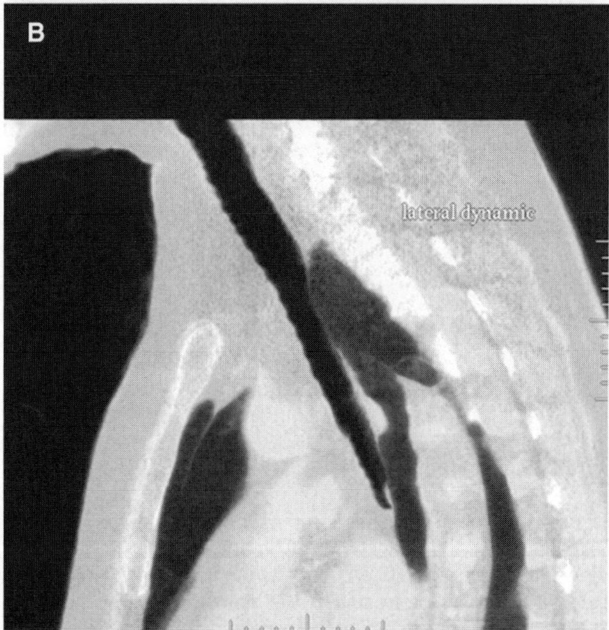

Figure 5 Multiplanar reformation images. Sagittal multiplanar volume reformations at end-inspiration (**A**) and dynamic expiration (**B**) demonstrate longitudinal length of tracheomalacia, involving entire intrathoracic trachea with extrathoracic sparing.

Obviously, in the setting of severe malacia, in which there is near complete collapse of the airway lumen during expiration, the diagnosis can be confidently made based on visual analysis of the images. Interestingly, about half of patients with acquired tracheomalacia will demonstrate an expiratory "frown-like" configuration, in which the posterior membranous wall is excessively bowed forward and parallels the convex contour of the anterior wall with <6 mm distance between the

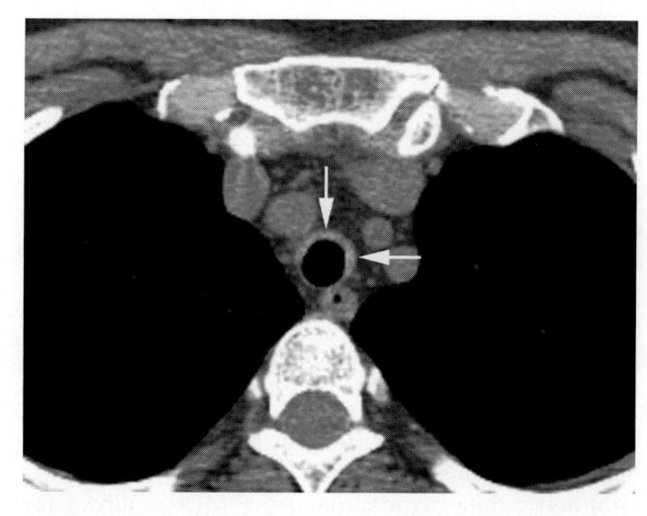

Figure 6 Relapsing polychondritis. Axial CT image demonstrates thickening of the anterior and lateral tracheal walls (*arrows*) with sparing of posterior membranous wall.

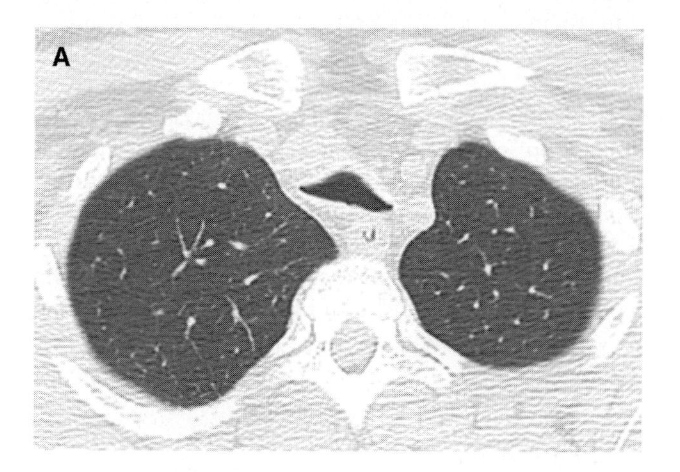

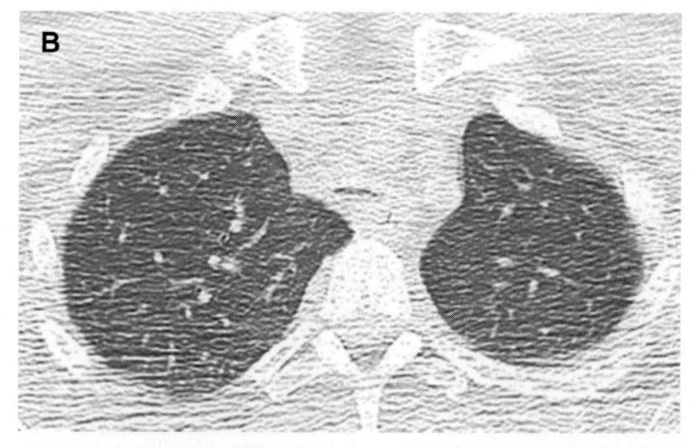

Figure 7 Lunate configuration of the trachea in a 39-year-old man with chronic cough, dyspnea, and recurrent respiratory infections. (**A**) Inspiratory CT image demonstrates widening of coronal diameter of trachea consistent with a lunate configuration. (**B**) Expiratory CT image demonstrates complete collapse of airway lumen, consistent with tracheomalacia. A small amount of air is incidentally noted in the esophageal lumen, but there is no visible tracheal lumen. Excessive image noise, most prominent posteriorly, relates to use of low-dose technique and large body habitus of the patient. *Source*: From Ref. 24.

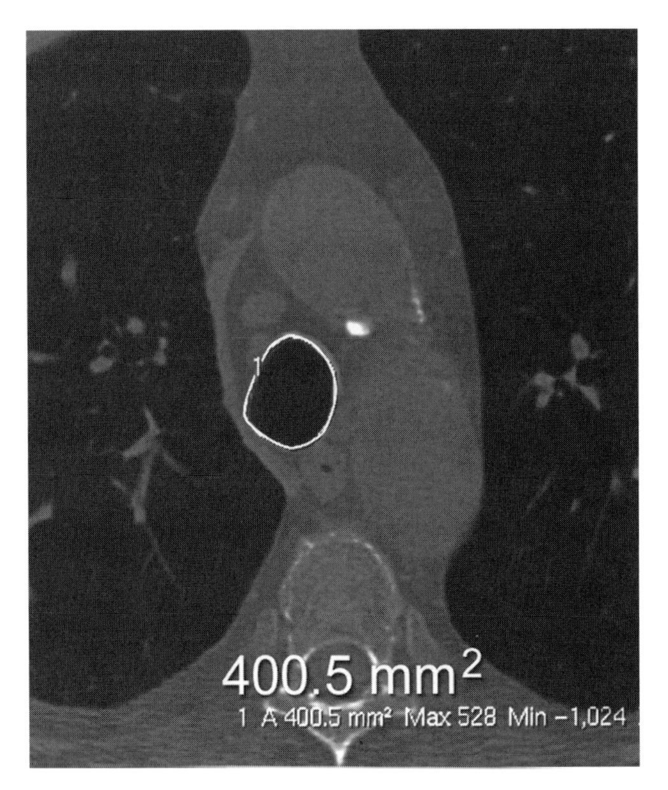

Figure 8 Example of electronic tracing method for measuring cross-sectional area of tracheal lumen at the level of the aortic arch. The tracing line has been electronically thickened to enhance visibility for photographic reproduction. *Source*: From Ref. 24.

anterior and posterior walls (Fig. 2B) (24). This appearance, which has been coined the "frown sign," is highly suggestive of tracheomalacia and has the potential to aid the detection of tracheomalacia when patients inadvertently breathe during routine CT scans (24). Ideally, however, the diagnosis of tracheomalacia should be confirmed and quantified by a dedicated study.

With regard to interpreting cine-coughing CT studies, they are ideally viewed in "cine" fashion at either a PACS workstation or 3D workstation. Quantitative measurements are obtained on individual static images in a similar fashion to the technique described for paired inspiratory–dynamic expiratory CT. As described earlier, >70% reduction in cross-sectional area during coughing is considered diagnostic. A commercial software program (Analyze 6.0, AnalyzeDirect, Inc., Lenexa, Kansas, U.S.) can also be used to provide automated measurement of changes in tracheal lumen cross-sectional area values during the cine sequence (18).

Beyond Diagnosis: Severity, Distribution, and Morphology

When interpreting functional CT scans of patients with tracheomalacia, it is important to report the severity, distribution, and morphology. These factors have an important impact upon treatment decisions, which are based upon a combination of symptoms, severity, and distribution of disease, and underlying cause of tracheomalacia (25).

Because there is not a single widely accepted scale for reporting the severity of tracheomalacia, it is important to report the quantitative degree of collapsibility rather than simply using a qualitative descriptor. A severity scale that has been employed by other investigators includes three grades of severity based upon the degree of airway collapse: (*i*) mild: 50% to 74%; (*ii*) moderate: 74% to 99%; and (*iii*) severe: 100% collapse (9,25). In contrast, at the authors' institution, a multidisciplinary team of physicians with experience in diagnosing and treating this condition considers >90% expiratory collapse as indicative of severe tracheomalacia.

Additionally, it is important to report the distribution of malacia. Murgu and Colt have recently proposed a functional class/extent/morphology/origin/severity (FEMOS) classification for tracheomalacia that combines a variety of factors (25). In their proposed classification, the distribution is considered focal if present in one tracheal region (upper, middle, or lower) or in one main or lobar bronchus; multifocal if present in two contiguous or at least two noncontiguous regions; and diffuse if present in more than two contiguous regions. From a practical perspective, accurate determination of distribution has implications for treatment. For example, focal areas of malacia may benefit from stenting, whereas diffuse disease is more amenable to tracheoplasty surgery.

Regarding morphology, one should describe whether the collapse occurs circumferentially, or if it occurs primarily due to either excessive bulging of the posterior membranous wall or collapse of the anterolateral cartilaginous structures. For example, patients with collapse primarily due to bulging and flaccidity of the posterior membranous wall are potential candidates for tracheoplasty surgery, a novel surgical technique in which in the posterior wall of the trachea is reinforced by a Marlex graft (26). Surgical reinforcement of the posterior membranous wall enhances the rigidity of this structure and makes it less susceptible to bowing during expiration.

Tracheoplasty: Preoperative and Postoperative Assessment

CT plays several potentially important roles in evaluating severely symptomatic tracheomalacia patients who are undergoing evaluation for curative tracheoplasty surgery (26). Preoperative roles include: (*i*) precise characterization of airway shape and determination of which parts of the airway wall

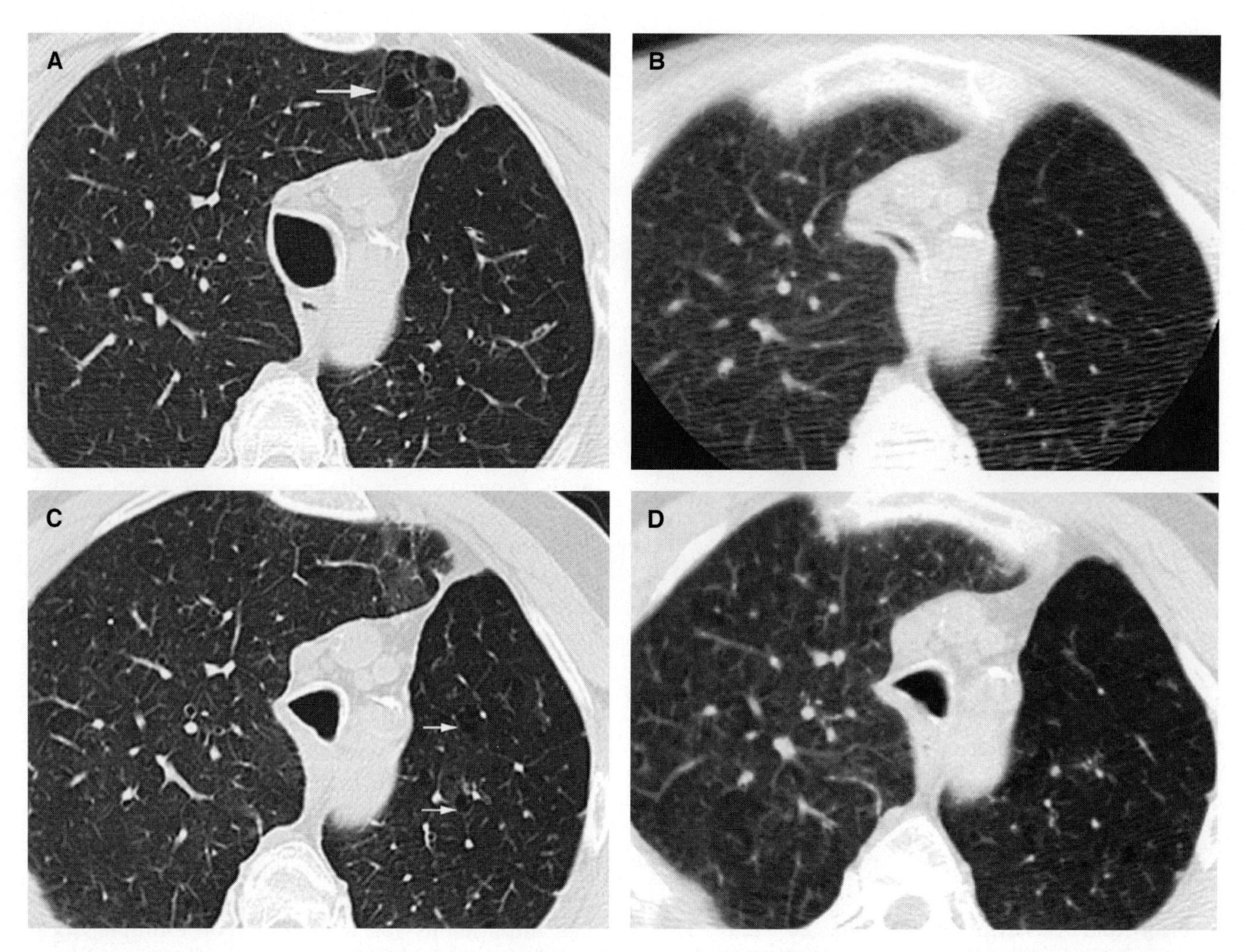

Figure 9 A 62-year-old man with tracheobronchomalacia treated by tracheoplasty: comparison of pre- and postoperative dynamic CT scans. Before surgery, the trachea has a biconvex ("fish mouth") shape at end-inspiration (**A**), and it shows a marked collapse at dynamic-expiration (**B**), acquiring a "lunate" shape. After tracheoplasty, the trachea has a normal, horseshoe shape at end-inspiration (**C**), which persists at dynamic-expiration despite a mild degree of collapse (**D**). *Source*: From Ref. 26.

contribute to excessive airway collapsibility; (*ii*) evaluation for airway wall thickening and calcification (in combination with airway malacia, these findings suggest polychondritis, a disorder that is not treated surgically); (*iii*) evaluation for extrinsic paratracheal masses, which may preclude surgery; (*iv*) baseline measure of airway collapsibility by which to compare postoperative scans for evaluating response to surgery. In the postoperative setting, CT provides a noninvasive method for assessing for postoperative complications and noninvasively quantifying the degree of improvement in airway collapsibility. Finally, CT has the unique ability to visualize the characteristic thickening of the posterior wall of the airways after surgery, which may serve as a clue for one to suspect that tracheoplasty has been performed (Fig. 9).

At the author's institution, surgeons and pulmonologists have found a combination of subjective symptomatic improvement and quantitative reduction in airway collapsibility at CT to be the most helpful measurements of determining response to surgery (26). Our preliminary findings comparing preoperative and postoperative scans showed that tracheoplasty resulted in a decrease in the degree of airway collapse that was accompanied by a qualitative improvement of respiratory symptoms (26).

SUMMARY

Recent advances in MDCT imaging afford the opportunity to noninvasively diagnose tracheomalacia with similar sensitivity to conventional bronchoscopy by using either paired inspiratory–dynamic expiratory CT or cine-coughing techniques. CT plays an important role in diagnosing tracheomalacia. CT also provides important information regarding disease severity, morphology, and distribution that aids management decisions. Future studies are necessary to define normative values of tracheal collapsibility and to better define threshold values for diagnosis.

REFERENCES

1 Carden K, Boiselle PM, Waltz D, Ernst A. Tracheomalacia and tracheobronchomalacia in children and adults: an in-depth review of a common disorder. Chest 2005; 127:984–1005.
2 Johnson TH, Mikita JJ, Wilson RJ, et al. Acquired tracheomalacia. Radiology 1973; 109:576–80.
3 Jokinen K, Palva T, Sutinen S, et al. Acquired tracheobronchomalacia. Ann Clin Res 1977; 9:52–7.
4 Boiselle PM, Feller-Kopman D, Ashiku S, Weeks D, Ernst A. Tracheobronchomalacia: evolving role of dynamic multislice helical CT. Radiol Clin North Am 2003; 41:627–36.
5 Palombini BC, Villanova CA, Araujo E, et al. A pathogenic triad in chronic cough: asthma, postnasal drip syndrome and gastroesophageal reflux disease. Chest 1999; 116:279–84.
6 Ikeda S, Hanawa T, Konishi T, et al. Diagnosis, incidence, clinicopathology and surgical treatment of acquired tracheobronchomalacia. Nihon Kyobu Shikkan Gakkai Zasshi 1992; 30:1028–103 [Japanese].
7 Hasegawa I, Boiselle PM, Hatabu H. Bronchial artery visualization on multislice CT in patients with acute PE: comparison with chronic or recurrent PE. AJR 2004; 182:67–72.
8 Lee KS, Ernst A, Trentham D, Lunn W, Feller Kopman D, Boiselle PM. Prevalence of functional airway abnormalities in relapsing polychondritis. Radiology 2006; 240:565–73.
9 Gilkeson RC, Ciancibello LM, Hejal RB, Montenegro HD, Lange P. Tracheobronchomalacia: dynamic airway evaluation with multidetectorCT. AJR 2001; 176: 205–10.
10 Zhang J, Hasegawa I, Feller-Kopman D, Boiselle PM. Dynamic expiratory volumetric CT imaging of the central airways: comparison of standard-dose and low-dose techniques. Acad Radiol 2003; 10:719–24.
11 Lee KS, Sun ME, Ernst A, Feller-Kopman D, Majid A, Boiselle PM. Comparison of dynamic expiratory CT with bronchoscopy in diagnosing airway Malacia. Chest 2007; 131:758–764.
12 Brasch RC, Gould RG, Gooding CA, Ringertz HG, Lipton MJ. Upper airway obstruction in infants and children: evaluation with ultrafast CT. Radiology 1987; 165: 459–66.
13 Kao SC, Smith WL, Sato Y, Franken EA, Kimura K, Soper RT. Ultrafast CT of laryngeal and tracheobronchial obstruction in symptomatic postoperative infants with esophageal atresia and tracheoesophageal fistula. AJR Am J Roentgenol 1990; 154:345–50.
14 Heussel CP, Hafner B, Lill J, Schreiber W, Thelen M, Kauczor H-U. Paired inspiratory/expiratory spiral CT and continuous respiration cine CT in the diagnosis of tracheal instability. Eur Radiol 2001; 11:982–9.
15 Baroni R, Feller-Kopman D, Nishino M, et al. Tracheobronchomalacia: comparison between end-expiratory and dynamic-expiratory CT methods for evaluation of central airway collapse. Radiology 2005; 2:635–41.
16 Wilson TA, Rodarte JR, Butler JP. Wave speed and viscous flow limitation. In: Macklem PT, Mead J, eds. Handbook of Physiology: The Respiratory System. Vol 3, Mechanics of Breathing, part 1. Bethesda, MD: The American Physiological Society, 1986:55–61.
17 Hein E, Rogalla P, Hentschel C, Taupitz M, Hamm B. Dynamic and quantitative assessment of tracheomalacia by electron beam tomography: correlation with clinical symptoms and bronchoscopy. J Comput Assist Tomogr 2000; 24:247–52.
18 Boiselle PM, Lee KS, Lin S, Raptopoulous V. Cine CT during coughing for assessment of tracheomalacia: preliminary experience with 64-multidetector-row CT. AJR 2006; 187:438.
19 Stern EJ, Graham CM, Webb WR, Gamsu G. Normal trachea during forced expiration: dynamic CT measurements. Radiology 1993; 187:27–31.
20 Aquino SL, Shepard JA, Ginns LC, et al. Acquired tracheomalacia: detection by expiratory CT scan. J Comput Assist Tomogr 2001; 25:394–9.
21 Mayo JR, Aldrich J, Mller NL. Radiation exposure at chest CT: a statement of the Fleischner Society. Radiology 2005; 228:15–21.
22 Boiselle PM, Ernst A. State-of-the-art imaging of the central airways. Respiration 2004; 70:383–94.
23 Boiselle PM. Multislice helical CT of the central airways. Radiol Clin North Am 2003; 41:561–74.
24 Boiselle PM, Ernst A. Tracheal morphology in patients with tracheomalacia: prevalence of inspiratory "lunate" and expiratory "frown" shapes. J Thorac Imag 2006; 21:190–6.
25 Murgu SD, Colt HG. Recognizing tracheobronchomalacia. J Respir Dis 2006; 27:327–35.
26 Baroni RH, Ashiku S, Boiselle PM. Dynamic-CT evaluation of the central airways in patients undergoing tracheoplasty for tracheobronchomalacia. AJR 2005; 184:1444–9.

Index